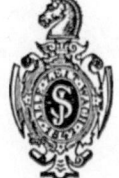

Recent Results in Cancer Research

Fortschritte der Krebsforschung

Progrès dans les recherches sur le cancer

3

Edited by

Editor in chief

P. Rentchnick, Genève

Springer-Verlag Berlin Heidelberg GmbH 1966

Occupational and Environmental Cancers of the Respiratory System

W. C. Hueper

With 48 Figures

Springer-Verlag Berlin Heidelberg GmbH 1966

Dr. W. C. Hueper, 9307 Rockville Pike, Bethesda, Md. 20014/USA

Sponsored by the Swiss League against Cancer

ISBN 978-3-642-87687-5   ISBN 978-3-642-87685-1 (eBook)
DOI 10.1007/978-3-642-87685-1

Introduction

Since the advent of the modern industrial era some 150 years ago, a large and growing number of diverse man-made chemicals have been introduced in increasing amounts into the occupational and general environmental air. This development of industrial atmospheric pollution, while first rather mild and locally restricted, has assumed during recent decades with the growing industrialization of the human economy, regional proportions which encompass in some cases large portions of entire States and countries covering them especially in their metropolitan areas, with an almost permanent cloud of chemical effluents. Many of these chemical wastes contaminating the environmental air of industrial establishments and communities and composed of constantly changing mixtures of identified and non-identified chemicals are to varying degrees, irritants to the respiratory mucosa in which they elicit by chemical action or by mechanical trauma, a variety of functional and anatomic disease manifestations (chronic laryngitis, tracheitis and bronchitis, emphysema, chemical pneumonitis, bronchiectases, pneumoconiosis).

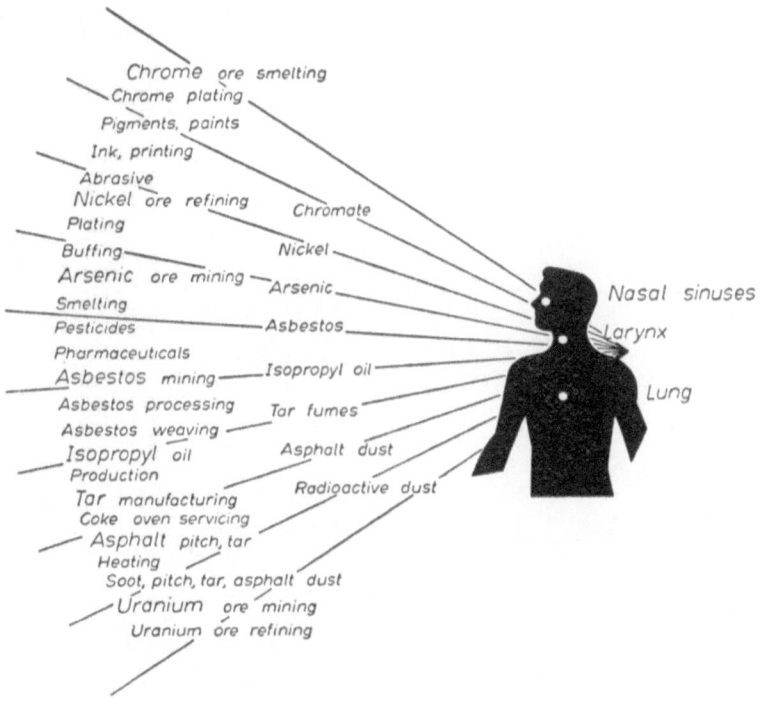

With the rapid rise in the frequency of lung cancers in all industrialized countries observed since the turn of the century, this progressive industry-related contamination of the atmosphere with a great variety of dusts, fumes, mists, vapors, and gases has become the subject of increasing interest as one of the causes underlying the recent developments in the respiratory cancer panorama. Diverse chemical atmospheric pollutants of industrial origin have been incriminated as specific and nonspecific respiratory carcinogenic irritants.

Table of Contents

A. Nonspecific Industrial Irritants 1

    Pneumoconiosis 2

        a) Mineral Dust Pneumoconiosis 2

           α) Anthracosis 2

           β) Silicosis 2

        b) Vegetable and Animal Dust Pneumoconiosis 6

           α) Tabacosis 6

           β) Shellac Pneumoconiosis 7

        c) Chronic Chemical Pneumonitis and Bronchitis 7

B. Specific Industrial Respiratory Carcinogens 7

    1. Significance of Specific Industrial Carcinogenic Irritants 8

        a) Classification of Occupational Respiratory Carcinogens 9

        b) Route of Exposure 11

    2. Occupational Respiratory Cancer and Smoking 13

    3. Epidemiology of Occupational Respiratory Cancers 15

    4. Pluripotentiality of Respiratory Carcinogens 21

    5. Carcinogenic Symptom Complex 21

    6. Sex distribution 22

    7. Occupational „Neighborhood" Cancers 23

    8. General Periplant Dissemination 23

    9. Carcinogenic Potency and Attack Rates of Industrial Respiratory Cancers . . 24

    10. Age Distribution 24

    11. Latent Period 27

    12. Histologic Types 28

C. Specific Occupational Cancers and Their Environmental Counterparts 28

    1. Arsenic 30

        a) Non-occupational Sources of Exposure to Arsenicals 31

           α) Atmospheric Urban Pollutants 31

           β) Water Pollutants 31

           γ) Foodstuff Contaminants 31

           δ) Soil Contaminants 32

           ε) Tobacco Contaminants 32

        b) Arsenicals as Carcinogens 32

        c) Respiratory Arsenic Cancers 33

        d) Experimental Arsenic Cancer 38

2. Asbestos 38
   a) Technologic Data 38
   b) Epidemiologic Data on Asbestos and Carcinoma of the Lung 41
   c) Clinicopathologic Relations 47
   d) Epidemiologic Data on Mesotheliomas of the Pleura and Peritoneum . . . 50
   e) Age Distribution of Asbestosis Cancers 52
   f) Sex Distribution of Asbestosis Carcinomas of the Lung 53
   g) Anticarcinogenic Action of Asbestos 53
   h) Syncarcinogenesis in the Production of Asbestosis Cancers 54
   i) Exposure Time and Latent Period 54
   k) Experimental Production of Cancers with Asbestos 54
   l) Causative Mechanism of Asbestos Carcinogenesis 55

3. Chromium 56
   a) Technologic Aspects 57
   b) Epidemiologic Cancer Aspects 59
   c) Special Aspects 64
   d) Histologic Types of Chrome Cancers of the Lung 65
   e) Clinical Aspects 70
   f) Chromium Content of Tissues, Blood and Urine 70
   g) Atmospheric Neighborhood Pollution 72
   h) Atmospheric Intraplant Pollution 75
   i) Chromate Carcinogenesis and Smoking Habits 75
   k) Experimental Production of Chrome Cancers 76
   l) Causative Mechanism of Chromium Carcinogenesis 80
   m) Preventive Measures 82
      α) Technologic Measures 83
      β) Medical Prophylactic Measures 84

4. Nickel 85
   a) Technological Aspects 85
   b) Epidemiology 86
   c) Pathology 89
   d) Etiology 89
   e) Experimental Production of Nickel Cancers 91
   f) Carcinogenic Mechanism 93
   g) Prophylaxis of Nickel Cancer Induction 93

5. Iron 93
   a) Technological Aspects 93
   b) Epidemiology 94
   c) Experimental Iron Carcinogenesis 97
   d) Etiology 98

6. Beryllium 99
   a) Technological Aspects 99
   b) Epidemiology 99
   c) Beryllium Cancers 101
   d) Etiology 102

7. Mustard Gas — Yperite-Lost — Beta, beta'-dichlorodiethyl sulfide — Bis(beta-chloroethyl) sulfide 103
   a) Technological Aspects 103
   b) Epidemiology 103
   c) Experimental Mustard Cancers 105
   d) Etiology 105

8. Isopropyl Oil 105
   a) Technological Aspects 105
   b) Epidemiology 106

9. Coal Tar, Tar Oils, Soot, and Other Combustion Products of Coal 107
   a) Technological Aspects 107
   b) Epidemiology 108
   c) Experimental Respiratory Carcinogenesis 114

10. Petroleum — Mineral Oil — Wax — Asphalt — Petroleum Carbon — Carbon Black — Methylated Naphthalene — Combustion Products — Shale Oil and Derivates 118
    a) Technological Aspects 118
    b) Epidemiology 120

11. Ionizing Radiations 125
    a) Technological Aspects 125
    b) Epidemiology 126
       α) Respiratory Cancers in Radioactive Ore Miners and Millers 127
          αα) Radioactive, Non-Uranium Miners 127
          αβ) Lung Cancer in Schneeberg Miners 127
          αγ) Radioactive Lung Cancer Hazard in a Fluorspar Mining Community in Newfoundland 131
          αδ) Miscellaneous Non-Uranium Mines 133
       β) Uranium Ore Miners 136
          βα) Lung Cancer in Joachimsthal Miners 136
          ββ) Lung Cancers in Uranium Ore Miners of the Colorado Plateau . . 138
       γ) Lung Cancer Hazards for Employees of Uranium Ore Refineries, Radium Laboratories, Nuclear Installations and Power Plants and Similar Establishments 142

12. Miscellaneous Respiratory Carcinogens 147
    a) Isonicotinic Acid Hydrazide (Isoniacid) 148
    b) Nitrosamines 149
    c) Nitroquinolines and Related Nitro- and Amino-Compounds 150
    d) Carbamates 151
    e) Chlorinated Hydrocarbons 151
    f) Formaldehyde 152
    g) Natural and Man-Made Polymers 152

D. Prevention and Control of Occupational Respiratory Cancer Hazards 153

References 155

Subject Index 208

A. Nonspecific Industrial Irritants

The "chronic irritation theory" of cancerigenesis proposed by Virchow around the middle of the past century forms the scientific basis for the often-repeated claim that the inhalation of nonspecific irritative air pollutants, especially those encountered in certain industries and occupations, represents a significant cause of cancers of the respiratory system.

In support of such allegations, it is argued that any air pollutant (dust, fume, mist, vapor, gas) exerting a prolonged but nonspecific irritating effect upon the respiratory mucosa would stimulate in this tissue epithelial proliferations and metaplasias which ultimately would lead to cancerous developments (SCHMORL; HAMPERL; SEYFARTH; DUGUID; BROCKBANK; KREYBERG; STAEMMLER) and that, therefore, people employed in "dusty" work were more liable to develop lung cancers than people with "open-air" occupations and "housework" (KREYBERG). In agreement with such statements are the observations that there seems to exist, according to statistical studies, a positive association between previous respiratory diseases of chemical or parasitic nature (chronic bronchitis, chronic fibrosing pneumonia, bronchiectais, tuberculosis, influenza, etc.) and the subsequent appearance of lung cancers (RÖSSLE; WOODRUFF and NAHAS; FINKE; CASE and LEA; CAMPBELL and LEE; CUNNINGHAM; NASSAU and WALTER).

In fact, chronic inflammatory processes in this organ system, especially chronic bronchitis, regardless of their infectious or chemical etiology, have been proposed as furnishing the principal basis for subsequent cancerous developments in the lung (PASSEY; LÖHR and WAGNER). The existence of such correlations has been advocated particularly in England, where industrial air pollution, chronic bronchitis and cancer of the lung are most prevalent (NATIONAL SURVEY; STOCKS; PEMBERTON FAIRBAIRN and REID; BURGESS and SHADDICK; CAMPBELL and LEE; KUSCHNER), although BRETT recently was unable to demonstrate any statistically significant associations between lung cancer and previous respiratory disease. A similar connotation regarding the existence of interrelations between chronic fibrosing processes of the lung, regenerative bronchiolar epithelial proliferations in their periphery and the subsequent development of pulmonary cancers from such lesions is incorporated in the concept of scar cancers of the lung proposed by RÖSSLE; FRIEDRICH; LÜDERS and THEMEL; and others. BALO, JUHASZ and TEMES suggested that a part of the recent increase in lung cancer might be attributable to the formation of lung cancers around pulmonary infarcts, since there has been a rise in embolic processes during recent years due to the increase in cardiovascular diseases. Since STANTON and BLACKWELL failed to induce experimentally cancers of the lung near infarcted areas unless a specific carcinogenic chemical was also administered, it is unlikely that scar formation as such predisposes to the development of lung cancers and that for this reason the concept of traumatic cancers of the lung has any scientific and medicolegal validity (HUEPER). This interpretation of the available evidence is supported by the following specific observations.

Pneumoconiosis

Chronic fibrosing processes in the lungs of benign or progressive character are often the result of an occupational inhalation of foreign materials in the form of particles or droplets, which are in part retained in the lung (STOFER). While some investigators have claimed that such exposures and their anatomic sequelae might ultimately lead to the development of pulmonary cancers, this concept is not supported by the majority of the epidemiologic facts on hand for most of these conditions (anthracosis, aluminosis, silicosis, barytosis, resinosis, suberosis, byssinosis, etc.) (TELEKY; KOELSCH; HUEPER). There is so far only a single case on record in which a cancer of the lung developed in a worker who had suffered from bagassosis (ONUIGBO). The most comprehensive and convincing data on the absence of such associations exist for the two most common pneumoconiosis, namely, anthracosis and silicosis.

a) Mineral Dust Pneumoconiosis

α) Anthracosis

Various epidemiologic studies of the frequency of lung cancers among coal miners often affected with anthracosis which were conducted in several countries have shown that members of this population group have not an excessive liability to this type of cancer, and that in fact their lung cancer mortality rate, as a rule, is lower than the standard rate for the entire population and is similar to that of the rural population, which generally is the lowest of all occupational and socio-economic groups investigated (KENNAWAY and KENNAWAY; JAMES; DYER; FEIL; VERSLUYS; GERBE; SCHULZ; ALLEN; SCHULTE). The bronchitis rate for coal miners, on the other hand, was found to be highly excessive (STOCKS). Anthracosis which is a nonprogressive type of pneumoconiosis, therefore, does not exert any demonstrable favorable influence on the induction of pulmonary cancer.

β) Silicosis

Silicosis has been in the past and to somewhat lesser extent still is a rather common occupational disease occurring among members of several large worker groups, such as especially hard rock miners, foundry workers, anthracite miners, stone masons and granite cutters. The relationship of silicosis to cancer of the lung covers three aspects (HUEPER; WEISSMAN).

A. The occurrence of large densities observed on x-ray film of the chest in individuals suffering from tuberculosilicosis may be mistaken for carcinoma of the lung.

B. It has remained controversial whether silicosis favors the development of lung cancer, hinders it, or does not exert any influence on this process.

C. Since the exposure to several established or suspected occupational respiratory carcinogens (radioactive substances, iron, arsenic) is complicated in some occupations by a simultaneous contact with silica, the role of silica and silicosis on the action of the specific carcinogens and on the cancerization process, respectively, has remained a subject of dispute.

The difficulties not infrequently encountered in the clinical diagnosis of cancer of the lung, whenever chronic inflammatory conditions prevail in this organ, are common experience and are likely to be aggravated in the presence of a tuberculosilicosis (KERGIN; SCHAUTZ and KLEIN; BRADSHAW and CHODOFF). A definite diagnostic decision in some such cases may be possible only through an autopsy. The degree of diagnostic uncertainty which may be created under in vivo conditions may be judged by the fact that the diagnosis of cancer of the lung was found either to be incorrect or not justified by the clinical evidence presented in approximately 40% of several hundred cases in which cancer of the lung was listed on the death certificate as the cause of death. Epidemiologic studies on the association of silicosis and carcinoma of the lung based solely on clinical criteria have evidently only limited scientific value and may even yield misleading information.

Under the influence of the theory incriminating chronic irritation as a major cause of cancer through stimulating a typical regenerative cell proliferation, silicosis was considered by various investigators as a condition favoring through mechanical, physical or chemical irritation, the development of lung cancer (ADAMO; MOREL et al.; PIAZZA; GROSSE; EHRHARDT; BOSSI; TAKEDA et al.; AHLENDORF; ASTORRI; FINE and JASO; DIBLE; ANDERSON and DIBLE; KLOTZ and SIMPSON; RACUGNO and CARTA; SCHAUTZ and KLEIN; CHIURCO; DIKSHTEIN; PUCCINI; GHISLANDI and FINULLI; KLOTZ; KIKUCHI and KODAMA). In support of this claim, SCHAUTZ and KLEIN as well as PUCCINI and DIKSHTEIN, cited the occurrence of epithelial metaplasias in the bronchial mucosa of individuals with silicosis coexisting with bronchogenic carcinoma. They asserted that the development of such precancerous changes in the bronchial mucosa were stimulated by the chronic bronchitis which according to these authors is regularly associated with even minor silicotic pulmonary changes. PAUL, on the other hand, noted a very low incidence of chronic bronchitis (0.1%) in Rhodesian copper miners among whom silicosis is prevalent. A similar connotation has the observation of CHATGIDAKIS who reported that the enlarged bronchial glands with excessive mucous secretion and dilated ducts found among white South African gold miners with silicosis was a phenomenon commonly seen also among elderly male non-miners. These lesions, therefore, were regarded by him as causally not related to the silicotic state.

In contrast to KAHLAU, who contended that only minor silicotic lesions furnish a favorable soil for subsequent cancerous developments, SCHAUTZ and KLEIN claimed that the close topographic relation between fibrotic silicotic scarred areas in the lung and carcinomas of this organ indicated the existence of positive associations between the two conditions. This concept of silicosis carcinoma of the lung proposed in recent years again by ROESSLE and BALO, is closely related to the concept of cancer of the lung forming in the marginal areas of old tuberculous and syphilitic scars and of infarcts.

It is possible that pulmonary scars with their locally disrupted vascular supply and their phagocytic accumulations may indeed favor the development of cancers from the surrounding tissue because of their tendency to arrest and store foreign matter which is either inhaled or after ingestion or parenteral introduction has entered the circulating blood (HUEPER). Since such substances retained in and around pulmonary scars may possess carcinogenic properties, such as soot, the occurrence of cancerous reactions near fibrous silicotic nodules is conceivable provided that an associated exposure to some specific carcinogen takes place (RACUGNO and CARTA). The carcinogenic effect under such circumstances would not depend upon any non-specific irritative action of silica or be the result of some mysterious deviation of regenerative cellular proliferations but would be the result of some secondary and independent carcinogenic exposure for which the silicotic scar tissue acts in the role of a localizing and preparatory focus.

The bulk of the available epidemiologic evidence on the association of silicosis and lung cancer supports the view of a mere coincidental role of silicosis in this combination. Several large statistical analyses performed on autopsy material derived from several occupational groups with silicosis hazard confirm this conclusion (Table 1), which is, moreover, shared by many experienced investigators (VORWALD

Table 1. *Frequency of Carcinoma in Lungs with Silicosis*

Author	No. of Silicotic Lungs at Autopsy	No. of Carcinomas of Lung in Series	Percentage of Lung Cancers
KLOTZ, 1932	50	4	8.00
GOLDING, 1946.	270	—	0.70
	170	3	
SPOERLEIN, 1952	81	1	1.20
	383	7	1.80
FINE and JASO, 1938 . . .	22	1	4.54
MEIKLEJOHN, 1950	210	4	1.90
FRUEHLING et al., 1953 . .	186	10	5.37
LEICHER, 1948	256	12	4.68
SLADDEN, 1933	60	2	3.33
RUETTNER, 1949	2204	32	1.50
SWEANY et al., 1936	40	1	2.50
EHRHARDT, 1949	804	4	0.50
LAVENNE	358	7	1.95
VORWALD and KURR, 1935.	1438	10	0.73
MITTMANN, 1959	5951	440	8.00
BECKER, 1958	439	13	3.00
Total	12,922	551	3.11

and KARR; SCHULZ; SCHULTE; KENNAWAY and KENNAWAY; MEREWETHER; FAULDS; MITTMANN; FRUEHLING and OPPERMANN; BRAUN; JAMES; MULLER, MARCHAND-ALPHAND, CUALLACCI, NADIRAS and MULLER; ALLEN; RUETTNER; SCHOCH; BERBLINGER; WEDLER; FISCHER; FISCHER-WASELS; HOLSTEIN; STAEMMLER; JOHNSTONE; CHARR; WAETJEN and others).

The concept that silicosis may even exert a certain protective effect against the development of lung cancer, especially during advanced stages of the disease, has found several proponents because they could show, that an inverse relation seems to exist between the grade of silicosis and the relative liability to cancer of the lung (SPOER-LEIN; SCHOCH; MITTMANN; BAUER; MEIKLEJOHN). Additional support for this claim is received by observations made by ROSTOSKI and SAUPE on SCHNEEBERG miners, since cancers of the lung among these miners were found to be exceptional if a severe silicosis existed. Similar correlations were recorded by BONSER, FAULDS and STEWART; and FAULDS to exist for the silicotic changes and lung cancers seen in English hematite miners (Table 2).

Table 2. *Distribution of Lung Cancer in Relation to Grade of Silicosis*
(MITTMANN) *(1950—1957)*

	Minimal Silicosis	Light Silicosis	Medium Silicosis	Severe Silicosis	Total
Silicosis with Lung Cancer					
Cases	165	154	81	40	440
Percentage.	37.5	35.0	18.4	9.1	
Silicosis without Lung Cancer					
Cases	1,515	1,769	1,480	1,187	5,951
Percentage.	25.5	29.7	24.9	19.9	

The available data on the age distribution at death of individuals suffering from silicosis and cancer of the lung are rather scanty and do not reveal any striking or significant changes from the ordinary age distribution of lung cancer (Table 3), unless

Table 3. *Age Distribution at Death from Silicosis Lung Cancer*

Years	30—39	40—49	50—59	60—69	70 & over	Total
Cases	1	7	16	12	1	37

the observations of FRUEHLING *et al.* can generally be applied. These authors recorded an average age of 53.36 years at death for silicotics with lung cancer, while this age stood at 62.87 for individuals with lung cancer without silicosis. It is proposed that the silicotic complication accounts for this distinct shift into an earlier age group. It does also not appear that the distribution pattern of histologic types of lung cancers found in coexistence with silicosis presents any deviations from the norm (Table 4). Lung cancers in silicotics likewise seem to be located more often at the

Table 4. *Histologic Types of Lung Cancers in Silicotics*

Squamous Cell Carcinoma	Round- and Oat Cell Carcinoma	Adeno-carcinoma	Total
16	20	1	37

hilum and in the upper lobes than in the lower lobes, where the majority of asbestosis cancers are situated.

Attempts to produce cancers of the lung in experimental animals (mice, guinea pigs) by exposing them to dust of silica or silicon carbide, respectively, have yielded equivocal results since adenomatoid formations in both species occur also on a "spontaneous" basis (CAMPBELL; WILLIS and BRUTSAERT). Of more definite significance in regard to carcinogenic properties of quartz, a macromolecular silicon oxide, are the experiments of DRUCKREY and SCHMAEHL. These investigators observed the development of four (4) sarcomas in the abdominal cavity in 29 rats intraperitoneally implanted with finely powdered quartz sand, and interpreted this result as an indication of a weakly carcinogenic action of quartz. Sarcoma formation apparently did not occur in rats following a subcutaneous deposition of quartz sand and after an intraperitoneal and subcutaneous implantation of powdered glass, indicating thereby that a chronic mechanical irritation alone does not provide a carcinogenic stimulus (HUEPER and PAYNE; DRUCKREY and SCHMAEHL; HUEPER).

From the evidence on hand it appears that a well developed or advanced silicosis does not seem to furnish a favorable soil for the subsequent development of cancer of the lung. It is likely that any extensive fibrosis and hyalinization is likely to interfere with an adequate action of chemical carcinogens which might be embedded in such an oligocellular or acellular matrix. There exists, moreover, the possibility that any microcarcinomas formed in such an ill-vascularized tissue may find it difficult to proliferate or to survive especially in the face of a progressive fibrosis, such as that characterizing silicosis. Whether or not the concept of KAHLAU, that an incipient silicosis provides a more suitable soil for carcinogenesis deserves further consideration as a part of the general problem of carcinogenesis occurring in the vicinity of pulmonary scars (DI BIASI).

b) Vegetable and Animal Dust Pneumoconiosis

Among the numerous occupational activities associated with an inhalation of dusts of vegetable and animal matter (cotton, hemp, sisal, cork, sugar cane, wood paper, silk, wool, animal hair, feathers, shellac), some of which give rise to progressive fibrosing pneumoconioses (byssinosis, bagassosis, etc.), only tabacosis has been related by epidemiologic evidence to cancer of the lung, while the possibility of such associations deserves consideration for shellac pneumoconiosis.

α) *Tabacosis*

Because of the numerous claims made especially during recent years concerning carcinogenic chemicals present not only in tobacco smoke but also in processed tobacco leaves and responsible for the induction of cancers of the respiratory system and of the oral cavity, it is noteworthy that several decades ago dust of tobacco leaves inhaled during the cultivation, harvesting and curing was incriminated on statistical grounds of causing cancer of the lung in cigarette makers (ENGER; ROTTMANN; BRINKMANN; KOUWENAAR; KOELSCH; SEYFARTH). In commenting on such claims, LEHMANN noted that persons engaged in the tobacco trade are usually heavy smokers, and that this habit is more likely to be the causative mechanism than the inhalation of tobacco dust.

Since more recent epidemiologic studies on the frequency of lung cancer among American workers employed in cigarette factories have failed to show any excessive liability to lung cancer for these individuals, the supposition of LEHMANN lacks factual evidence. It is moreover a reasonable suspicion that the chewing of tobacco leaves, particularly when forming a part of the betel nut quid and khaini quid furnishes the main carcinogenic principle responsible for the high incidence of cancer of the oral cavity prevalent among populations in South-East Asia. Apart from any natural carcinogens present in tobacco leaves, consideration also must be given to the fact that such leaves are contaminated frequently with arsenical and chlorinated hydrocarbon pesticide residues and with soot from burnt wood or heavy petroleum oils used during the curing process.

It is at present uncertain whether any of these materials or some others are responsible for the excessive frequency of lung cancer among English grain dockers (DUNNER and HICKS).

β) Shellac Pneumoconiosis

In view of the repeatedly reported abnormally high lung cancer incidence among painters (MÜLLER; DUBLIN and VANE; FULTON; WYNDER and GRAHAM), it is of interest that the inhalation of shellac used in lacquers and varnishes and often applied with a spray gun, may elicit a chronic indurative and progressive fibrosing pneumonitis (HIRSCH and RUSSEL). After purification, shellac consists mainly of hydroxy acids of aromatic and aliphatic hydrocarbons jointed together by lactone and various internal ester linkages. While it will be wise to include shellac in any assessment of cancer hazards to the lung among painters and cabinet makers, members of these trades sustain occupational exposures to various additional respiratory carcinogens, such as chromates, nickel, arsenic, carbon black, aniline dyes used as pigments, solvents and paint removers of coal tar and petroleum derivation, etc. which presumably are more carcinogenic than shellac, if such should be the case.

c) Chronic Chemical Pneumonitis and Bronchitis

Similarly negative epidemiologic observations exists concerning causal relations between various types of chemical pneumonitis and the liability to bronchial cancers in individuals thus affected (acid workers, alkali workers, cement workers, synthetic fertilizer producers, manganese and cadmium smelter workers, epoxy resin producers, etc.), although some workers in such occupations (acid workers, alkali workers, cement workers) develop perforated nasal septa through the corrosive action of the inhaled dust or mist. They thus display exposure stigmata similar to those seen in workers with occupational contact to several specific chemical dusts and fumes implicated in the production of cancers of the respiratory tract (arsenicals, chromates) (KOELSCH). The negative evidence on such association available for alkali workers refutes the allegation of MORGAN that the respiratory cancers observed in nickel refinery workers are attributable to the inhalation of alkali dust generated in the calcining process.

There is likewise no valid epidemiologic evidence supporting the claim that workers exposed to fumes and mists of mineral acids have an excessive liability to respiratory cancer. The large scale use of such acids (sulfuric acid, hydrochloric acid, nitric acid, fluoric acid, etc.) for a large variety of industrial operations resulting in an occupational exposure of many workers to these agents has not yielded any incriminating evidence (KOELSCH; KIKUTH; LICKINT; ADELHEIM). These observations are not only of practical but also of scientific importance, because these agents have been accused of arresting the ciliary movement of the bronchial epithelium thereby decreasing the natural forces of resistance of this tissue to the action of inhaled carcinogens (KUSCHNER; FALK, TREMER and KOTIN).

B. Specific Industrial Respiratory Carcinogens

The evidence concerning an etiologic role in the induction of cancers of the respiratory organs is a great deal more reliable, definite, and comprehensive, on the other hand, for a number of specific occupational respiratory carcinogens. Many of them are, moreover, introduced into the general atmosphere in the form of industrial and industry-related effluents and enter the home environment in the form of consumer goods and economic poisons (Table 5).

Table 5. *Recognized Occupational Respiratory Carcinogens*

Agents	Sites:			
	Lung	Larynx	Nares	Nasal Sinuses
Arsenic	+	+	+	+
Asbestos	+			
Chromium	+	+	+	+
Nickel	+		+	+
Isopropyl Oil	+	+		+
Mustard Gas	+	+		
Coal Tar	+	+		
Mineral Oil	+	+		
Radioactive Chemicals	+			+

1. Significance of Specific Industrial Carcinogenic Irritants

Although the knowledge of specific industrial carcinogenic agents affecting the skin dates back to almost 200 years, the recognition of occupational carcinogens

Table 6. *The Time Table of Discoveries of Occupational Cancers*

Name of Agent	Date	Discoverer	Target Organ	Type of Contact
Chemicals-Organic				
Coal Soot.	1775	POTT	Skin	Occupational
Coal Tar (lignite) . . .	1876	VON VOLKMANN	Skin	Occupational
Coal Tar (Bitumen) . .	1892	BUTLIN	Skin	Occupational
Coal Tar (Anthracite) .	1910	ZWEIG	Skin	Occupational
Coal Tar (fumes) . . .	1936	KAWAHATA	Lung	Occupational
Creosote Oil	1920	O'DONOVAN	Skin	Occupational
Anthracene Oil	1908	OLIVER	Skin	Occupational
Paraffin Oil				
(Shale)	1876	BELL	Skin	Occupational
(Petroleum).	1910	SCHAMBERG	Skin	Occupational
Petroleum Coke	1890	DERVILLE and GUERMONPREZ	Skin	Occupational
Lubricating Oil				
(Petroleum).	1930	HELLER	Skin	Occupational
(Shale)	1910	WILSON	Skin	Occupational
Benzene	1928	DELORE and BORGOMANO	Bone Marrow	Occupational
Hydrogenated Coal				
Oil (Bergius)	1960	SEXTON *et al.*	Skin, Mouth	Occupational
Isopropyl Oil	1947	NALE and HUEPER	Nasal Sinus, Larynx, Lung	Occupational
Mustard Gas	1959	YAMADA	Larynx, Lung	Occupational
Chemicals-Inorganic				
Arsenic	1822	PARIS	Skin	Occupational
	1887	HUTCHINSON	Skin	Medicinal
	1930	SAUPE	Lung	Occupational
Asbestos	1935	LYNCH and SMITH	Lung	Occupational
Chromates	1935	PFEIL-ALWENS	Lung	Occupational
Nickel	1932	GRENFELL	Nasal Cavity and Sinuses, Lung	Occupational
Radiations				
Ultraviolet Rays	1894	UNNA	Skin	Occupational
Roentgen Rays	1902	FRIEBEN	Skin	Occupational
Radioactive Chemicals .	1879	HÄRTING and HESSE	Lung	Occupational

acting upon the organs of the respiratory system is only 35 years old, despite the fact that some of these respiratory carcinogens had been known for many decades to cause skin cancers. The pace of discovery of respiratory carcinogens of industrial derivation has been accelerated during recent years and has resulted in the establishment of a list of suspected and potential chemical carcinogens, some of which doubtlessly will subsequently be found to be carcinogens to the human respiratory organs (Table 6).

a) Classification of Occupational Respiratory Carcinogens

Depending on the amount and quality of evidence incriminating occupational environmental agents in the causation of cancers of the respiratory system, these etiologic factors can be classified into the following three groups:

Recognized respiratory carcinogens
Suspected respiratory carcinogens
Potential respiratory carcinogens

1. Recognized respiratory carcinogens are those agents for which the available medical, epidemiologic, pathologic and experimental evidence is adequate for establishing reliably causal relations between occupational exposures to such agents and the subsequent development of cancers of the respiratory system in man.

The following agents fulfill such requirements:

Arsenicals (inorganic)
Asbestos
Chromates and Chrome Pigments
Nickel
Isopropyl Oil
Mustard Gas
Coal Tar
Mineral Oil
Radioactive Substances

Since occupational cancers are non-intentional experimental cancers obtained in man, they should be assessed in regard to their etiologic significance on the same level as evidence obtained in experimental animals. They in fact provide even more weighty evidence than experimental animals as far as the existence of specific human cancer hazards is concerned because they demonstrate the carcinogenic effectiveness of particular environmental agents in the species man. This consideration is specifically applicable in adjudging arsenicals as recognized human carcinogens despite the equivocal nature of the experimental evidence on hand.

2. Suspected Respiratory Carcinogens are those agents for which the human evidence is at present not entirely conclusive although the available experimental evidence support directly or indirectly the existence of causal reactions of such agents to the development of cancers of the respiratory system in man.

Environmental Agents which belong to this group are:

Beryllium
Benzidin
Iron Oxide
Soot — Incomplete Combustion Products of Carbon, Petroleum, Wood, Gas
Chemicals Contained in Gasoline and Diesel Engine Exhausts
Thermic Tobacco Derivatives (Tobacco Combustion Products and Volatilized Normal and Artefactual Constituents).

Table 7. Suspected and Potential Respiratory Carcinogens

Agents	Species	Route	Lung	Skin	Subcut. Tissue	Bone	Bladder	Liver	Kidney	Hemat. Tissue	Miscellaneous
Iron	Man	Respiratory	+								
(Iron-polymer Complex)	Mouse, Rat Hamster				+?						+
Beryllium	Rat	Respiratory	+								
	Rabbit	Intravenous				+					
Carbamate	Mouse	Parenteral	+								
	Rat	Oral	+								
Dimethylaminostilbene	Rat	Oral	+	+ +				+ +	+	+	+
Benzidine	Man	Respiratory, Oral	+				+	+		+	+
Nitrosamines	Rat	Cutaneous	+				+				
	Dog		+				+				
	Guinea pig										
Acetylaminofluorene	Rat	Oral	+				+	+ +	+ +		+
Isoniacid	Rat	Oral						+		+	+
	Mouse	Oral?	+								
	Man	Subcut.	+?								
Diesel & Gasoline Motor Exhaust	Mouse	Respiratory	+		+						
	Man	Respiratory	+								
	Mouse	Cutaneous		+							
Oxydized Vaporized Gasoline	Mouse	Respiratory	+		+						
	Mouse	Cutaneous		+ +							
Atmospheric Soot	Mouse	Cutaneous		+							
	Mouse	Parenteral									
	Man	Respiratory	+								
4-nitroquinoline-l-oxide	Rabbit	Cutaneous		+							
	Rat	Subcut.	+		+						
Silicosis, Bagassosis, Byssinosis	Man		+								
Tobacco Tar	Mouse	Cutaneous		+	+						
	Dog	Bronchial	+								
Aliphatic and Aromatic Epoxides	Mouse	Subcut., Cutaneous		+	+						

3. Potential Respiratory Carcinogens are those agents for which the incriminating evidence is predominantly restricted to observations made in experimental animals exposed to these agents being components of local or general human environments incriminated by suggestive epidemiologic evidence in man (Table 7).

Environmental Agents included in this group are:
Carbamates
Nitrosamines
Isoniacid
Carbon Polymers (PVP, PVA, Polymethane, Epoxy Resins, Carboxymethyl-cellulose, etc.)
Oxidized aliphatic and aromatic hydrocarbons (epoxides and peroxides) generated in heated vegetable oils and animal fats and by photooxidation of evaporated gasoline
Silicosis
Byssinosis, Bagassosis and related Organic Pneumoconioses
Acetylaminofluorene

Table 8. *Cancers in Non-Respiratory Organs Elicited by Occupational Respiratory Carcinogens*

Agents	Route of Contact	Connective Tissue	Skin	Liver	Hemato-poietic Tissue	Bones	Alimentary Tract
Arsenic	Cutaneous Oral Respiratory		+	+			+
Coal Tar	Cutaneous		+				
Mineral Oil	Cutaneous Parenteral Oral	+	+				+
Radioactive Chemicals	Cutaneous Oral Parenteral	+	+ +	+	+	+	

b) Route of Exposure

While the majority of respiratory carcinogens enter the respiratory tract as pollutants (dust, fumes, spray, mist, vapor, gas) of the inhaled air, a few may apparently become active on the pulmonary tissue when introduced into the body of man or animals through non-respiratory routes, i.e., by ingestion, penetration of the skin, or parenteral introduction (arsenicals, benzidine, nitrosamine, acetylaminofluorene; carbamates), or even by transplacental penetration (ethyl carbamate). Some of the carcinogenic atmospheric pollutants are rather stable (chromates, nickel, arsenic, radioactive substances, asbestos), whereas others are changed and inactivated by chemical and photochemical reactions to which they are subjected in the air (polycyclic aromatic hydrocarbons, such as 3,4-benzpyrene). Climatic conditions and associated non-carcinogenic pollutants (particulate and gaseous) influence the quality and quantity of the atmospheric carcinogenic spectrum and its individual components.

Although some of the respiratory carcinogens have been constituents of the human environment for thousands of years, most of them are products of modern industrialism and all of them have been polluting the air to an increasing degree during the past century. Three fundamental types of respiratory exposure to these carcinogens can be distinguished:

1. Occupational exposure to specific carcinogens in specific industrial operations. Since the degree of exposure is, as a rule, more severe under these conditions than under any other ones, incidence rates of respiratory cancers among some of the exposed worker groups are also higher than those noted from any other types of exposure. All recognized respiratory carcinogens are involved in the production of occupational respiratory cancers and have, moreover, furnished the bulk of the epidemiologic evidence incriminating exogenous agents in the production of respiratory and nonrespiratory cancers in man. The first discovery of occupational cancers of the lung dates back as early as 1879 when the high incidence of lung cancer among Schneeberg miners was traced to, at that time, non-definable occupational factors.

An occupational contact with carcinogens is not necessarily restricted to workers who produce, process or handle directly such agents but not infrequently exists also for workers employed only temporarily in such operations (maintenance and repair men) or who work near such operations, such as yardmen, truckers, packers and loaders, or who are employed in other jobs near carcinogenic operations carried on in the same room or building or in nearby buildings.

2. Atmospheric pollutants of local and general distribution provide the second type of exposure to respiratory carcinogens. Carcinogens disseminated in the general atmosphere originate from various chemical and radioactive effluents emitted from smokestacks, chimneys of plants, houses, and ships, from exhaust pipes of automobiles, busses, trucks and railroad locomotives, from dust of oiled, asphalted and tarred roads, from radioactive fallout of atom bomb explosions and from chemical fallout of pesticide drift. Local carcinogenic effluents may be found within the vicinity of plants in which carcinogenic materials are produced, used, processed, and handled and along the roads on which they are trucked. Locally restricted air pollution of carcinogenic nature may be connected with the use of chromates and carcinogenic mineral oils in air conditioning equipment and of anticorrosive chromates in the water of steam heating plants of homes and office buildings, with the employment of asbestos in insulating material in homes and the use of carcinogenic pesticides and herbicides in homes and on lawns. Local or general types of carcinogenic respiratory exposure are connected with the dietary consumption of foodstuffs contaminated with arsenical pesticide residues or other carcinogenic contaminants of foodstuffs.

3. Habitual exposure to carcinogenic air pollutants of a personalized type, which in contrast to the two previously mentioned ones is voluntary, is associated with the smoking of tobacco, especially in the form of cigarettes. Similar voluntary exposures to the inhalation of respiratory carcinogens may be connected with the spraying or nebulizing of hair lotions and hair lacquers containing carcinogenic ingredients, such as 8-hydroxyquinoline, creosote, arsenicals, and various carbon polymers, such as polyvinyl pyrrolidone and polyvinyl alcohol. A voluntary type of carcinogenic exposure is associated also with the consumption of arsenicals and mineral oils for certain medicinal reasons. A similar iatrogenic mechanism may account for the

marked and increasingly often reported cancers in tuberculous lungs of patients treated with antituberculous chemicals (isoniacid).

It is apparent from this classification of exposure types that during recent decades technologic developments have spread respiratory carcinogens originally mainly active among members of restricted occupational groups not only to ever larger and more general industrial worker groups but also have disseminated such in part highly potent agents through industrial and industry-related wastes from occupational environments into local and general environments where they have contact with the population particularly its urban and industrialized components.

2. Occupational Respiratory Cancer and Smoking

During the past decade numerous investigators have attempted by comprehensive biostatistical studies and experimental investigations to determine the relative causal role which cigarette smoking allegedly plays in the induction of cancer of the lung, larynx and several non-respiratory organs such as the oral cavity, esophagus, stomach and bladder, and has contributed within the last 50 years to the alarming rise in frequency of lung cancers. A rather modest effort has been made during this period, on the other hand, of ascertaining equally comprehensive and pertinent information on the same etiologic and epidemiologic aspects of respiratory carcinogenesis as they apply to the various recognized environmental carcinogens which, in part are evidently not only considerably more potent than those apparently present in cigarette smoke but which have also much more prolonged and intense contact with large portions of the general population. An exposure to such atmospheric factors often lasts 24 hours a day and starts with the most susceptively neonatal age period and lasts throughout the entire life-time. This quantitatively and qualitatively disproportionate etiologic information on respiratory carcinogens available for these factors has tended to produce a distorted assessment of the relative significance of the various carcinogens in etiologic and epidemiologic respects and has interfered with the development of an over-all balanced programmatic approach to an effective prevention of respiratory cancer hazards of all types and from all sources.

This interpretation of the prevailing situation is supported by the following observations. Critical analyses of the causal environmental background of the excessive incidence of lung cancers among chromate workers, employees in asbestos plants and trades, and radioactive ore and hard rock miners, have demonstrated that such phenomena could not be attributed to cigarette smoking as a predominant etiologic factor, but were due to occupational exposures to specific chemicals (BIDSTRUP and CASE; SELIKOFF, CHURG and HAMMOND; WAGONER et al.; PARSONS, DE VILLIERS, BARTLETT and BECKLAKE). Symptomatic and epidemiologic evidence supporting this view in connection with lung cancer in chromate workers is contained in the reports of ALWENS et al.; FISHER; and GAFAFER et al.

ALWENS et al., in an early publication on the subject of chromate cancers of the lung, pointed out that an abuse of tobacco could not be demonstrated in most of his patients. GAFAFER et al. recorded that 81.1% of the chromate workers with lung cancers and that 79.4% of the foundry workers used as controls had been smokers These investigators noted, moreover, that the white chromate workers smoked more heavily than the colored ones.

On the other hand, the lung cancer liability of the colored workers was considerably higher (80-fold of standard rate) than that of the white workers (40-fold increase); in the brief report of FISHER, mention was made of the fact that among the 38 chromate producers with lung cancer, two (2) were non-smokers, three (3) smoked pipe and/or cigar, three (3) smoked less than one pack of cigarettes per day, nineteen (19) smoked between 1 and $1^1/_2$ packs per day, and five (5) smoked two (2) packs.

The most valid analysis on this matter has been provided by BIDSTRUP and CASE who came to the following conclusion: "Thus even if the smoking habits of the chromate workers were so changed from those of the general population that all of them fell into the category of heavy smokers, the increase of carcinoma of the lung that then would be expected would not satisfactorily account for the increase which we have observed. In fact, we have no reason to believe that their smoking habits are different from those of the general population, and an explanation based on a hypothesis of altered smoking habits would need to be supported by satisfactory evidence of such alteration before it could be seriously considered".

The recent allegation of OETTEL that lung cancers in chromate workers were found only in individuals who smoked cigarettes thus appears to be an expedient subterfuge and skillful device helpful to industrial management for escaping their legal and moral obligations toward their employees and the human society. Such fanciful contentions have obviously no scientific basis in fact and belong to the pseudoscientific propaganda emanating during the last decade to an increasing degree from some scientific guardians of commercial interests.

According to KREYBERG, workers breathing the air of a Norwegian gas plant inhale during a 40-hour-work-week, an amount of 3.4-benzpyrene which is equivalent to that present in 5,000 cigarettes (200 to 730 micrograms per 100 cbm of air) (ECKARDT). The general population of London, which has one of the highest worldwide lung cancer rates, sustains a daily exposure to 3.4-benzpyrene inhaled with the polluted air which corresponds in degree to an amount of this chemical present in 5 packages of cigarettes (SAWICKI et al.).

SELIKOFF, CHURG and HAMMOND commenting on this aspect in connection with their study of an excessive liability to lung cancer in asbestos cement workers came to the following conclusion: "From this we may conclude, that even if all our asbestos workers had smoked a pack or more of cigarettes a day (and, indeed, from our sample we know they did not), and if exposure to asbestos were of no significance, then their lung cancer death rate would have been about 3.4 times as high as the rate in the general US male population. Clearly, the smoking habits of the asbestos workers cannot account for the fact that their lung cancer death rate was 6.8 times as high as that of white males in the general population.

The epidemiologic and etiologic evidence on hand justifies the conclusion that occupational cancers of the respiratory system, like those of other organs and tissues, doubtlessly escape proper recognition and recording in many, if not most cases. They are included under these circumstances either among the cancers of so-called "spontaneous" or more correctly, "cryptogenetic" origin or are attributed during more recent years to cigarette smoking as the allegedly most important, most wide-spread and most universal environmental carcinogen.

It should be obvious that any wide acceptance of such scientifically unsound and socially irresponsible claims concerning the principal role of cigarette smoking in the causation of cancers, especially respiratory cancers, would paralyze not only a legitimate and urgently needed pursuit into the various environmental factors inducing such cancers, particularly the many industry-related pollutants of the urban air, but has provided already effective legal arguments before civil courts and compensation boards for denying justified claims for compensation of occupational respiratory cancers to the victims of such hazards as well as to their widows and orphans (HUEPER and CONWAY; HUEPER; HUEPER, KOTIN, TABOR, PAYNE, FALK and SAWICKI).

3. Epidemiology of Occupational Respiratory Cancers

The distinct caution which should be exercized at present in quantitating the relative role which individual factors or groups of factors assume in the causation of respiratory cancers and in their marked rise in frequency is indicated by the prevailing inability of assigning any reliable figures to the number of occupational respiratory cancers as well as to their industry-related environmental counterparts induced by atmospheric pollutants. Despite the definite shortcomings of the available epidemiologic data for both groups of respiratory cancers, the available evidence nevertheless clearly indicates that occupational and industry-related industrial factors are distinctly more important than this is conceded by the proponents of the cigarette theory, which is moreover defective in several important biologic characteristics of environmental carcinogenesis.

The highly fragmentary nature of the presently available epidemiologic data on occupational respiratory cancers is documented by the following facts:

Existing epidemiologic information is restricted to data obtained from surveys of relatively small industrial operations or special moderately sized and specialized industries with highly excessive respiratory cancer risks. No country possesses any large scale, systematized and current information on such matters for entire, large industries producing, processing, handling and using one or several of the known respiratory carcinogens and employing sometimes thousands, if not millions of workers sustaining occupational contact with these carcinogens to varying degrees and durations. Such conditions, for instance, exist in the United States for the steel and iron industries, for the power industry, petroleum industry, metal ore smelting and refining industries, metallurgical industries, chemical and rubber industries, plastic industries, asbestos industry, nickel and chromate industries, transportation, shipping, railroad and aviation industries, and paper and textile industries.

Even where some fragmentary epidemiologic data exist they scarcely ever cover those workers who have left for some reason the hazardous occupation and often have become employed in other companies or industries, while having carried along their specific occupational cancer liability to their new jobs (BIDSTRUP and CASE; HUEPER). Since work in many such operations is objectionable to the workers employed because it is dirty and inductive to toxic effects, the labor turnover is frequently considerable creating thereby a large number of effectively exposed workers escaping proper surveillance for their delayed cancerous manifestations.

Rarely any attempt has been made to ascertain the number of occupational respiratory cancers which occurred previous to the discovery of the cancer hazard in an industrial operation. It is intriguing to speculate about the number of lung cancer which were elicited in chromate producers in a plant which at the time of the discovery of this hazard showed a lung cancer frequency of 40 times the standard rate among white workers and 80 times such a rate among colored workers, considering the fact that this plant had been engaged in this type of manufacture for over 5 decades. It is also provocative to contemplate the medical diagnosis of the cause of death for workers dying from a pulmonary ailment after being employed in an asbestos brake lining factory, before it was found upon post mortem examination of such workers that 50 per cent of those who came to autopsy with the diagnosis of asbestosis were also suffering from cancer of the lung. Additional experiences with the peculiar nature of present-day industrial and public health practices on occupational respiratory cancer hazards are contained in the discussion of the various specific respiratory carcinogens (coal tar, petroleum oils, radioactive ores, etc.). They throw a revealing light on a recent comment made by a high medical official of the U.S. Public Health Service in regard to the evidence pertaining to environmental lung cancer hazards as they relate especially to cigarette smoking when he asserted that no additional research is anymore necessary for the establishment of the facts (July 27, 1965).

The distinct inadvisability of adopting a public health policy of the blocked mind toward the diconcerting problem of lung cancer etiology with its many complex aspects awaiting satisfactory solution is further demonstrated by the numerous observations indicating the action of occupational and industry related environmental agents in the causation of these tumors in industrialized as well as economically underdeveloped societies.

Several comprehensive epidemiologic studies on the frequency of lung cancer among members of different socio-economic classes and of large occupational or industrial groups have demonstrated the existence of definite differences in the rela-

Table 9. *Standardized Mortality Ratio* [1] *at Ages 35—65 in Each Social Class from Cancer of Various Sites*
Dicennial Supplements 1921 and 1931 (Registrar General)

Social Class	1921—1923				Males	1930—1932				
	I	II	III	IV	V	I	II	III	IV	V
All sites	80	92	99	96	123	83	92	99	102	114
Lip	30	50	70	140	170	—	56	68	147	183
Tongue	48	73	95	100	165	78	60	98	110	143
Tonsil	25	88	94	106	163	(86)	6	93	97	147
Pharynx	89	78	100	160	161	(76)	83	99	87	130
Oesophagus	76	91	104	88	130	74	87	98	94	130
Stomach	60	82	100	106	130	55	83	98	111	122
Upper alimentary canal	58	80	99	102	140	63	80	97	109	129
Lower alimentary canal	105	105	100	93	98	98	103	102	100	95
Larynx	72	96	93	96	135	60	81	98	90	143
Skin	63	73	100	120	150	(59)	75	95	116	133
Lung	100	109	97	79	124	107	96	101	91	112

[1] Registered percent of calculated deaths.

tive liability of such members to contract cancers of the lung (REGISTRAR GENERAL; STOCKS; COHART; MANCUSO and COULTER; HERDAN; CLEMMESEN and NIELSEN;

GRAHAM, LEVIN and LILIENTHAL; KENNAWAY). While the criteria used by the English investigators represent somewhat arbitrary groupings of the surveyed population on socio-economic and occupational characteristic reflecting a decreasing scale of income as well as types of occupation, American and Danish investigators have

Table 10. *Standardized Mortality of Males in 1949—53 by Social Class and in Farm and Mine Workers for Lung and Bronchus*

| Social Class | (P. STOCKS) | | | | | | | | | |
| | SMR at Ages 20—63 | | | | | PMR at Age 65 & over | | | | |
	I—II	III	IV—V	Farm	Mine	I—II	III	IV—V	Farm	Mine
Lung and Bronchus	82	107	104	55	79	95	105	99	47	55

The specification of the social classes and sub-classes is as follow:

Class	I	Professional and similar occupations
	II	Intermediate
	III	Skilled occupations
		(i) Mineworkers
		(ii) Transport workers
		(iii) Clerical workers
		(iv) Armed forces
		(v) Others in III
	IV	Partly skilled occupations
		(i) Agricultural workers
		(ii) Others in IV
	V	Unskilled occupations
		(i) Building and dock labourers
		(ii) Others in V

Table 11. *Lung Cancer Death Rates in 3 Districts of Connecticut* (GRISWOLD)

| District | Occupational Character | Standard Lung | | Cancer Rates |
		Males	Females	Both
Naugatuck Valley Area.	Rubber, metal, machinery, chemical	85.02	14.87	48.01
Northeast Area	Textile, paper, agriculture	69.24	21.69	45.01
Rural	Agriculture Industry, agriculture	30.60 85.02 38.65	— 17.35 14.87	15.00 50.54 26.53

Table 12. *Standardized Incidence Ratios in United States Cities and Standardized Mortality Ratios in England and Wales for Cancers of Lung and Bronchus Among Men* (BUELL, DUNN and BRESLOW)

| Primary Site | Ten United States Cities, 1947, Standardized Incidence Ratios by Income Class (All Ages) | | | | | England and Wales, 1949—1953 Standardized Mortality Ratios by Social Class (Ages 20—64) | | | | |
	I[1]	II	III	IV	V[2]	I[3]	II	III	IV	V[4]
Lung, bronchus	67	78	99	118	134	81	82	107	91	118

[1] High income.   [2] Low income.   [3] Professional workers.   [4] Unskilled workers.

Source: - U. S. data from DORN and CUTLER, England and Wales data from Registrar-General's report.

employed rent and income or residence in different quarters of a community as a gradient, which in turn also reflects differences in occupational activities of the groups, in addition to living habits, medical care, and social activities. There is general agreement in these studies that relative lung cancer liability exhibits a distinct social class gradient (Tables 9, 10, 11, 12 and 13) (Griswold; Buell, Dunn and Breslow).

Table 13. *Socioeconomic Distribution by Region of Cancer of the Lung in New Haven, 1935—1949* (E. M. Cohart)

Region	Male Cases			Female Cases			Total Cases		
	Obser-ved	Expected	Ratio of P O to E	Obser-ved	Expected	Ratio of O to E	Obser-ved	Expected	Ratio of P O to E
I	52	58.77	0.88	11	16.97	0.82	66	75.74	0.87
II	58	68.85	0.84	11	16.77	0.66	69	83.62	0.81
			<0.05			>0.05			<0.01
III	125	107.38	1.16	31	22.26	1.39	156	129.64	1.20
Total	235			53			291		

The circumstantial epidemiologic evidence supporting a major role of occupational factors in the induction of respiratory cancers is provided by statistical analyses of lung cancer rates in large industrial worker groups and of members of various occupations and trades. (Mancuso; Morrison; Breslow; Lew; Registrar General;

Table 14. *Mortality from Lung Cancer and All Causes. Specific Occupations* With Significantly Divergent S. M. R.'s for Lung Cancer in California Men, Ages 20 to 64, 1949 to 1951

Social Class	Occupation	Lung Cancer Deaths			All Causes S. M. R.
		Observed	Expected	S. M. R.	
Lung Cancer S.M.R. Above 100					
I	Authors, etc.	11	6.3	175	107
III	Bookkeepers	12	6.4	188	100
III	Carpenters	108	74.7	145	89
III	Machinists, etc.	44	32.1	137	122
III	Plumbers, pipefitters	27	18.5	146	110
III	Stationary engineers	29	15.4	188	145
IV	Mine workers	29	11.6	250	225
V	Sailors, deck hands	11	3.8	289	272
IV	Taxicab drivers	16	7.4	216	139
IV	Cooks (not private)	44	24.4	180	184
V	Fishermen	11	5.6	196	106
V	Laborers (not farm or mine)	155	118.7	131	162
Lung Cancer S.M.R. Below 100					
I	College faculties	1	4.8	21	30
I	Civil engineers	4	10.9	37	89
I	Electrical engineers	1	5.8	17	72
II	Teachers (n.e.c.)[1]	4	12.5	32	64
II	Managers, trade	92	140.5	65	82
III	Other clerical workers	80	98.7	81	82
V	Janitors	33	47.1	70	78
V	Other specified laborers (mainly gardeners)	16	31.5	51	64

[1] N. e. c., not elsewhere classified.

Kennaway and Kennaway.) The data presented in the several Tables (Tables 14, 15, 16, 17 and 18) prepared by various investigators in different countries on the lung cancer death rates of members of various occupations trades, professions and industries illustrate this point. Such fluctuations in the relative liability to lung cancer

Table 15. *Cancer Mortality by Occupation; Persons Insured Under Ordinary Policies —* *Special Studies: Occupations with Probably Higher-Than-Average Death Rates* *from Cancer* (E. A. Lew)

Occupational Group	Deaths from Cancer	Ratio of Acutal Deaths from Cancer to Expected Deaths Measured by Average, Mortality Ratio ± Probable Error %	Period Covered by Study
Waiters in hotels, restaurants, and club	14	125 ± 22	1915—1927
Waiters in hotels, restaurants, and clubs (male, no liquor served)	32	200 ± 24	1925—1936
Cooks, hotel, restaurant, and domestic.	13	136 ± 25	1915—1927
Cooks in hotels, restaurants, and clubs	23	123 ± 17	1925—1936
Domestic cooks	10	200 ± 42	1925—1936
Hotel keepers, etc. (not at bar)	78	176 ± 13	1915—1927
Guards, watchmen, and doorkeepers, exclusive of those at penal institutions	22	233 ± 33	1915—1927
Janitors and sextons	24	125 ± 17	1915—1927
Stationary firemen	22	131 ± 19	1925—1936
Brick and stone masons	11	150 ± 30	1915—1927
House painters and varnishers	31	173 ± 21	1915—1927
Grinders of metals	11	220 ± 44	1925—1936
Furnacemen and puddlers in iron and steel works	11	172 ± 35	1915—1927
Blacksmiths	20	150 ± 22	1915—1927
Tailors (ages 40 and over)	33	150 ± 16	1915—1927
Semiskilled operatives in clothing manufacture (ages 40 and over)	18	175 ± 20	1915—1927
Spinners, weavers, and winders in cooton mills	22	165 ± 23	1925—1936
Enlisted men (Army, Navy, Marine Corps) . .	12	160 ± 31	1925—1936
Laborers in nonhazardous occupations	18	180 ± 28	1925—1936
Section and track foremen on railroads	11	247 ± 49	1915—1927
Proprietors, foremen, and semiskilled workers in production of nonalcoholic beverages . . .	14	300 ± 53	1915—1927
Junk and rag dealers	18	175—28	1915—1927

Table 16. *Lung Cancer Death Rates per 1,000 Deaths from All Causes for 7* *Industrial Groups in Ohio, 5,309 Males, 1947* (Mancuso)

Industry	Death Rate
Nonferrous metal	3.22
Transportation	2.91
Rubber and plastics	2.34
Iron and steel	2.18
Mining and quarrying . . .	1.53
Agriculture	0.82
Stone, clay, glass	0.66
Rate for all industries listed	1.76

among such diverse population groups cannot justly be attributed to differences in the biologic constitutional composition of their membership to contract cancer of the lung. They can only be ascribed to quantitative and qualitative variations in the exposure conditions to mainly still unidentified environmental and occupational respiratory carcinogens.

Additional evidence on differences in occupation-related differences of lung cancer mortality rates have been recorded by WYNDER and GRAHAM; BERNDT; POCHE, MITTMANN, and KNELLER; TURNER and GRACE, and others. It appears

Table 17. *Standard Mortality Rates of Malignant Neoplasms of the Respiratory System in Occupational Classes in Scotland* (MORRISON)

Occupational Code No.	Occupation	SMR: Above 130
160—164	Platers, riveters, shipwrights	183
231—249	Electrical apparatus makers, electricians	170
131, 132	Moulders	162
589	Masons and stone cutters	162
134—138	Foundry workers, etc.	161
681	Dock laborers	157
912	Crane drivers	150
600—609	Painters, decorators	132
		Below 70
019, 021, 029	Farm workers	25
010, 011, 018, 020	Farmers, etc.	27
110—119	Foremen & overlookers in metal manufacture	54
013—015	Market or other gardeners	56
620—629	Managers or industrial under-takings other than managers of office departments	69

Table 18. *Mortality from Lung Cancer and All Causes. Standardized Mortality Ratios by Major Occupation Groups in California Men, Aged 20 to 64, 1949 to 1951*

Major Occupation Group		Lung Cancer		All Causes S. M. R.	Occupation Reporting Bias[1]	
Number	Title	Deaths	Actual S. M. R		Number	Ratio
	All reported occupations		99	96		
1	Professionals, etc.	151	84	90	24/18	133
3	Managers, etc.	269	76	83	17/17	100
4	Clerical, etc.	97	86	82	14/14	100
5	Sales	152	103	97	22/23	96
6	Craftsmen, etc.	567	120	95	92/82	112
7	Operatives, etc.	278	105	93	36/47	77
8—9	Service workers	202	110	109	44/55	80
11	Laborers	203	119	142	33/32	103
2	Farmers	111	94	93	11/6	183
10	Farm laborers	61	54	90	4/10	40

[1] Number on death certificate divided by number according to occupational history. Histories were obtained by interview with hospitalized lung cancer patients who were subsequently traced on routine state death records (BRESLOW).

from these studies that workers employed in the metallurgical industry, painters, decorators, and mechanics are distinctly more often affected by lung cancer than farmers and agricultural laborers as well as coal miners. There is no evidence nor is it conceivable that such variations in lung cancer frequencies for different worker groups are in any way causally associated with demographic differences in cigarette smoking habits. This argument is applicable with equal force to the etiologic factors responsible for the occupational lung cancers of women working in smoke filled kitchens or inhaling smoke from braziers who develop lung cancer at a high rate, such as the Mexican women in Southern California (STEINER; BUECHLEY, DUNN, LINDEN and BRESLOW) or at a rather young age, such as the Bantu women in South Africa (HURWITZ).

4. Pluripotentiality of Respiratory Carcinogens

Respiratory carcinogens display to a remarkable degree pluripotential properties. This phenomenon is in part due to the fact that carcinogenic agents inhaled with the environmental air come in contact not only with the mucosal lining of the respiratory tract, but invariably also with that of the alimentary tract by being swallowed with the saliva and nasal secretion, as well as with the epidermis of the skin. The observation of cancers in non-respiratory organs in individuals exposed to atmospheric carcinogens, therefore, should serve as a warning of simultaneously existing cancer hazards to the respiratory system. The experiences obtained in the past with the discovery of occupational lung cancer hazards related to previously recognized skin carcinogens furnishes an adequate illustration in support of such correlations. It can be expected that this pattern of multiple target organs of respiratory carcinogens applies also when presently available observations are restricted to the respiratory organs. It is remarkable therefore that this biologic principle generally valid for occupational carcinogens does not hold apparently for exposures to cigarette smoke. Despite the fact that there exist definitely many more heavy cigarette smokers than coal tar workers and cobblers who have developed cancer of the fingers and hands from exposure to carcinogenic tar and pitch, cancers of the fingers often deeply brown stained by a prolonged and intense contact with cigarette tar have not been observed in chain smokers. A similar discrepancy exists regarding the apparent absence of cancer of the lip in cigarette smokers whose labial mucosa is constantly bathed in the tarry juice oozing from the tip of the cigarette. Lip cancers, on the other hand, have been recorded in tar workers as well as in fishermen keeping the tarry threads and the tar contaminated needle used during the repair of nets between their lips (HUEPER). It is improper to invoke as an explanation for such differences in action between cigarette tar and coal tar a hypothetical variation in tissue susceptibility especially since cigarette tar is capable of inducing cancer of the skin in mice, and as claimed, is present in a concentrated form in the butt of cigarettes.

5. Carcinogenic Symptom Complex

All known respiratory carcinogens elicit in man in addition to cancers in different part of the respiratory system also a complex of symptoms which in part is characteristic for a particular carcinogen and which reflects its toxic action on the respiratory mucosa as well as other tissues.

Arsenic: Perforated nasal septum, bronchitis, metaplastic changes in bronchial mucosa, chronic dermatitis, melanosis of the skin, leukoderma, hyperkeratoses of palmar and plantar surfaces, neuritis, cirrhosis of the liver, obliterative arteritis in lower extremities, multiple cancers of the skin, liver, lung, esophagus, etc.

Asbestos: Asbestos warts of the hands and forearms, bronchitis, progressive fibrosis of lung of diffuse character and involving lower lobes first, focal emphysema, adenocystic degeneration of bronchioli, thickening and calcification of pleura, asbestos bodies in sputum, squamous cell metaplasia of bronchial mucosa, atypical carcinosis of abdominal cavity, peritoneal mesothelioma, mesothelioma of pleura, carcinoma of lung.

Chromates: Chronic dermatitis with chrome holes (indolent ulcers) on hands and forearms, perforated nasal septum, chronic rhinitis, chronic ulcerative bronchitis, chronic laryngitis, chromitosis of lung, chronic chemical pneumonitis, chronic ulcerative gastritis and colitis, cancer of lung.

Nickel: Chronic dermatitis, chronic bronchitis, chronic chemical pneumonitis, adenocystic degeneration of bronchioli, chronic rhinitis, carcinoma of nares and paranasal sinuses.

Radioactive Chemicals: Chronic bronchitis, radiation pneumonia, anemia and leukemia, hypoplastic and hyperplastic changes in bone marrow, cancer of lung, cancer of nasal sinuses.

Coal Tar: Chronic dermatitis, tar warts, melanoderma, cornified horns on exposed skin, chronic rhinitis with loss of sense of smell and taste, bituminosis of lung, chronic bronchitis, papillomas and cancers of skin, cancer of lung.

Mineral Oil: Chronic dermatitis, melanoderma, warts, papillomas, chronic chemical pneumonitis (lipoid pneumonia), cancer of the skin at sites of principal exposure (hands, forearms, face, neck, scrotum, feet, lower extremity), cancer of the larynx, cancer of the lung.

Crude Isopropanol: Chronic sinusitis, nasal polyps, cancer of the larynx, nasal sinuses, lung.

Mustard Gas: Chronic dermatitis, chronic rhinitis, laryngitis, and pneumonitis, emphysema, bronchiectases, cancer of the lung, larynx and nasal sinuses.

These etiology specific symptom complexes represent in part exposure stigmata. They occur in many but not all individuals with these occupational cancers. Their appearance may precede often by many years the manifestation of the cancer.

6. Sex Distribution

With the exception of asbestos cancers of the lung and cancers of the nasal sinuses after exposure to radioactive gases or dust in luminous dial painters, the occurrence of all other occupational cancers of the respiratory system has been limited so far to members of the male sex. This sex distribution reflects and is the result of the exclusive employment of males in the various occupations with respiratory cancer hazards. Whenever females were equally exposed to occupational respiratory carcinogens, they exhibited a liability to cancer comparable to that seen in males.

7. Occupational "Neighborhood" Cancers

Recent observations on individuals living in the vicinity of industrial operations with occupational respiratory cancer hazards (coal tar fumes, chromate fumes, asbestos dust, beryllium dust) (FIRKET; GROSS; WAGNER et al.; KIMINA; SARUTA et al.; FERSHTUDT; BOURNE and RUSHIN; WALTERS; WEBSTER; THOMSON; EISENBUD et al.), have revealed that industrial respiratory cancer hazards were spread into the immediate environment of plants in which such chemicals were produced or handled and were found along the roads on which industrial carcinogens were transported. Characteristic pulmonary lesions (asbestosis, berylliosis) were found in environmental residents as well as in consumers using such materials in their household and also in animals living in such environments (NIEBERLE; WEBSTER, KIVILUOTO). Industrial carcinogens thus have produced not only endemic "neighborhood pneumoconioses and cancers" but presumably also nonoccupational "household cancers of the lung".

As the result of general intraplant contaminations of the air, occupational lung cancers have been seen, moreover, in workers who were not directly employed in carcinogenic operations but were engaged only transitorily in such operations for repair and maintenance work or were employed in adjacent buildings, or did yard work in the vicinity of such buildings (GROSS) or performed work of non-carcinogenic nature, but were brought in direct contact with carcinogenic chemicals handled by other workers in the same operation (SELIKOFF et al.). The existence of such "occupational association" exposures has rarely been considered in past epidemiologic investigations on an occupational causation of cancer in man.

Equally important in this respect should prove more comprehensive epidemiologic studies on the scatter pattern of occupational respiratory cancers in worker populations, as well as in the general population, along the lines of the known "traffic pattern" of specific carcinogens. Such studies should start with the original production operations of the carcinogens. They should follow them through the consuming industries and trades and finally be applied to the home environment of the ultimate public consumer as well as to the local and regional general environment. The ultimate consumer becomes exposed to these agents not only when they are present as ingredients, impurities and contaminants of consumer goods but also when they pollute water, air, soil, fauna, and flora (HUEPER; KIVILUOTO; WAGLER; MUELLER and ANSPACH; NEWHOUSE).

8. General Periplant Dissemination

The existence of respiratory cancer hazards in the immediate intraplant and extraplant environment has been demonstrated by the presence of several types of respiratory carcinogens in such areas. The spread of occupational cancer hazards in accordance with their known "traffic pattern" has also been proven. It stands to reason therefore that a similar, while mitigated effect, of the various occupational and industry-related respiratory carcinogens present in the general air, especially of cities and industrialized regions, accounts for a significant portion of the respiratory cancers occurring in the general population. There are good reasons for assuming that industrial atmospheric pollutants are responsible in part, not only for the alarming increase of lung cancers during recent decades but also for the distinctly higher lung cancer rates in urban populations over rural ones (COMMINGS; HAMPELN; HUEPER; KOTIN and FALK; STOCKS; STOCKS and CAMPBELL; HAMMOND; CURWEN, KENNAWAY and KENNAWAY; PYBUS).

9. Carcinogenic Potency and Attack Rates of Industrial Respiratory Cancers

The high carcinogenic potency of most industrial respiratory carcinogens is reflected in the highly excessive attack rates of respiratory cancers affecting various parts of this system (nares, paranasal sinuses, larynx, bronchi) according to observations in various circumscribed and usually severely exposed worker populations (Table 19). This fact receives additional support from the evidence that the carcino-

Table 19. *Attack Rates of Occupational Respiratory Carcinogens*

Chemical	Site of Cancer	Incidence in Population in Risk	% of All Cancer Deaths	Attack Rate Morbidity Rate per 100,000	Attack Rate Mortality Rate per 100,000
Arsenic	Lung	—	—	—	145.7 males (10.9 normal)
Asbestos	Lung	—	—	12 × normal	(13.2—50.0% of all autopsies on asbestotics) (1 normal)
Chromium	Lung	—	—	42 × normal	146—338
Nickel	Nares, Paranasal Sinuses	329:100,000 574:100,000	—	20 × normal	—
Radioactive Chemicals	Lung	—	—	—	(50—80% of all deaths)
Crude Isopropanol	Paranasal Sinus, Larynx	10:100	—	134.5 (normal 6.5)	—
Coal Tar	Lung	500:100,000	45%	—	—
Mineral Oil	Lung	2,000:100,000	55%	—	—

gens involved are capable of producing in most instances, cancers in several organs and in several species when introduced into experimental animals by the same or different routes.

10. Age Distribution

It is a well-established experience in occupational and experimental chemical carcinogenesis that optimal exposures to potent carcinogens sustained at an early adult period of life often lead to a shift of the age peak of cancers produced into an earlier period of life than that seen with the same type of cancer found in the general population which is often less intensely exposed to same agents.

The data recorded indicate that there is a distinct shift toward younger age groups demonstrable only for cancers of the lung induced by exposures to chromates and chrome pigments and to radioactive chemicals (Table 20). Most occupational lung

Table 20. *Age Distribution of Occupational Cancers of the Lung, Nose, Larynx, and Pleura in Percentage of Total Number*

Years	0—29	30—39	40—49	50—59	60—69	70 and over	Total number of cases
Carcinogen			Percentages				
Arsenic	1.2	3.6	22.2	45.7	21	6	81
Asbestos: Carcinoma .	0	6.6	19.0	32.0	21.3	3.2	122
Mesothelioma		23	31	23	23	0	40
Chromium	0.8	15.7	25.5	33.3	22.5	2.2	102
Nickel: Lung	0	1	6	50	41	2	75
Nose		0	0	41	55	4	29
Coal Tar	0	9	24	20	25	22	58
Mineral Oil	0	0	0	58	42	0	12
Mustard Gas	0	5	15	47	33	0	19
Radioactive Chemicals .	7	36	27	19	11	0	83
Controls General . . .	6	12	24	34	21	3	1,792
Silicosis	0	2	21	43	32	2	100

cancers do not differ in this respect from those allegedly caused by excessive cigarette smoking and seen in the general population.

It is likely that the absence of a distinct shift in the age distribution of the majority of industrial respiratory cancers is related to the fact that the age of onset

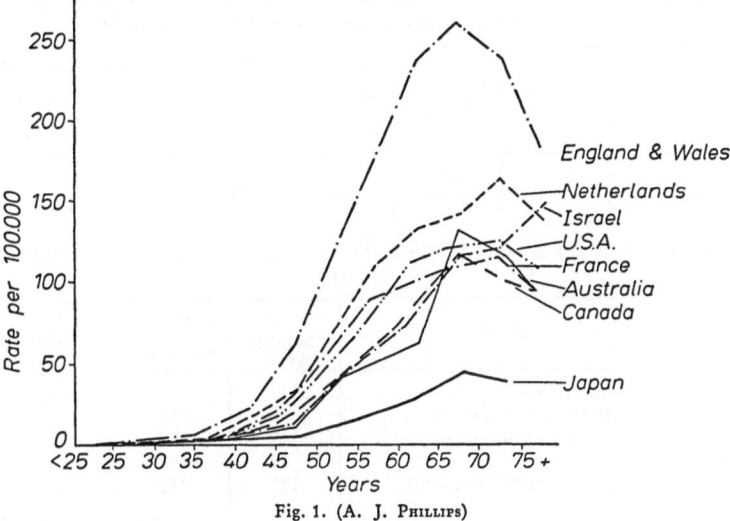

Fig. 1. (A. J. Phillips)

of exposure to the occupational carcinogen is, as a rule, at an adult age and that the degree of exposure to the various carcinogens is not sufficiently high for shortening significantly the length of the latent period. Observations on chimney sweep cancer of the scrotum (Hueper) and on occupational aromatic amino cancer of the bladder

(GOLDBLATT and GOLDBLATT), on the other hand, indicate that the age at entrance into a hazardous occupation determines to a demonstrable degree the age of manifestation of the cancer. Since PHILLIPS recently recorded a shift of the age-peak of pulmonary cancers in the English population by one decade, into a younger age group than that seen in other Western countries, it seems to be unlikely that such a

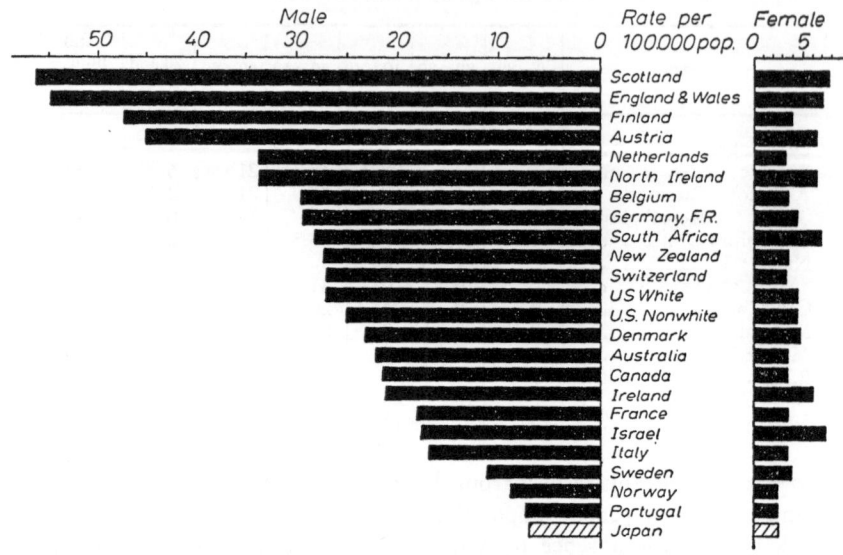

Fig. 2. Malignant neoplasm of lung and bronchus trachea 1956—1957 (M. SEGI)

Table 21. *Observed and Expected Death Rate of Lung Cancer According to Place of Birth*
A. New Zealand and Great Britain (D. F. EASTCOTT, 1956)

Birthplace	Observed No. of Deaths	Expected No. of Deaths	Age at Time of Immigration from Great Britain			
			Observed	Expected	Observed	Expected
			Under 30 years of age		Over 30 years of age	
New Zealand . .	632	721.8	—	—	—	—
Great Britain . .	369	279.8	201	229.2	168	139.8

B. Lung Cancer Death Rates Among White Males in South Africa, 1947—1956, per 100,000
(G. DEAN)

Country	Age Periods	
	54 — 64 Years	65 + Years
South Africa:		
Native Male Whites . .	50	112
British Immigrants . . .	112	172
Others	67	152
England and Wales, 1951 .	135	219

shift can justly be attributed to any intensification of exposure to carcinogenic respiratory agents for occupational and habitual reasons occurring during the last 50 years, but is more likely due to enhanced pollution of the atmosphere with carcinogenic chemicals which were inhaled to an increasing degree during this period starting with an early age (Fig. 1). The age shift thus is the result of a progressively intensified and extraordinary exposure of the children of England to carcinogenic air pollutants. This phenomenon evidently accounts also for the greater part of the unusually high lung cancer rates among the English population (SEGI) (Fig. 2) as well as for the excessively high pulmonary cancer liability of British immigrants to New Zealand, South Africa and the United States (EASTCOTT; DEAN; MANCUSO) (Tables 21, 22 and 23).

Table 22. *Death Rates of Lung Cancer in Male Immigrants, 25—64 Years of Age Per 100,000 Population in Ohio*
(T. F. MANCUSO)

Population of	Death Rate	Immigrants in Cuyahoga County from	Death Rate
Cuyahoga County 1947—1951, Native White Americans	28.75	All Foreign Countries 1947—1951	38.11
England and Wales, 1950	55.48	England and Wales 1947—1951	31.75
Italy, 1951	16.26	Italy, 1947—1951	18.61

Table 23. *Inhalation of 3,4-Benzpyrene in Urban and Rural Regions*
(SAWICKI *et al.*, 1960)

Estimated Amount of Bzp Inhaled by a Male Non-Smoker Living in	Micrograms per Year
Missouri State Forest	0.1
San Francisco . . .	14.0
Detroit	110.0
London	320.0

11. Latent Period

The average length of latent period of occupational cancers of the respiratory tract ranges from 10 to 30 years (Table 24). It may be much shorter in some cases

Table 24. *Latent Period of Occupational and Environmental Cancers of the Lung*

Carcinogenic Chemical	Average Latent Period in Years	Range of Latent Period in Years
Asbestos	18	15—21
Chromates	15	5—47
Nickel	22	6—30
Coal Tar Fumes . .	16	9—23
Ionizing Radiations	15—35	7—50

and considerably longer in others. While often the length of the latent period is equal to the exposure period, the exposure time may be much shorter than the latent period and after cessation of exposure to a carcinogen may be followed by a symptomless "lag" period of several months to many years. In some cases of asbestos carcinoma of the lung, for instance, the exposure time was only six months, while the first evidence of a pulmonary cancer in an asbestotic lung appeared in these individuals some 10 to 15 years later. In most cases of asbestos mesothelioma of the pleura, on the other hand, the average latent period was 30 to 40 years which included a lag period of some 20 years. Similar observations on a much delayed appearance of occupational and industry-related lung cancers have been made among chromate producers and among individuals living near asbestos mines and mills (HUEPER; WALTER; WAGNER *et al.*). It is obvious that workers once exposed adequately to an occupational respiratory carcinogen carry their excessive liability to an occupational cancer along into later life and into occupations which may be free from such hazards.

12. Histologic Types

Claims have recently been advanced that specific etiologic factors, such as cigarette smoke, determine the histologic type of lung cancers (KREYBERG). Hence, it should be emphasized that adequate and reliable experiences with a variety of occupational respiratory carcinogens attest to the histologic nonspecificity of the ensuing cancerous responses (HUEPER). These carcinogens induce pulmonary carcinomas of any types in man and experimental animals. In fact, they may elicit in the same lung multicentric cancers of different histologic type and, in animals, also sarcomas (Table 25). The reasons for such different histologic responses of the bronchial mucosa are

Table 25. *Histologic Types of Lung Cancers in Man Induced by Several Occupational Carcinogens*

Carcinogen	Squamous-Cell Ca.	Histologic Types of Lung Cancers		
		Round-Cell Ca.	Adeno Ca.	Total Number
Arsenic	19	24	4	47
Chromium.	46	66	11	123
Asbestos	45	40	19	104
Silica (Control). . .	16	20	1	37
Ionizing Radiation .	14	16	0	30
Coal Tar	3	0	2	5
Nickel (Nares) . . .	3	13	0	16
Mustard Gas . . .	11	8	0	19
Controls-Males (DORN and CUTLER)	29.3%	61.2%	9.5%	100%

obscure, although it is conceivable that adenocarcinomas are more likely to evolve from the adenocystic bronchial proliferations commonly found in asbestotic lungs, while squamous cell carcinomas probably develop from focal squamous cell metaplasias. The observations on the histologic types of occupational pulmonary cancers do not support the allegation that adenocarcinomas have a genetic origin and thus differ fundamentally in etiology from their squamous cellular or round cellular counterparts (KREYBERG).

C. Specific Occupational Cancers and Their Environmental Counterparts

The preceding critical appraisal of the characteristics of occupational respiratory carcinogens has demonstrated definitely that occupational respiratory cancers can be induced by a variety of chemical agents. Occupational respiratory cancers and their industry-related and etiologically identical environmental and medicinal counterparts provide conclusive evidence of the polyetiology of respiratory cancers. The data presented have shown moreover that some of the occupational respiratory carcinogens are widely distributed in the general atmosphere especially in urban and industrialized regions and in some metropolitan communities, such as London and New York, contaminate the air and therefore are inhaled by their residents in amounts considerably higher than those inhaled by the majority of smokers and reached only exceptionally by the most heavy smokers. It has been noted also that the carcinogenic potency of many of the occupational respiratory carcinogens is distinctly higher according to human and experimental evidence than that demonstrable for cigarette smoke even when applied as a tar condensate under most severe experimental conditions. While pluripotential carcinogenic properties of cigarette smoke has been deduced from circumstantial statistical evidence on man, these qualities have been established beyond any doubt in man and animals for various occupational carcinogens. Human experience with the majority of the occupational respiratory carcinogens indicates furthermore that these agents are capable of inducing cancers in different parts of the respiratory tract, including the nasal cavity and nasal sinuses. The latter parts so far have as yet not been incriminated as susceptible to the alleged carcinogenic action of cigarette smoke. There exists also adequate clinical and experimental evidence which demonstrates that cancers of the lung and nasal sinuses follow not only by an inhalatory introduction of respiratory carcinogens but also upon an ingestive and parenteral one. More recent observations on the carcinogenic action of a large series of nitrosamines by DRUCKREY and associates, and others, have brought out the fact that the chemical structure of these compounds some of which are widely used in industry directs their action toward specific target organs, including the lung and nasal sinuses for some of these substances.

With these facts on hand, it is rather surprising that the results of the numerous recent statistical analyses on the causation of lung cancers and their remarkable increase during recent decades either have totally failed to obtain evidence incriminating to any significant degree occupational carcinogens and their environmental counterparts in such matters or have relegated them to a minor and negligible role (Surgeon General's Report on Tobacco and Health). The misleading and deceptive argument that the epidemiologic evidence in support of the cigarette theory of lung cancer is even more conclusive than that which supported the contagious causation of smallpox when prophylactic measures were introduced reveals more crusading fervor than sound and sober medical judgment, since smallpox are due to a well defined and single infectious agent, while respiratory cancers are attributable to a considerable number of different causal agents. Because lung cancer rates are continuing to rise despite the various measures adopted to reduce the consumption of cigarettes, it may be proper to consider the introduction of preventive and protective measures against the various additional and factually proven causes of respiratory cancer.

The following detailed descriptions of the various recognized, suspected and potential occupational respiratory cancer hazards should provide sufficient and valid evidence for justifying a widening of the medical, public health and technologic approaches aimed at a preventive control of cancers amenable by past experience in industry to such measures.

1. Arsenic

Sites of Arsenic Cancers: Recognized: Skin, Lung, Liver; Suspected: Mouth, Esophagus, Larynx, Bladder.

Exposure Stigmata: Dermatosis, Neuritis, Arteritis, Gastroenteritis, Liver Cirrhosis; Laryngitis, Perforated Nasal Septum, Bronchitis, Anemia.

Compounds of Economic Importance (tri- and pentavalent): Arsenic metal and alloys, Ores of Silver, Gold, Copper, Tin, Lead, Cobalt, Nickel, Antimony, Iron (Pyrite), Realgar, Orpiment Arsenic acid, Arsenious acid, Arsenic trioxide, Arsenic pentoxide, Sodium arsenite, Calcium arsenate, Copper arsenate, Lead arsenate, Cupric Acetoarsenite (Paris Green), Cupric arsenite (Scheele's Green), Schweinfurt Green, London purple, Wolman's salt, Arsine (Arseniuretted Hydrogen), Arsanilic acid, Cacodylates, Arsphenamines, Lewisite, etc. Tryparsamide; Carbasone; Stovarsol.

Operations and Products with Contact to Arsenic for Producers, Processers, Users, Consumers, Residents: Copper alloy; lead shot; dust, fumes, mist, vapors in and around *metal ore smelters and refineries; dust and water draining off slag heaps* of mines and smelters; *water from arsenic containing rock;* pigments in paints, ink, glazes, glass, soap, and dyes of textiles and paper; decolorizer of glass; mordant; *preservative of wood, pelts, fur hides;* dehairing agent of pelts; *herbicide;* antisprouting agent; *pesticide* (cattle and sheep dip, grasshopper and mosquitoc bait, insecticide of potato beetle, Japanese beetle, cotton boll weevil, codling moth, gypsy moth); amebicide, algicide rodenticide; gas purification by Thylox process; war gases (Lewisite, etc.); hair lotion; animal feed additive; *pharmaceuticals* (tonics, antianemic preparations, Fowler's solution, Donovan's pills, Asiatic pills, cacodylates, arsphenamines, caustic ointments, etc.).

Population Groups with Occupational and Environmental Exposure to Arsenic Occupational Groups: Airplane pilots, arsenic roasters, artificial flower makers, book binders, bronze workers, cannery workers peeling fruit treated with insecticides, citrus fruit orchard workers, cotton plantation workers, cut-glass workers, dyers, dyestuff makers, electroplaters, enamelers, *farmers, fur handlers and preparers,* galvanizers, gardeners, glass mixers, glass workers, glue manufacturers, gold refiners, ink manufacturers, *insecticide makers, insecticide sprayers and dusters,* Japan makers, jewelers, lead factory workers, lead shot workers, linoleum color workers, lithographers, *miners of arsenic, copper,* zinc, silver, lead ores, oil cloth manufacturers, oil refinery workers, paper (colored) makers, paper glazers, paper hangers, paper printers, pelt and hair factory workers, pencil (colored) makers, pharmaceutical workers, photographers, poison bait makers, pottery decorators, pottery plant glaze dippers and mixers, printers, pyrites burners, rotogravure workers, rangers, rubber compounders, mordant mixers, rubber pressors, rubber tire manufacturers, sealing wax makers, seamstresses handling fabrics dyed or treated with arsenicals, *sheep dip manufacturers, smelter workers,* sulfur burners, sheep wool cutters, sulfuric acid workers, stevedores, tannery workers, taxidermists, textile printers, tinners, tobacco processers, velvet makers, *vinery workers, vineyard workers,* war gas manufacturers, weavers of yarns dyed with arsenical pigments, weed killer producers, wire drawers, wood preservers, wax goods manufacturers, zinc mixers, zinc smelter chargers, felt hat carroters, ferro-silicon workers.

Non-occupational Groups: Residents in vicinity of metal smelters and of orchards, fields and woods dusted and sprayed with arsenical pesticides; *individuals consuming drinking water and foodstuffs contamined with arsenical algicide* and insecticide residues; individuals smoking tobacco with arsenical residue; and inhaling arsenical air pollutants from burnt coal; *veterans with war gas poisoning; patients given prolonged treatments with arsenical preparations* (anemia, psoriasis, syphilis, trypanosomiasis, etc.); inhabitants of rooms with arsenic containing wall paint or wallpaper.

The world production of arsenic in 1955 was 37,000 short tons of which 10,800 were produced in the U.S.A. and of which were used 18,000 tons.

Arsenic and its compounds are widely distributed in nature and are practically ubiquitous. For this reason arsenic is found in traces in most inanimate and animate matter. Exposure to arsenicals from non-occupational sources is therefore common and accentuates that from occupational ones. The wide spread use of arsenicals as pesticides and herbicides as well as of feed additives furnishes and additional avenue of human contact because of the thereby conditioned contamination of foodstuffs with residues from such materials. Inorganic and organic arsenicals are moreover employed for various medicinal uses in tonics, antianemics, amebicides, and spirocheticides. Arsenicals are moreover released into the air and bodies of water with the effluents of non-ferrous metal smelters and of coal burning furnaces. Since exposures from these sources often complicate occupational contacts with arsenicals, a brief listing of data regarding quantities of arsenic in various environmental media is presented.

a) Non-occupational Sources of Exposure to Arsenicals

α) Atmospheric Urban Pollutants

DAFF and KENNAWAY (1950) and GOULDEN, KENNAWAY and URQUHART (1952) recorded the following information on the arsenic content of the air of several English communities

Beckton (London)	0.132 micrograms As_2O_3 per cbm of air
Bilston	0.075
Manchester	0.073
Liverpool	0.068
Sheffield	0.065
County Hall (London)	0.058
Hull	0.054
Bristol	0.037

While the effluents from the stacks of one copper smelter in U.S.A. were said to emit only about 10 per cent of the arsenic originally present in the flue dust and fumes, the balance being retained by electrostatic precipitators, in a second American smelter about 50% of the arsenic was released into the general atmosphere from the stacks. The arsenic content of soot of English factories was given by SOWDEN (1927) to be 500 ppm, while SILVERSTEIN (1962) noted that 0.015 to 0.100 mgm. of arsenic was contained in one cbm. of air.

β) Water Pollutants

The arsenic content of sea water was found to be 0.0006 to 0.03 ppm, whereas that of water of estuaries into which industrial wastes are being drained was 0.14 to 1.0 ppm (VALLEE, ULMER and WACKER, 1960). The development of dietary arsenic cancers of the skin in persons consuming fresh water contaminated industrially or naturally with arsenic was observed when the water contained the following amounts: Reichenstein, Silesia: 1.22 mg. per 100 cc. (GEYER, 1898); Cordoba (Argentina): 0.28 to 5.45 mg. per 100 cc. (ARGUELLO et al., 1938; TELLO, 1951); Taiwan (China): 0.8 to 2.5 ppm (How and YEH, 1963). For comparison it may be stated that the maximal official dose of FOWLER's solution contains 5 mg. As in 0.5 cc.

γ) Foodstuff Contaminants

The maximal allowed concentration of arsenic in vegetables and fruits in the United States is 1.4 mg. As_2O_3 per kg. and stands at 2.65 mg. per kg. of animal tissue. Seafood has naturally a relatively high arsenic content varying between 3 mg. of As/kg for oysters and 174 mg. for prawns.

Arsenic in fruits and vegetables is mainly derived from pesticides residues and, locally, also in part from chemical fallout of smelters, pesticides factories and similar establishments. Milk, meat, liver, eggs, etc. may retain some of the arsenic contained in organic arsenical feed additives.

δ) Soil Contaminants

SMALL and McCANTS reported that the soil from farmland not treated with arsenical pesticides in North Carolina had an arsenic content of 1 to 5 ppm., while it stood at 2.8 ppm. after arsenic application. Crops raised on such a soil translocated arsenic from the soil into roots and stems of crops.

ε) Tobacco Contaminants

While the arsenic content of human food is usually regulated by law, that of tobacco is not. Arsenical pesticides have been used freely on tobacco crops for several decades in most countries. Smoking tobacco therefore contains arsenic in amounts which have varied from 2 parts per million to 170 ppm. depending upon the type of tobacco tested and the year of examination. Arsenic in cigarette tobacco has been considered by some investigators to represent a significant factor in the causation of lung cancer among smokers (DAFF and KENNAWAY; HOLLAND et al.; SATTERLEE; and others).

There are numerous reports on the occurrence of acute and chronic arsenic poisoning from contact with arsenic from non-occupational sources (HUEPER). Such effects have not remained restricted to man but have been observed also in domesticated and wild animals, especially when exposed to arsenic containing smelter fumes (cattle, sheep, horses, goats, hogs, bees, deer, foxes, hares, fish) (PRELL; KAY; NIEBERLE; HUEPER; HARKINS and SWAIN) (Germany, Canada, U.S.A., France; Japan).

b) Arsenicals as Carcinogens

During recent years several American industrial investigators challenged the widely held conclusion that arsenicals are definite human carcinogens inducing cancers in the skin and various internal organs, including those of the respiratory tract (SNEGIREFF and LOMBARD; VALLEE, ULMER and WACKER; JOHNSTONE and MILLER; FROST; ECKARDT). This allegation has been applied not so much to the causation of cancers of the skin from a medicinal use of inorganic arsenicals, as to the existence of such associations particularly in regard to cancers of internal organs following contact with inorganic arsenicals for occupational reasons. There exists a voluminous literature on occupational, medicinal, dietary and environmental arsenic cancer effecting mainly the skin and less often other organs (NEUBAUER; HUEPER; HUEPER and CONWAY), refuting definitely such unfounded contentions. Some uncertainty still exists regarding a carcinogenic effect of organic arsenicals mainly used for medicinal purposes and as feed additives. Since organic arsenicals produce toxic symptoms identical with those elicited by inorganic arsenicals, it would be surprising indeed if the two types of arsenicals should differ in carcinogenic respects. In fact, several reports have indicted several medicinally used organic arsenicals as being responsible for the development of multiple cancer of the skin (NEUBAUER). The high incidence of uterine cancer among Danish protistutes was tentatively also related to the arsenical antisyphilitic treatments often received by these individuals. A similar suspicion has been entertained regarding an arsenical causation of the oral and pulmonary carcinomas found in the presence of syphilis (DÖRKEN).

There is no established carcinogenic dose for arsenicals. The German vintners with dietary arsenic cancers analyzed by ROTH who developed multiple cancers of the skin, liver, lung and other organs ingested over a twelve year period a total of 53,682 mgms. of arsenic at an average (minimum 18.6 mgm.; maximum 88,764 mgm.). NEUBAUER noted a variation of arsenic intake in individuals with medicinal arsenic cancers involving mainly the skin which ranged from 190 mgm. to 121,000 mgm. The average was about 28,000 mgm. Little valid information exists regarding the minimal exposure time of arsenic cancers (NEUBAUER; ROTH; KOELSCH; CURRIE).

c) Respiratory Arsenic Cancers

The development of cancers of the respiratory system has been noted following an occupational, medicinal and dietary introduction of inorganic arsenicals by inhalation and ingestion (ROTH; CALNAN; SEMON; WILLIAMSON; MONTGOMERY; SOMMERS and McMANUS; DANBOLT and FOSS; HOPKINS and SUDDIFORD; RUSSELL and KLABER; and others). In an appreciable percentage of these cases their occurrence was preceded or associated with the appearance of additional primary cancers in other organs, especially the skin. They were often but not always accompanied by the presence of symptoms of chronic arsenic poisoning, thereby establishing to some extent their arsenical origin (DOIG).

Epidemiologic studies on the frequency of lung cancer in workers occupationally exposed to arsenicals are available for insectidide producers (HILL and FANING), copper smelter workers (SNEGIREFF and LOMBARD; LULL and WALLACH), vintners using arsenical insecticides (ROTH), nickel refinery workers (ROCKSTROH) and gold miners (OSBURN) (Table 26, Fig. 3). Additional cases of lung cancer in similarly

Table 26. *Lung Cancer Mortality in Several Counties of Montana 1947—1948*
(LULL *and* WALLACH)

County and Total Population 1940	Major Industry	Numbers Lung Cancers Male	Female	Total	Total Cancer Death	Percent Lung Cancer Male	Female	Annual Lung Cancer Death Rate per 100,000 Male	Female
Deer Lodge 13,627	Copper Smelting	21	0	21	98	30.8	0.0	145.7	0
Silver Bow 53,207	Copper Mining	27	2	29	259	22.6	1.5	48.6	3.9
Cascade 41,499	Copper Mining Smelting	20	5	25	299	12.7	3.5	46.3	12.3
Gallatin 18,269	Agri- culture	1	0	1	81	3.0	0.0	5.2	0

The estimated crude death rate for lung cancer among white males in the entire United States in 1947 is 10.9 per 100,000 population.

The workers employed in copper ore mining and smelting inhale dust and fumes of arsenic contained in the ore and released as a by- and waste-product during the smelting process. The copper ores mined in Montana contain about 5 per cent of arsenic.

exposed workers are listed in Table 27. There is moreover a certain likelihood that the excessive liability of hard rock miners in the Rocky Mountains, recently reported by WAGONER *et al.* are attributable in part to the arsenic content of the ore dust inhaled by them. The apparent lack of similar observations among Swedish copper miners and millers handling arsenic containing ores (RINGERTZ; FORSSMAN; HOLM-QUIST) is perhaps due to the fact that such mining operations in Sweden started only in 1928. Information on the occurrence of arsenic cancers among metal miners in Mexico and Chile is lacking (ABELIUK *et al.*).

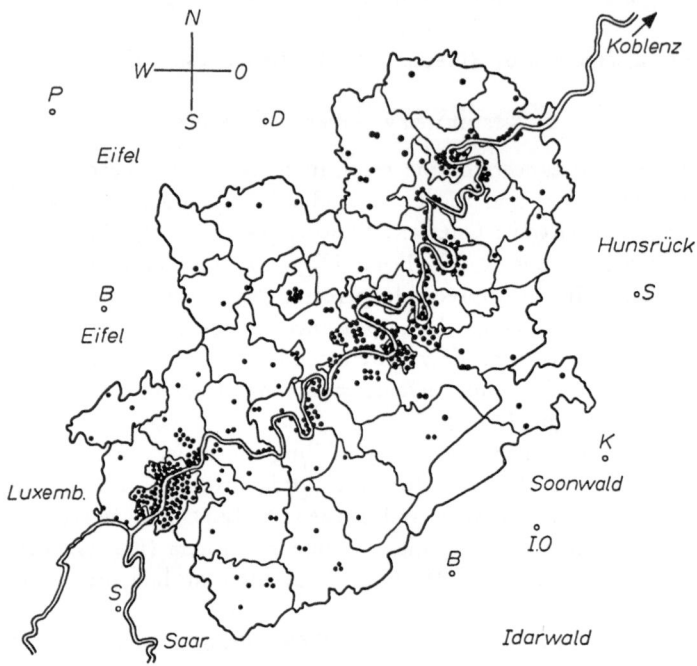

Fig. 3. Moselle from Trier to Cochem. Regional distribution of cases of lung cancer (ROTH)

Table 27 lists a total of 155 cancers of the lung probably or definitely attributable to an occupational contact with arsenicals. Arsenical dermatoses coexisted in 82 cases and cancers of the skin in 17 cases. The exposure period which often was equivalent to the latent period varied widely and ranged from 3 to 45 years. The lag period varied between 8 and over 10 years. The occurrence of arsenic cancers of the respiratory organs was not entirely restricted to members of the male sex, since ROTH mentioned their occurrence in seven female vintners, who died with clinically diagnosed bronchiogenic carcinoma. In addition to 155 cancers of the lung, there were reported 3 cancers of the larynx and 2 cancers of the nasal sinuses.

SNEGIREFF and LOMBARD noted seven deaths from lung cancer among American copper ore smelter workers in a total of 18 deaths from cancer of all sites. OSBURN recorded 19 lung cancers among 34 cancers of all sites observed among African gold ore miners (Negroes), i.e. a frequency rate of lung cancers among African Negroes which is threefold that of American males. ROTH reported that lung cancers were found in 42 per cent of German vintners who came to autopsy with symptoms of chronic arsenic poisoning. He compared this figure with that of 44.4 per cent of lung cancer noted by BEHOUNEK and FORT obtained in an autopsy series of uranium miners of Joachimsthal. ROTH, moreover, pointed out that the lung cancer rate among German vineyard workers of the Moselle valley applied to a rural and agricultural population which as a rule has a low lung cancer rate. The 45 lung cancers described by ROCKSTROH occurred among a plant population of nickel refiners averaging 111 workers during the years 1932 to 1953. These and other observations

Table 27. *Occupational Arsenic Cancers of the Lung, Larynx and Paranasal Sinuses*

Sites and Numbers							
Lung	Larynx	Nares and Nasal Sinuses	Coexisting Keratoses	Skin Cancers	Exposure Period	Occupation	Author, Year
7						Copper Smelter	SNEGIREFF and LOMBARD, 1951
19			1		5	Gold Ore Miner	OSBURN, 1957
	1					Pesticide Producer	DEROBERT and HADENGUE, 1952
9			9	4	17	Vineyard Worker	BRAUN, 1958
1					36	Cobalt Smelter Worker	KRUG, 1959
19	1	2	19	9		Vineyard Worker	ROTH, 1956, 1958
2						Arsenic Smelter Worker	SCHMORL, 1928
1				1		Farmer	MONTGOMERY and WAISMAN, 1941
1					43	Arsenic Worker	CURRIE, 1947
2					37	Pesticide Worker	BRIDGE et al., 1939
17					20	Copper Ore Miner	AKAZAKI, 1960
8			6		3—8	Vineyard Worker	HESS, 1956
45			45		8—45	Nickel-Cobalt Ore Smelter Worker	ROCKSTROH, 1959
5	1					Pesticide Producer	HILL and FANING, 1948
2						Sheep-dip Producer	HENRY, 1934
4					37—43	Sheep-dip Producer	MEREWETHER, 1944
1			1	1		Vineyard Worker	v. PEIN, 1943
1				1		Vineyard Worker	LIEBEGOTT, 1950
8						Vineyard Worker	KOELSCH, 1958
1						Furrier	FROMMEL, 1927
2			1	1		Pesticide Sprayer	HUEPER, 1961

155 Total

justified the recognition of occupational arsenic cancers of the lung before German courts, when they were brought to litigation (LIEBEGOTT; MEESSEN; BAUER; VON PEIN). The recently reported occurrence of three cases of lung cancer associated with cutaneous arsenic dermatosis among French wine growers indicates the general applicability of this concept (LATARJET).

Arsenic cancers of the lung involve, according to KOELSCH, more often the upper lobes than the lower ones and resemble in this respect pulmonary cancers of unknown causation. The age distribution of individuals at time of death from arsenic cancer of the lung exhibits a moderate shift toward younger age groups (Table 28).

Table 28. *Age Distribution of Arsenic Cancers of the Lung*

Year	0—29	30—39	40—89	50—59	60—69	70 and over	Total
Cases	1	3	18	37	17	5	81
Percent	1.2	3.6	22.2	45.7	21	6	

The distribution of histological types of lung cancers of occupational arsenic causation did not differ fundamentally from that found in cancers of this organ in general (Table 29).

Table 29. *Histological Types of Lung Cancers of Arsenical Etiology*

Squamous Cell Carcinoma	Round Cell and Anaplastic Carcinoma	Adeno-Carcinoma	Total
19	24	4	47

In two cases of ROTH, two primary carcinomas were present in the same lung which differed in their histologic structure. Considering the fact that at times different parts of the same carcinoma of the lung may exhibit carcinomatous structures of differing morphology, such observations made in multicentric pulmonary cancers are not unusual. One of ROTH's cases had moreover a cancer of the larynx and a cancer of the skin, while the second one was associated with a cancer of the skin. Combinations with 1 to 4 cancers of the skin were recorded for 6 of 16 bronchiogenic carcinomas of the lung seen by ROTH in German vintners, who had also cirrhosis of the liver. Similar heteroorganic multiplicity of arsenic cancers, some involving the lung, has been reported also after a medicinal administration of arsenicals.

There is evidence that both trivalent and pentavalent inorganic arsenicals possess carcinogenic properties. Pentavalent arsenic is reduced in the body to the trivalent form. Although some uncertainty still remains concerning the carcinogenic potency of organic arsenicals of the two valencies. The occurrence of only few cutaneous cancers usually of multicentric type has been related to such compounds (arsphenamines, cacodylates). Such an action must be anticipated since organic arsenicals are metabolically degraded in the body with the release of arsenic (NEUBAUER). An oral or respiratory occupational exposure to either type of arsenical, therefore, should be considered as significant in constituting a lung cancer hazard.

Little reliable and valid information is available concerning the minimal dose and minimal duration of exposure to arsenicals required for causing a cancerous reaction in any organ, including those of the respiratory system (NEUBAUER; ROTH; KOELSCH; CURRIE). As a rule, like with other occupational cancers, contact with the carcinogenic agent was prolonged in arsenic cancers of the respiratory organs, extending over many months or years. Exposure, on the other hand, did not need to be continuous but was often intermittent. Because arsenic is relatively readily excreted through various channels from the body (Table 30), this fact is important for medicolegal and diagnostic reasons. Chemical analyses for arsenic in the urine, hairs, nails, etc. performed years after arrest of contact, therfore, may not show amounts of arsenic above the "normal" level, which, on the other hand, may vary within a wide range because of the common environmental exposure to arsenicals

Table 30. *Arsenic Content of Biological Materials of Man*

"Normal" Arsenic Content:		
PRIEST (1961)	Blood	0—60 mg per 100 grams
SZEP (1941)	Hair	24—77 mg per 100 grams
	Nail	150—520 mg per 100 grams
CAMP and GANT (1949)	Hair	25—88 mg per 100 grams
FRANK (1950)	Skin	200 mg per 100 grams
FORDYCE et al. (1923)	Milk	0—900 mg per 100 grams dry weight
SCHRENK and SCHREIBEIS (1958)	Urine	10—160 per liter
COX (1925)	Urine	0—200
SULTZZBERGER (1943)	Urine	30
KINGSLEY and SCHAFFERT (1951)	Urine	46—200
SMALES and PAGE (1952)	Urine	13—330
J.A.M.A. (1942)	Urine	5—8
Washington, D.C., Residents	Urine	60—65
THRONE and MYERS (1935)	Blood	8
Exposed Persons:		
PRIEST (1961)	Blood	140 mgm. per 100 grams
JHAVERI (1959)	Hair	209 ppm
	Nail	564
J.A.M.A. (1942)	Urine	80—190 micrograms per 100 cm^3
		300 Consumers of sprayed apples
SILVESTRINI (1962)	Urine	5—550
KUENKELE (1940).	Urine	100 or more indicates poisoning
THRONE and MAYERS (1935)	Hair	300 or more indicates poisoning
	Urine	30 abnormal
PINTO and McGILL (1953)	Urine	820
KUENKELE (1940)	Urine	150
	Hair	120 per gram
BUTZENGEIER (1949)	Urine	100 per liter
FORDYCE et al. (1923)	Urine	670—3111
FRANK (1950)	Skin	300 to 106, 700 per 100 gm
CRISTOL et al. (1939)	Skin	150,000
	Hair	1000 per kg
	Nails	3000 per kg

Arsenic is retained in bones (BOOS and WERBY, 1935).

from many natural and manmade sources including footstuffs, cigarette smoke and air (TELLO; HOFMANN; GOULDEN, KENNAWAY and URQUHART; FOOD STANDARDS COMMITTEE; EDITORIAL; ARGUELLO, TELLO, MACOLA and MANZALO; ARHELGER and KREMEN BAILEY; BAILEY, KENNAWAY and URQUHART; BOHNENKAMP; BUTZENGEIGER; DAFF and KENNAWAY; HOLLAND et al.; JHAVERI; PINTO and McGILL; SATTERLEE).

KOELSCH stated that a daily intake of 3 to 4 mg. of arsenic causes the development of chronic arsenic poisoning. In analogy with observations made on many human and experimental carcinogens, it may be assumed that the carcinogenic dose of arsenic is well below this level and that, therefore, the demonstration of symptoms of chronic arsenic poisoning are not essential and obligatory for concluding on an arsenical causation of a respiratory cancer.

The etiologic significance of arsenic in the production of occupational respiratory cancers is supported by the following evidence:

1. The occupational history demonstrates an exposure to arsenicals.

2. The clinical symptoms of a chronic arsenicosis (melanosis, hyperkeratoses especially of the trunk, palmar and plantar surfaces; solitary and multiple cancers of the skin, cirrhosis and cancer of the liver, perforated nasal septum, chronic bronchitis, toxic neuritis, neurovascular disorders) in many individuals with respiratory cancer having such an occupational history provide medical evidence of the toxic and carcinogenic effects of the exposures sustained. Such symptoms represent prodromal and, in part, precancerous and cancerous manifestations as well as occupational stigmata of an arsenic cancer syndrome observed in single individuals and groups of individuals exposed to arsenicals.

3. Respiratory cancers in individuals with such a history and syndrome have developed respiratory cancers following an exposure of adequate intensity and duration, and after lag- and latent-periods conforming with observations made with other recognized occupational cancers of the respiratory system.

4. The demonstration of excessive amounts of arsenic in the excreta, blood, hair and nails of individuals belonging to such occupational groups when performed during such exposures or soon after their cessation, provides factual evidence of the biologic effectiveness of such contacts.

5. The unusually high frequency of multicentric cancers affecting either the same organ or different organs observed in individuals after occupational, medicinal and dietary exposure to arsenicals, supplies additional evidence of the primary carcinogenic action of this chemical.

6. A similar connotation must be ascribed to the predominant localization of arsenic cancers in the organs of primary contact or of secondary metabolism and excretion or of prolonged deposition.

7. In view of the abundant and reliable evidence in man, the past failure of producing unequivocally cancers in experimental animals does not furnish any valid evidence against the conclusion that arsenic is a human carcinogen.

d) Experimental Arsenic Cancer

Despite frequent attempts to induce cancer in experimental animals (mice, rats, chickens, rabbits) by the administration of various arsenicals by various routes (cutaneous, oral, parenteral), a reliable and consistently repeatable production of experimental arsenic cancers has not been achieved as yet (LEITCH and KENNAWAY; SCHINZ; RAPOSO; LIPSCHUTZ; HUEPER and ITAMI; HUEPER and PAYNE; BOUTWELL BARONI, VAN ESCH and SAFFIOTTI). The recent production of liver cancers in rainbow trout fed carbasone by HALVER and ASHLEY, if confirmed, may provide, however, this long sought evidence.

2. Asbestos

a) Technologic Data

Among the many chemicals inhaled by inhabitants of modern industrialized and chemicalized countries for environmental and occupational reasons asbestos plays a rapidly increasing role because of the phenomenal growth of the asbestos mining and consuming industries and the therewith connected great rise in the use of consumer goods containing asbestos in some form (Fig. 4). Asbestos is a complex magnesium-silicon polymer containing varying amounts of aluminum and iron oxide. The bulk of the asbestos commercially used (95%) is chrysotile which is mined in Canada; U.S.A.; U.S.S.R.; South Africa and many other countries. Chrysotile has an iron content ranging from 0.1 to 11.0 per cent and a magnesium oxide content ranging

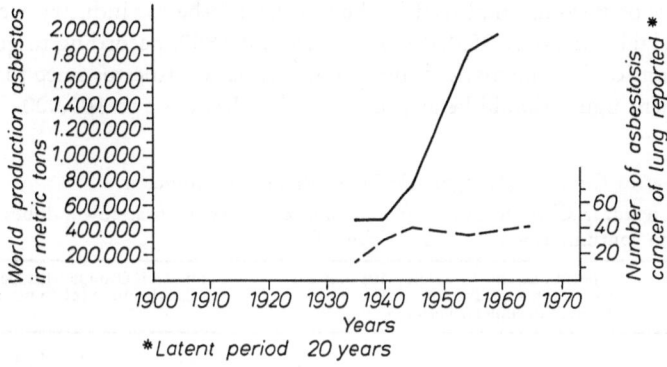

Fig. 4. World production of asbestos and asbestosis carcinoma of the lung

from 39 to 44 per cent. Crocidolite mainly mined in South Africa, on the other hand, consists of sodium iron silicate which contains from 34 to 44 per cent iron oxide and from 1 to 7 per cent magnesium oxide. The different types of asbestos vary also in their fibrillar structure among each other. While chrysotile felts when in contact with water, blue Cape asbestos (crocidolite) retains its fluffy consistency and therefore its insulating qualities. The fibrillar polymerized molecule of asbestos assumes either a band-like structure or a chain-like structure (Fig. 5) (PARKES). During recent years organic silicones of poly-merized nature have been produced synthetically, such as Silastic, which is a polymerized dimethyl siloxane. They are used as lubricants, coating agents, and rubber. When silastic latex is vul-canized for its conversion into rub-ber, it assumes a sponge structure. Ex-periments with implants of silastic latex and rubber have shown that this material is cancerigenic when implanted into rats (HUEPER).

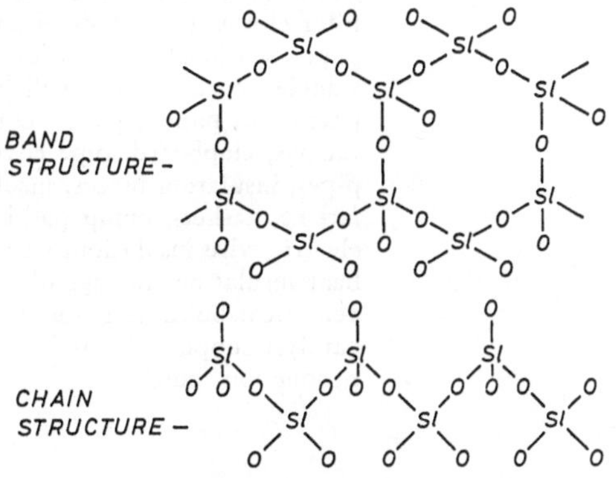

Fig. 5. Asbestos; fibrous polymerized silicate

Detailed data on the origin, pro-duction and industrial application of asbestos are contained in the monographs of ROSATA and of SINCLAIR.

The rapid growth in employment in the asbestos industry and the phenomenal increase in the number of products in which asbestos is used is well illustrated by data supplied by LEATHART and SANDERSON. The number of workers employed in the English asbestos industry stood in 1935 at 10,000 persons. It had risen to 18,700 by 1958. While the amount of asbestos cement products expressed in tons was 105,720 in 1930, it had increased to 461,700 by 1958. While 2070 tons of cement insulation was used in 1930, this figure stood at 42,500 in 1958. About 2200 tons of asbestos were used for asbestos brake lining in 1935, while approximately 10,000 were employed in the production of brake lining in 1958.

The number of persons employed in the American asbestos industry was estimated to be in the neighborhood of 35,000 workers around 1950, according to governmental statistics. Considering the marked increase in the use of asbestos since that time, the total employment figure should be at present in the U.S. close to 100,000.

Sites of Asbestos Cancers: Recognized: Lung, Pleura, Peritoneum

Exposure Stigmata: Chronic fibrosing pneumonia involving first lower lobes (asbestosis), asbestos bodies in sputum, asbestos warts of skin (fingers.)

Compounds of Economic Importance	Operations and Products with Contact to Asbestos for Producers, Processers, Users, Consumers, Pesidents	Population Groups with Occupational and Environmental Exposure to Asbestos
Chrysotile, Amphibole, Amosite, Crocidolite Tremolite Containing Magnesium, Aluminium, Calcium, Iron, Silica	Asbestos rock mining, loading, shipping, crushing, milling; *asbestos spinning, weaving,* mixing, cutting, pressing, molding, plastering, cementing, spraying of steel construction, under-coating of automobiles, insulating pipes, etc. clothes, cloths, sheets, blankets, curtains, brake linings, yarns, cords, ropes, twines, ribbons, artificial snow, filler in rubber goods, plastics and roof coatings, filter cloths, filter pads, filter paper, artificial wood, tiles, shingles, card boards, wall boards, partitions, panels, paper, clutch facings, clapboard, pipe coverings, pipes, insulation blocks, insulation jackets, gaskets, pump packings, electric wire insulation, structural heat insulation, facings of acoustical building materials, catalyst supports in sulfuric acid production, putties	*Occupational Groups:* *Asbestos rock miners, loaders truckers, crushers, millers; asbestos spinners, weavers;* electrical appliance and wire manufacturers, masons, carpenters, heating equipment workers, rubber workers, shingle and tile manufacturers, building material manufacturers, filtering material manufacturers, molders of asbestos products, asbestos-asphalt makers, putty manufacturers, asbestos cement makers, asbestos paper cardboard and *brake-lining producers, asbestos felt insulation worker,* asbestos sound insulation worker, asbestos insulator, pipe coverer, *asbestos tube wrapper,* asbestos cork insulation worker; construction workers, automobile makers, garage attendants
		Nonoccupational Groups: Residents in vicinity of asbestos processing, asbestos cement and textile mills inhaling plant effluents polluted with asbestos dust and individuals living and working along roads on which asbestos is trucked; inhabitants of houses with asbestos insulation.

b) Epidemiologic Data on Asbestos and Carcinoma of the Lung

Since cancers of the lung, pleura and peritoneum are directly related to occupational and environmental exposures to asbestos dust and to the development of asbestotic reactions in the lung, the delay encountered in the discovery of asbestosis in modern times and the difficulties in its diagnosis represent important features in the epidemiology of asbestos cancers. Despite the fact that the use of asbestos as a textile fiber and the knowledge of asbestosis date back to antiquity (DEMY), it was rather recent that this occupational pneumoconiotic hazard was rediscovered (MURRAY, 1900). The first cases of asbestosis complicated by pulmonary carcinomas were described several decades later (1933) by LYNCH and SMITH and by GLOYNE.

Although some investigators still maintain that asbestosis is a rather rare occupational disease, the actual known facts are quite different (HUEPER). The enormous increase in the production and industrial use of asbestos during recent decades has been followed by a growing number of reports on the occurrence of occupational asbestosis observed in many countries (United States, Canada, Mexico, Great Britain, France, Germany, Belgium, Switzerland, U.S.S.R., Sweden, Denmark, Finland, Italy, South Africa). Epidemiologic and pathologic evidence obtained during the last few years moreover indicates that exposure to asbestos of a non-occupational basis may have become quite common, because asbestos bodies and mild to severe asbestosis have been observed rather frequently in individuals without demonstrable occupational contact with asbestos (TOTTEN and GROSS; THOMSON; WAGLER, MÜLLER and ANSPACH; WEBSTER; KIVILUOTO; NEWHOUSE; CORDOBA, TESLUK and KNUDTSON), affected in part also with carcinoma of the lung and mesothelioma of the pleura (NEWHOUSE).

The published records on asbestosis have remained rather defective for various reasons. Without any doubt a considerable number of cases of occupational asbestosis have been and still are incorrectly diagnosed as chronic pulmonary tuberculosis, silicosis, chronic fibrosing pneumonia and similar chronic pulmonary diseases. The diagnosis of asbestosis may be missed entirely during lifetime and this condition is then only discovered at autopsy (KÖNIG; THOMSON). Morbidity data on asbestosis based on clinical diagnoses only therefore tend to underestimate the frequency of this occupational disease.

Such diagnostic difficulties are sometimes accentuated by undesirable practices in the bona-fide recognition of asbestosis and of any cancerous lesions associated with it. DEMY recently noted: "One would think that would be enough, but medical obtuseness, industrial coyness, and labor's timidness unwittingly hoodwinked the law in a Department of Labor investigation in Canada, in 1912. The Commission could find no occupational damage in 600 asbestos workers. Even in 1918, HOFFMANN, in a U.S. Labor Bureau Statistics Bulletin, assured the insurance companies that the early deaths among asbestos workers were due to tuberculosis. It is a pretty exercise in medical history to consult textbooks of pathology from 1910 to 1930. They are uniformly blank on asbestosis. And even today, the descriptions smell of library paste."

The former astounding lack of medical and epidemiologic information has changed for the better in recent years, although it has remained rather defective in some countries (MITCHELL). Asbestosis is relatively common among asbestos workers of various occupations. MEREWETHER and PRICE noted in 1930 that 95 or 26.2% of 363 out of a total of 2,200 asbestos workers medically examined in England showed evidence of asbestosis. According to BOHLIG, JACOB and MUELLER, more than 33% of the approximately 10,000 German asbestos workers show signs of asbestosis (1960). BOEHME, on the basis of radiologic evidence, obtained on 132 German asbestos workers, arrived at an attack rate of asbestosis of 29%. The rate increased with the duration of employment, being 5% among individuals employed less than 3 years and 79% among those exposed for over 10 years. Data from Finland and Sweden by WEGELIUS and NORO on 476 and 167 workers, respectively, recorded a frequency of asbestosis in members of these groups of 30 and 65%, respectively, following the discovery of the first case of occupational asbestosis in Sweden as late as 1953 (AHLBORG and HANSSON). Among 31 Danish workers employed for over 20 years in asbestos work, 9 exhibited signs of asbestosis (30%) (FROST et al.). ALVA-RADO et al. recorded the occurrence of asbestosis in 6 out of 8 Mexican asbestos workers studied. While LANZA stated in 1936 that between 1928 and 1936 only 12 deaths from asbestosis among about 10,000 exposed asbestos workers were recorded in the U.S.A., and that the Metropolitan Life Insurance Company was notified during the period of 1924 to 1936 that asbestosis was a contributory cause of death in 17 of its policy holders, LYNCH and CANNON published observations made between 1931 and 1948 on 40 cases of asbestosis seen at autopsy among workers employed in one medium-sized textile plant. An identical number of asbestosis cases were seen between 1940 and 1960 by O'DONNELL and MANN at post mortem examinations of patients coming from a small town with a large asbestos brake lining plant. It should be obvious from even these fragmentary data that asbestosis is still a frequent and often fatal occupational disease among workers of many countries, even if comprehensive and long-term medical and pathological studies on the large and growing worker populations having occupational contact with asbestos dust are lacking.

Since the presence of asbestosis has usually been considered the prerequisite for the subsequent development of a carcinoma of the lung or of a mesothelioma of the pleura or of the peritoneum, these deficiencies in the available information tend to impair a clear demonstration of the real scope of the existing associations between the two conditions. A second difficulty encountered in reliably assessing the extent and degree of lung cancer hazards of asbestotics is represented by the fact that there has occurred in the past a confusing duplication in reporting cases of asbestosis cancers. In the following (Table 31) an attempt has been made to eliminate this error as far as possible by critically analyzing the various published reports, relating to asbestos carcinoma of the lung.

The reports of the authors were evaluated in the preparation of this table:

United States: ANDERSON and CAMPAGNA; EGBERT and GEIGER; HOLLEB and ANGRIST; HOMBURGER; LYNCH and SMITH; LYNCH and CANNON; LYNCH and PRATT-THOMAS; ISSELBACHER, KLAUS and HARDY; O'DONNELL and MANN; O'DONNELL; STOLL, BASS and ANGRIST; TELISCHI and RUBENSTONE; MANCUSO; SELIKOFF, CHURG and HAMMOND; DYSON and TENTRALANCE; CORDOBA, TESLUK and KNUDSON (Three (3) cases of carcinoma of the lung with asbestosis in shipyard workers under investigation by HUEPER and PAYNE were omitted).

Canada: DESMEULES, ROUSSEAU, GIROUX and SIROIS; LUTON and CHAMPEIX; CARTIER; ROUSSEAU; BRAUN and TRUAN (34 unpublished cases of asbestosis carcinoma of the lung in asbestos miners of Quebec and studied histologically between 1940 and 1955 by VORWALD and SCHEPERS at the Saranac Laboratories have not been included).

Great Britain: GLOYNE; SMITH; CURETON; OWEN; HUGH-JONES and HEARD; ELWOOD and COCHRANE; BUCHANAN; KEAL; MEREWETHER; DOLL; BONSER, FAULDS and STEWART; KENNAWAY and KENNAWAY (cases recorded by WYERS were omitted because they were apparently included in listings of MEREWETHER of 1947 and 1955).

Table 31. *Carcinomas of the Lung in Asbestotics: Reported Cases*

Country	Number	Sex	Age	Exposure Time	Latent Period	Lag Period	Site	Histological Type
USA	88	M 87	37—69	5—48	6—36	1—30	LL 29	S 18
		F 1	Av. 50	Av. 23	Av. 23		UL 10	R 18
								A 9
Canada	10	M 10	48—65	2—33	14—34	4—16		
			Av. 57	Av. 22.5	Av. 25	Av. 11		A 2
England	149	M 107	32—76	1—45	16—45	9—20	LL 4	S 16
		F 32	Av. M 55.2	Av. 16	Av. 23	Av. 3	UL 1	R 24
			F 44.6					A 3
			Av. 54					
Germany	58	M 44	35—79	3—34	4—40		LL 22	S 12
		F 7	Av. 52	Av. 28	Av. 28		UL 4	R 11
Finland	1							
Italy	3	M 2	46—54	17—26				
		F 1	Av. 49	Av. 29				S 1
France	2	M 1	53	10			LL	S 1
Switzerland	1	M 1	62	7	24	17	LL	A 1
Total	240	M 197	32—76	1—45	4—45	1—30	LL 53	S 45
		F 41					UL 7	R 40
								A 19

LL = Lower Lobe.
UL = Upper Lobe.
S = Squamous-Cell Carcinoma.
R = Round-Cell Carcinoma.
A = Adenocarcinoma.

Germany: LINZBACH and WEDLER; WELZ; WEDLER; BOHNE; BOEMKE; JACOB and BOHLIG; BOHLIG and JACOB; BOEHME; WERBER; BOHLIG, JACOB and MUELLER; HORNIG; KÖNIG.

Italy: PORTIGLIATTI-BARBOS; FRANCIA and MONARCA; ROMBOLA

France: HUREL, LAGUILLAUME, CHAMPEIX and JACQUEMENT

Finland: NORO

Switzerland: CHAUVET

The individuals affected by asbestosis cancer of the lung were asbestos miners, millers, crushers, loaders, sorters, grinders, cleaners, pipe laggers, cement mixers, packers, boiler coverers, mattress fillers, weavers, spinners, and cement workers.

The epidemiologic-statistical data supporting the existence of causal relations between exposure to asbestos dust and the subsequent development of asbestosis of the lung and carcinoma of the lung are in part derived from observations of post mortem material in part they are obtained by population studies. The first and still most frequent data indicating an excessive liability of asbestotics to develop cancers of the lung were gathered from autopsies. Although this material is a selective one, its significance as evidence supporting such a liability is attested by the consistency of the evidence showing a highly excessive frequency of lung cancer in individuals with asbestosis in all countries in which such studies were made (Table 32). KÖNIG in a recent publication noted a lung cancer rate for male asbestotics of 46.1% against one in the general autopsy series of 11.6%, and one for female asbestotics of 21.7% against one in the general autopsy material of 2.1%. CORDOBA et al. found that 33% of their series of 20 cases of occupational asbestosis had lung cancer, and WAGNER placed it at 20%. In an analysis of 549 cases of asbestosis recorded between 1924 and

Table 32. *Frequency of Cancers of the Lung in Autopsies of Asbestotics*

Author	Sex	Number of Autopsies of Asbestotics	Number of Lung Cancers	Percentage of Lung Cancers
MEREWETHER . . .	Males	222	48	22
	Females	143	17	12
	Both	365	65	17.8
WYERS		115	17	14.8
DOLL		105 (asbestos workers)	18	17
GLOYNE		121	17	13.2
O'DONNELL and MANN		40	20	50
LYNCH		40	5	8.3
BECKER				14—15
WEDLER		92	15	16
BOEHME	Both	31	11	36
	Males	17	12	71
	Females	14	2	14

Controls
    BECKER (males over 20, average age at death, 61 years)   4
          (silicotics)   3.6
    MEREWETHER (6,884 post mortems on silicotics, 91 lung (cancers)   1.32
          (average age at death, 59.4 years)

1962 in England, BUCHANAN noted 99 carcinomas of the lung among 364 males with asbestosis and 22 such cancers in 185 female workers with this disease. Even in the methodologically rather crude epidemiologic survey of white male employees of selected asbestos products plants conducted in U.S.A. by ENTERLINE these workers had a respiratory cancer rate of 193.3.

An identical connotation as to an excessive incidence of carcinoma of the lung among asbestos workers and especially among workers with asbestosis, have the results of the epidemiologic studies of DOLL in England (Table 33). The association of lung cancer to employment in asbestos was 15-fold that of the standard population. In a similar study conducted on the worker population of an American asbestos brake lining plant, MANCUSO and COULTER obtained identical evidence confirming the occurrence of an excess of deaths from lung cancer (Table 34). SELIKOFF et al. noted that a lung cancer rate of 6 to 7 times the normal rate prevails among insulation workers.

The scientific value of these observations was recently challenged by BOHLIG, JACOB and MUELLER and by BRAUN and TRUAN in investigations on the morbidity from lung cancer among asbestos workers in Saxony and in the Province of Quebec, respectively. While Bohlig *et al.* maintained that the lung cancer morbidity rate of all German asbestos workers is not higher than that of a comparable general population (between 5 and 6 per 10,000), it is most doubtful whether this calculation reflects the actual conditions prevailing. Experiences made on the epidemiology of occupa-tional cancers of various types have clearly shown that the anatomic reactions to such hazards, as a rule, become manifest only in long-term workers who have sus-tained a prolonged and often severe exposure or in individuals for whom, following cessation of exposure, an adequate latent period elapsed which usually extended over

Table 33. *Causes of Death among Male Asbestos Workers Compared with the Mortality Experience of all Men in England and Wales* (Doll)

Cause of Death	Number of Death		Test of Significance of Difference between Observed and Expected (Value of P.)
	Number observed	Expected on England and Wales rates	
Lung cancer [1]	11	0.8	< 0.000001
Other respiratory diseases [2] and cardiovascular diseases:			
With mention of asbestosis	14	— }	< 0.001
Without mention of asbestosis	6	7.6 }	
Neoplasms, other than lung cancer	4	2.3 }	> 0.1
All other diseases [3]	4	4.7 }	
All causes	39	15.4	< 0.000001

[1] Including 1 case with pulmonary tuberculosis.
[2] Including pulmonary tuberculosis.
[3] Including 2 cases (benign stricture of esophagus and septicaemia) in which asbestosis was present but was not thought to have been a contributory cause of death.

Table 34. *Observed and Expected Deaths Due to Lung Cancers, 1940 through Mid-1960 Among a Cohort of White Male and Female Employees of Company C at Some Time in 1938 or 1939, Ages 25—64 Years at Death*

Site	Total		White Males		White Females	
	Observed Deaths	Expected Deaths	Observed Deaths	Expected Deaths	Observed Deaths	Expected Deaths
Lung, bronchus, trachea (162, 163)	18	5.29	14	5.11	4	0.18
Peritoneum (158)	3	0.10	2	0.08	1	0.01

(Medical Survey in an American Asbestos Brake Lining Plant)

10 to 25 years. Unless proper methodologic precautions in the collection and evalua-tion of epidemiologic data are taken, data of the type used by Bohlig *et al.* contain a dilution factor which a priori may negate and defeat the purpose and validity of such studies (Hueper).

While Bohlig *et al.* conceded from their calculations that the lung cancer expectancy of one thousand workers with asbestosis and a more than 20-year-employment in the industry showed a ten-fold increase over standard rates (50 per 10,000), they attempted to minimize the obvious significance of this finding by arguing that the observed number of lung cancers in this group should not be applied to the actual number of 1,000 asbestoses but instead to a hypothetical number of

3,300 cases which they assume have asbestosis. As pointed out before, such a supposition scarcely reflects the real conditions. It is likely from past experience with occupational cancers of the lung that a competent comprehensive post mortem study of the added number of 2,300 cases would increase considerably also the number of asbestosis cases showing a coexisting carcinoma. The argument of BOHLIG et al. therefore is incorrect and misleading especially as it must be suspected that the number of observed lung cancers in this series understated their actual number.

If BOHLIG et al., moreover, noted in confirmation of their negativistic concept that asbestosis cancers of the lung have not been reported from South Africa, they labor evidently under a serious lack of pertinent information on the subject.

Even more serious objections must be raised against the scientific merits of the claims made in this matter by BRAUN and TRUAN who studied asbestos miners and millers in the Province of Quebec, Canada. Some importance must be attached to the fact that the project reported by BRAUN and TRUAN was to be undertaken under the aegis of the National Cancer Institute of Canada (Annual Report, NCI Canada, 1955—56) according to the "consensus of opinion" arrived at a meeting of the statistician of the National Cancer institute of Canada, the medical director of the Johns-Manville Corporation, the medical director of the Industrial Hygiene Foundation (DR. BRAUN), the medical officer of the Thetford Mines and other medical and technical personnel. After this initial arrangement the industrial sponsors of the project apparently abandoned this cooperative scheme and proceeded independently, being financially aided through contributions from various asbestos plants in the U.S.A.

According to the data published, this study was based on a survey of about 6,000 individuals employed by the asbestos industry in the Province of Quebec. While there is a break down as to the degree of dust exposure and the number of individuals in each of three graduated groups, no data are offered as to the duration of exposure to asbestos dust for the individuals contained in these groups. Although there is a statement as to the number of smokers and non-smokers, the report is totally devoid of any information concerning the number of asbestotics among the population group analyzed. No information is available regarding the number of long-term workers and their relative liability to lung cancer. No mention is made in the report in regard to the autopsies which have been performed on members of this cohort who died during the period surveyed. This aspect appears to be particularly important, since BRAUN and TRUAN professed that only nine (9) "proven" cases of lung cancer were discovered to have occurred in the cohort analyzed. This is a rather surprising observation since during a somewhat longer period than that covering the survey, a histopathologic study of lungs from dead asbestos workers from Quebec by pathologists of the Saranac Laboratory under the sponsorship of industrial management, revealed a total of 34 cases of asbestosis cancers of the lung. It should be obvious from this observation that the epidemiologic investigation of BRAUN and TRUAN contains most likely only a fraction and possibly a minor fraction, of the cases which actually occurred, and that a thorough and critical analysis of the surveyed worker group for clinical and pathologic evidence of asbestosis and cancer of the lung would have yielded a result quite different from the reported one.

The conclusions reached by BRAUN and TRUAN concerning an absence of an excessive liability to lung cancer among Quebec asbestos workers are even incorrect if proper epidemiologic procedures are applied to their data as reported. While the statement of BRAUN and TRUAN that the annual rate of deaths from lung cancer in the asbestos cohort for the years 1950 to 1955 is only slightly higher than the rate for the inhabitants of the Province of Quebec would be correct under these conditions, this statement represents a peculiar type of statistical acrobatics which tends to obscure the real incriminating evidence on hand by using a highly biased population group as a "normal" standard.

It is a well known fact that urban populations in all industrialized countries have a decidedly higher lung cancer death rate than that prevailing for inhabitants of rural regions (HUEPER). Since the asbestos mines are situated in rural areas of Quebec and are not located within the fume zones of Quebec and Montreal where a high lung cancer rate prevails (Montreal rate 32.3), the lung cancer death rates of the asbestos miners which stands at 33.8 per 100,000, has to be compared with the rates present in rural counties of the Province of Quebec, which, according to the data provided on this point by BRAUN and TRUAN, stands at 9.4 and 9.8. The method of establishing the absence of a significantly higher lung cancer liability for asbestos miners used by BRAUN and TRUAN is, therefore, patently incorrect, grossly misleading, and results in obscuring the actual existence of an excessively elevated lung cancer rate for members of this worker group when proper standards of comparison are used.

While such statistical manipulations may benefit industrial interests, they are neither original nor singular and have been applied repeatedly in the past to other occupational cancers, such as amine-cancers of the bladder and lung cancers from the inhalation of radioactive gases and dust. They have never been successful in the long run in obscuring the correct facts and have always been detrimental to public health and scientific and general morals.

It must be maintained on the basis of the evidence provided by BRAUN and TRUAN that the members of this worker group have indeed an excessive liability to cancer of the lung in accord with all other information available on this subject from many additional sources throughout the world. Although cancer of the lung does not seem to be the most frequent fatal complication of asbestosis, it is evidently sufficiently frequent for elevating the lung cancer rate of asbestos workers as a group and therefore is a serious sequela of exposure to asbestos.

c) Clinicopathologic Relations

The diffuse pulmonary fibrosis characteristic for asbestosis and distinct from the nodular fibrosis in silicosis, starts usually in the lower lobe, where radiographic studies may reveal a thickening of the pleura and a bunching of the small bronchi with their ends turned back (JACOB and BOHLIG). The close causal relation between asbestosis and cancer of the lung is demonstrated by the fact that asbestosis cancers affect more often the lower lobes than the upper lobes (53 : 7) in contrast to the general type of lung cancer which involves more frequently the upper lobes.

Associated with this etiologically significant topographical peculiarity of asbestosis cancers are the various equally important metaplastic, precancerous and cancerous changes of the bronchial and bronchiolar epithelium which precede and accompany the development of lung cancers in asbestotic lungs.

In the fibrotic matrix of such lungs, the mucosa of the usually non-stenosed bronchi and bronchioli shows multicentric atypical epithelial foci as well as squamous cell metaplasias. Bronchioli are often distended to adenocystic formations exhibiting the above-mentioned metaplastic changes and containing in their lumens desquamated epithelial cells and asbestos bodies. Adjacent to such metaplastic and precancerous lesions, the fibrous matrix may contain multicentric cancerous formations with or without asbestos bodies in the neoplastic parenchyma and stroma (Figs. 6 to 10). The high frequency of atypical adenomatoid and adenocystic bronchiolar lesions found in asbestotic lungs appears to account for the fact that adenocarcino-

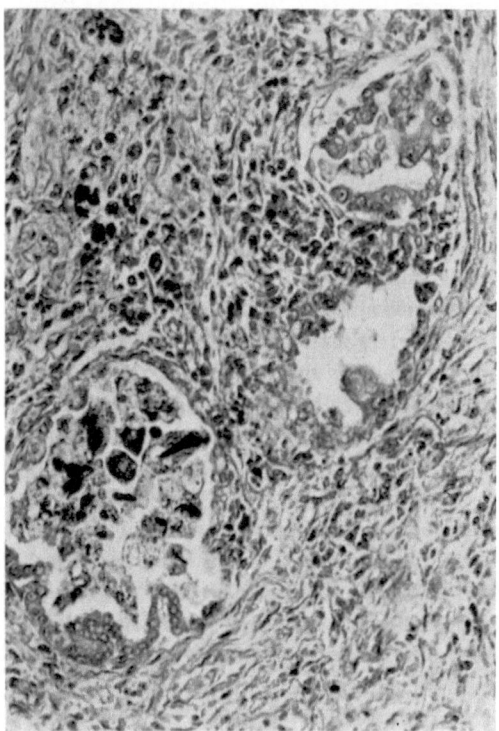
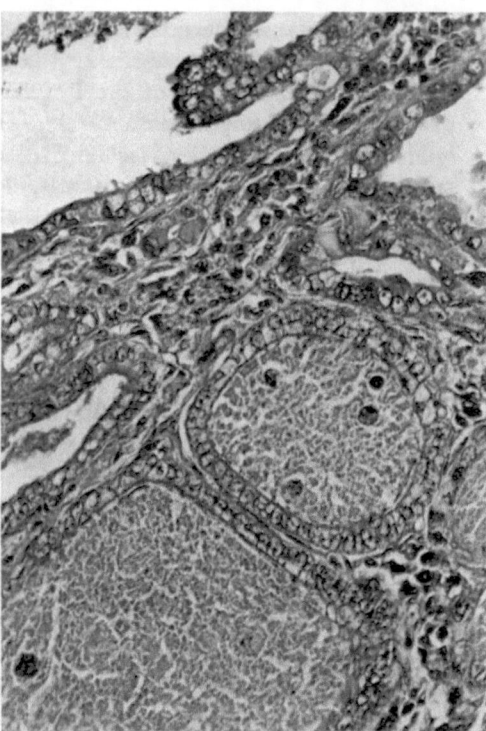

Fig. 6. Asbestotic fibrosis of the lung showing cystically distended bronchioli which contain in their lumens asbestos bodies. Asbestos textile worker

Fig. 7. Marked adenocystic transformation of bronchioli in the asbestotic lung of an asbestos textile worker

mas represent an unusually high percentage among asbestosis cancers (18% adenocarcinomas, 43% squamous cell carcinomas and 39% round-cell and anaplastic carcinomas). Also combinations of adenocarcinoma and squamous cell carcinoma have repeatedly been reported (Table 35) (BOHLIG, JACOB and MUELLER; LYNCH and SMITH). The commonly multicentric and widely distributed occurrence of the metaplastic changes in the bronchial mucosa of asbestotic lungs furnishes a plausible reason for the reported relatively frequent development of multicentric carcinomas in such lungs (GLOYNE; LYNCH and SMITH; BOEMKE). Although similar, while usually less marked, mucosal lesions are found in association with other occupational carcinomas

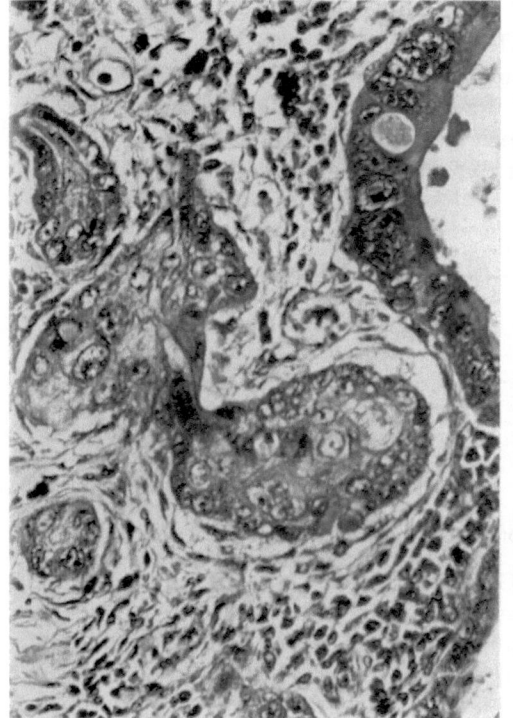

Fig. 8

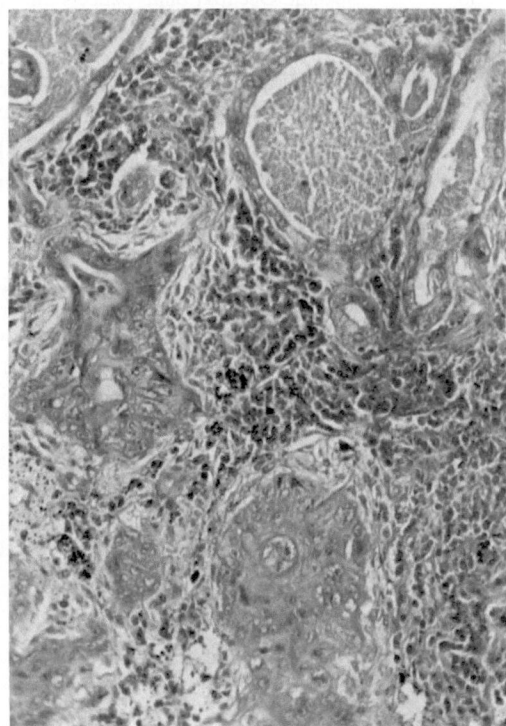

Fig. 9

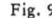

Fig. 10

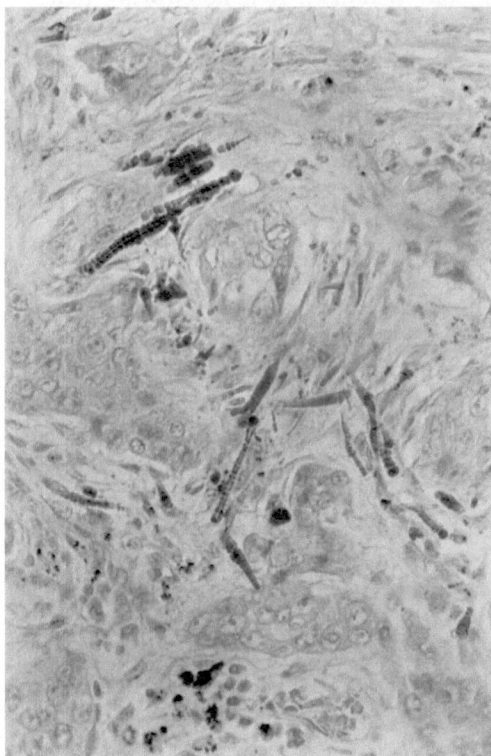

Fig. 8. Asbestotic fibrosis in the lung of an asbestos brake lining worker with atypical cellular lining of an adenomatus bronchiolar cyst and islands of metaplastic squamous cells suggesting beginning carcinomatous changes

Fig. 9. Squamous cell carcinoma and adenocystic bronchioli in the lung of an asbestos textile worker

Fig. 10. Squamous cell carcinoma with numerous asbestos body embedded in the carcinomatous tissue in a textile worker

4

of the lung (chromate, nickel), they are even less commonly encountered in lungs harboring the "spontaneous" variety of carcinoma.

The distinctive topographical distribution of asbestos carcinomas in the lower lobes as well as several special histopathologic properties of these neoplasms mentioned relate their development to the presence of asbestos and the pathologic changes incited in the lung by this mineral.

Table 35. *Distribution of Histologic Types of Pulmonary Carcinomas in Asbestotic Lungs*

	Squamous Cell Carcinoma		Round Cell and Undifferentiated Carcinoma		Adenocarcinoma	
	Number	per cent	Number	per cent	Number	per cent
Asbestos Series	45	43	40	39	19	18
Controls (DORN and CUTLER)						
Males		29.3		61.2		9.5
Females		13.6		59.7		26.7

d) Epidemiologic Data on Mesotheliomas of the Pleura and Peritoneum

Recent observations made in Germany, Great Britain, the United States, Canada, Italy, and South Africa strongly suggest that asbestosis is causally related also to the development of mesotheliomas of the pleura and peritoneum (CARTIER; MANCUSO and COULTER; BOHLIG; JACOB and MUELLER; KÖNIG; LEICHER; WEDLER; WEBSTER; OWEN; SELIKOFF, CHURG and HAMMOND; WAGNER; WAGNER et al; ENTICKNAP and SMITHER; SLEGGS, MARCHAND and WAGNER; DOLL; WEISS; KEAL; BONSER FRANCIA and MONARCA; THOMSON; FOWLER; SLOPER and WARNER). It is noteworthy that the occurrence of mesotheliomata in South Africa is restricted to the miners of the crocidolite (blue Cape asbestos) mines and to residents living in these mining districts (Fig. 11), either near asbestos mining operations or along the routes on which the

Table 36. *Mesotheliomas of the Pleura and Peritoneum in Asbestotics*

Country	Number	Sex		Age	Exposure Time	Latent Period	Lag Period	Site	
Germany	7	M	5	40—69	4—42	31—42	2—28	Pleura	6
		F	2	Av. 57	Av. 21	Av. 13	Av. 13	Peritoneum	1
Canada	2	M	2	65	10			Pleura	2
England	9	M	1	35—60	1—23	14—25	10—15		
		F	8	Av. 50	Av. 9	Av. 19	Av. 13	Peritoneum	9
USA	3	M	3	50—52				Pleura	1
								Peritoneum	2
Italy	1	M	1	46	17	30	13	Pleura	1
South Africa									
Occ.	16	M	15	36—68				Pleura	16
Res.	17	F	1	Av. 45				Pleura	17
		M	7	31—63					
		F	10	Av. 49					
Total	55	M	34	31—68	4—42	19—35	2—28	Pleura	43
		F	21	Av. 52	Av. 14	Av. 28	Av. 13	Peritoneum	12

asbestos was trucked (WAGNER). The occurrence of mesotheliomas in asbestos workers of many other countries indicates, however, that also chrysotile is capable of inducing these mesotheliomatous growths (Table 36).

The rather late discovery of these neoplastic sequelae to occupational and environmental exposure to asbestos may be attributable to three reasons. Although pleural
mesotheliomas have been considered by some investigators as pleural extensions of
pulmonary carcinomas, the recent observations on mesotheliomas in asbestos workers
show definitely that such pleural neoplasms may develop in the absence of carcinomatous growths in lungs with relatively minor asbestotic changes. Pleural and especially peritoneal mesotheliomas found in asbestos workers have moreover suffered

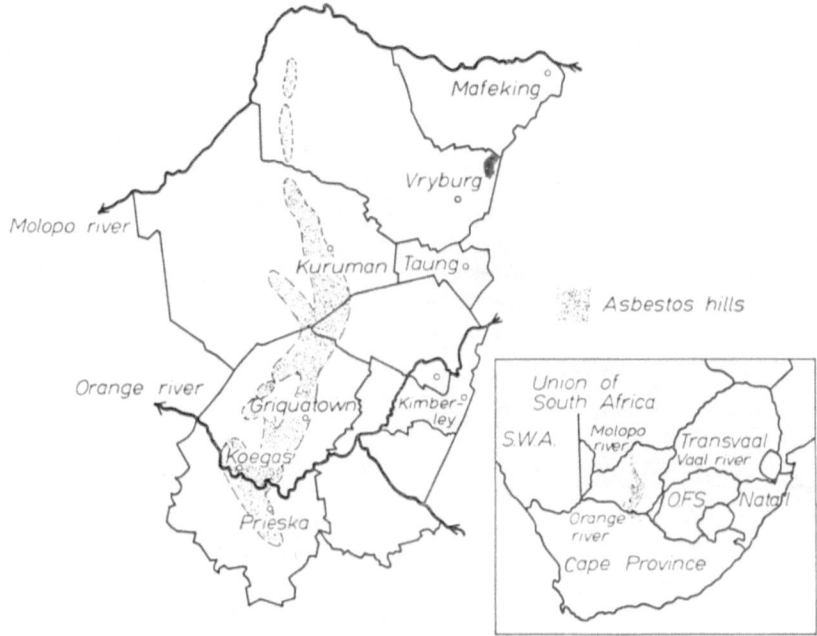

Fig. 11. Map of Griqualand west asbestos fields

from diagnostic misinterpretations, i.e. they have not infrequently been diagnosed as
adenocarcinomas of some glandular organ because of their frequent adenomatoid
components. The third reason for their late discovery is connected with their long
latent period, which often extends between 30 and 50 years and which may include a
lag period of several decades. From a diagnostic and etiologic standpoint, it is
important that the occurrence of asbestos bodies in cases of mesotheliomas was
restricted to the lungs (Figs. 12 and 13).

It is interesting to note that among the 11 intrathoracic cancers recorded by
König from Hamburg, 4 were pleural mesotheliomas. He noted moreover that
among the extrapulmonary cancers found in 36 asbestotics 3 were peritoneal mesotheliomas. These observations may be of historical as well as etiologic significance,
because the German shipbuilding industry was the first industry which soon after the
turn of the last century introduced the use of blue Cape asbestos, for which up to
that time no commercial use had been found.

The conclusion that definite causal relations exist between exposures to asbestos,
the presence of asbestos bodies in the lungs and the subquent development of meso-

theliomas of the pleura and peritoneum is supported by the fact that mesotheliomas, which ordinarily are rather rare tumors, represent, according to present observations, 15.1 per cent of all pulmonary cancers found in asbestotics, while this percentage stands for pulmonary cancers in general at about 4% (WALTHER). It is, moreover, significant that the number of mesotheliomas observed among a restricted population group specifically exposed in South Africa has been rising rapidly during recent years and that a similar epidemiologic phenomenon has occurred in workers of the English asbestos industry (WAGNER).

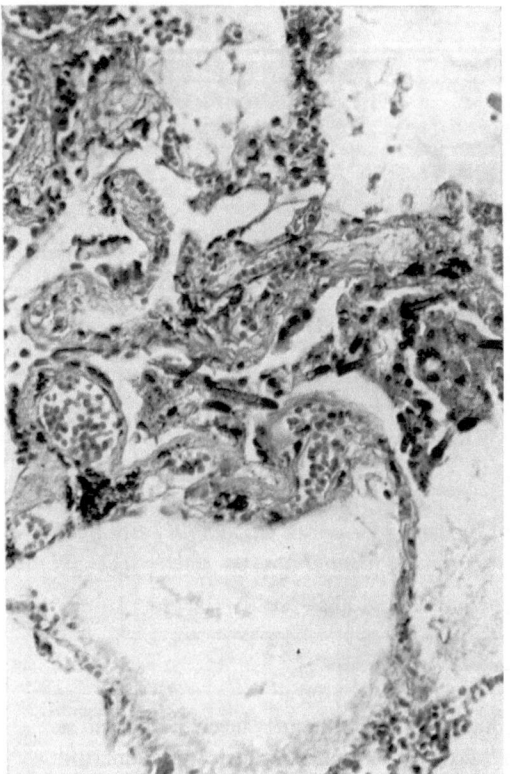

Fig. 12. Scattered minor deposits in the interstitial tissue of the lung of asbestos bodies in an asbestos worker with a mesothelioma of the peritoneum

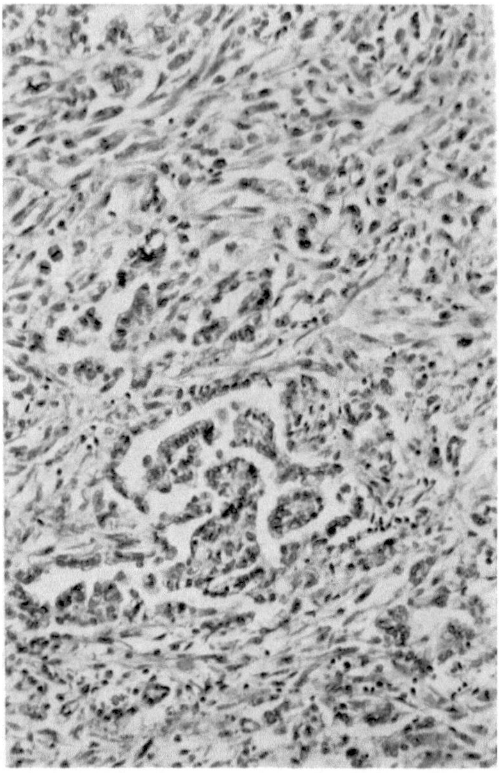

Fig. 13. Mesothelioma of the peritoneum of this worker showing pseudoglandular formations in a sarcomatoid matrix

e) Age Distribution of Asbestosis Cancers

It is noteworthy that asbestosis carcinomas of the lungs do not share with some other occupational respiratory cancers the frequently observed shift of the age distribution into younger age groups (Table 37). In fact, the mean age at death of

Table 37. *Age Distribution of Asbestosis Carcinomas of the Lung*

	Age in Years												Total
	10−30		31−39		40−49		50−59		60−69		70 and over		
	No.	%	No.	%	No.	%	No.	%	No.	%	No.	%	
Asbestos Series			10	8	28	23	47	39	32	26	5	4	122
Control (HUEPER)	99	6	222	12	444	24	609	34	356	21	62	3	1,792

asbestotics without lung carcinoma was 44.2 years (males 49.2 years, females 38), while that of asbestotics with lung cancer was 52.1 years (males 55.2, females 44.6) (MEREWETHER). Severe asbestosis seems often to kill before there is time for the development of a lung cancer.

The age distribution of pleural and peritoneal mesotheliomas seen in asbestotics and in individuals with occupational and environmental exposure to asbestos dust exhibits in comparison to the asbestosis carcinomas of the lung a distinct shift into younger age groups.

Table 38. *Age Distribution of Mesotheliomas of the Pleura and Peritoneum*

	Age in Years								Total
	30 – 39		40 – 49		50 – 59		60 – 69		
	No.	%	No.	%	No.	%	No.	%	
Cases	9	23	13	31	9	23	9	23	40

In the absence of reliable data on the age distribution in a sufficiently large control group of the general variety of mesotheliomas, it is uncertain whether the observed age shift has any etiologic significance.

f) Sex Distribution of Asbestosis Carcinomas of the Lung

In his first report on the sex distribution of asbestosis cancer of the lung based on a total of 31 cases and published in 1947, MEREWETHER noted a male-female sex ratio of 2.4 : 1 which contrasted significantly from the normal ratio of about 10 : 1 prevailing in recent decades. Assuming that all other conditions were equal, it could be concluded that with an equalization of a carcinogenic occupational exposure for male and female asbestos workers there resulted a tendency toward an equalization of a specific cancer hazard for the two sexes.

In a subsequent report by MEREWETHER published in 1955 and comprising 65 cases of occupational asbestosis cancer of the lung, the male-female sex ratio had risen to 3 : 1 (48 males, 17 females). This figure stands at 4 : 1 (194 males, 41 females) for the collective series of 235 cases recorded in this study. It seems, therefore, that the sex distribution, like the age distribution, is still in flux and displays a tendency toward a "normal" level (BOHLIG, JACOB and MUELLER). The apparent lower liability to female asbestos workers to develop cancers of the lung may be related to work in safer jobs.

However, as long as reliable information is lacking on the total number of asbestos workers of both sexes, their age distribution, their length and type of employment in asbestos occupations, and their degree and duration of exposure to asbestos dust, any definite conclusions on these points should best be kept in abeyance.

g) Anticarcinogenic Action of Asbestos

PELLER and others asserted that an antagonism or inverse relation exists between the development of cancers of the skin and that of internal organs in population groups exposed to cutaneous carcinogens. BOHLIG et al. recently claimed that a similar antagonistic relation seemed to be present between the relatively high liability to cancer of the lung, which represented 85% of all cancer deaths in the worker population furnishing 57 lung cancers, and the rather low cancer attack rate for other organs (10 cases). Apart from the fact that the validity of PELLER's thesis has been disputed by many investigators, especially those familiar with general cancer attack rates noted in various worker groups occupationally exposed to various carcinogens as well as in animals treated with physical and chemical carcinogens (coal tar, petroleum oils, polycyclic aromatic hydrocarbons, ionizing radiation) (HUEPER), the observation on which BOHLIG's claim is based was not confirmed by the results of the cohort study of MANCUSO. The expected total cancer death rate of the population group analyzed was 27.74, the observed one stood at 55. Although the abnormally high lung and peritoneal cancer rates contributed the main share to the excess, there was no distinct diminution in the incidence of cancer of other sites in this group. The brain tumor rate was even increased. It would be unreasonable to assume by applying PELLER's thesis in reverse that a carcinogenic action of asbestos on the pulmonary tissues protected the skin against a cancerous transformation of the cutaneous asbestos warts (DEWIRTZ; DREESSEN et al.; OLIVIER, MORAND and BRUN), which are as invariably benign as their silicotic counterparts (CROSSLAND). Whether asbestotics have an elevated cancer incidence of abdominal organs is still doubtful (MANCUSO and COULTER; KÖNIG; SELIKOFF; CHURG and HAMMOND).

h) Syncarcinogenesis in the Production of Asbestosis Cancers

BOHLIG et al. recently emphasized the important role which other occupational and environmental carcinogenic air pollutants, such as those contained in cigarette smoke, to which asbestos workers become exposed may assume in the causation of cancer of the lung. While it may be conceded that a synergistic action of several carcinogens has been demonstrated in experimental animals, such an effect between several carcinogens is by no means consistent. It may indeed be totally lacking or be of antagonistic nature (HUEPER). At any rate this concept should not be advanced for minimizing the fundamental carcinogenic importance of asbestos in the production of lung cancers and should not be offered or accepted as a valid medicolegal argument against awarding compensation in litigations on asbestosis cancer of the lung. SELIKOFF et al.'s findings did not support any significant accentuating role of cigarette smoking on asbestos carcinoma of the lung.

i) Exposure Time and Latent Period

In common with other occupational cancer hazards asbestosis cancers of the lung display an exposure time covering a wide range. These fluctuations reflect not only the importance of the intensity and duration of exposure but also the significance of the reaction of the host organism to the carcinogen in determining the occurrence and developmental speed of a carcinogenic response. A similar connotation is carried by the length of the latent period. Exposure time and latent period observed in asbestosis cancers, therefore, follow the general epidemiologic-biologic pattern of occupational cancers.

k) Experimental Production of Cancers with Asbestos

Attempts to produce cancers in experimental animals by the inhalation or parenteral introduction of asbestos have yielded contradictory results. NORDMANN and

SORGE who exposed mice to asbestos dust by inhalation and SCHMAHL who injected asbestos subcutaneously and intraperitoneally into rats, reported the development of cancers in the lung and subcutaneous tissue, respectively. Similar experiments by VORWALD, DURKAN and PRATT; LYNCH, McIVER and CAIN; WAGNER; and HUEPER, employing mice, rabbits, rats, guinea pigs, monkeys, and dogs gave, on the other hand, negative results, when various types of asbestos were inhaled or implanted parenterally. PEACOCK and PEACOCK, who injected asbestos into the axillary air sac of White Leghorn fowls observed carcinomas developing from the wall of the sacs in two of 30 chickens surviving for periods of a year or more. WAGNER succeeded in the production of pleural mesotheliomas in rats intrapleurally injected with powdered South African asbestos, and SMITH, MILLER, CHURG and SELIKOFF were equally successful in hamsters receiving asbestos by the same route. They found chrysotile and amosite effective in this respect.

The experimental evidence obtained favors the view that asbestos is not only carcinogenic to man but also to several animal species.

1) Causative Mechanism of Asbestos Carcinogenesis

Efforts to elucidate the carcinogenic mechanism active in the production of cancers in the lung and mesothelial tissues have yielded several in part contradictory concepts. Some investigators have proposed that the development of carcinomas in the asbestotic lung is a nonspecific neoplastic reaction to chronic inflammatory and fibrosing processes favoring an unlimited regenerative proliferation of bronchiolar epithelium. Since such chronic irritative reponses are minimal in the majority of the lungs of individuals suffering from asbestos mesotheliomas and since asbestos bodies have not been discovered within these tumors, this chronic irritative concept of asbestos carcinogenesis evidently is not applicable to asbestos mesotheliomas.

Observations on the decrease of particle size of asbestos bodies observed with the elapse of time after cessation of exposure by KÜHN and by KNOX and BEATTIE suggests that asbestos particles, especially chrysotile, to a lesser degree crocidolite, are decomposed in the lungs and that some degradation product of asbestos might furnish the carcinogenic stimulus. This concept receives support from observations made by HUEPER in connection with the carcinogenic action exerted by various maromolecular carbon and silicon polymers. It was shown in these experiments that some of these polymers were degraded especially when implanted as sponges into the abdominal cavity of rats. The implantation of polyurethane foam resulted in the development of sarcomas and of adenocarcinomas of the intestine as well as of peritoneal mesotheliomas. The neoplasms contained flaky degradation products of the sponges implanted. In an appreciable number of these animals the sponges were completely absorbed. These findings point to the operation of a chemical mechanism as the principal carcinogenic avenue in asbestos carcinogenesis.

Since asbestos bodies are surrounded by an iron-protein complex sheath and because most types of asbestos contain iron in appreciable amounts, the possibility of a specific carcinogenic action of iron was considered. The reported excessive frequency of lung cancer in English and French hematite miners and foundry workers was cited in support of this concept. It was also pointed out that HADDOW and HORNING had suggested that the iron in the carcinogenic irondextran complexes represented the actually active carcinogenic principle and not the dextran. Apart from the fact that a carcinogenic action of iron in man and experimental animals has not been established as yet by these observations, the well known lack of carcinogenic developments around iron deposits of old hemorrhages definitely discourages the acceptance of the iron concept of asbestos carcinogenesis (HUEPER). The same reluctance should apply to the suggestion that the protein-iron complex might be related to a specific immuno-chemical reaction as an essential phase in asbestos carcinogenesis (Editorial).

The recent demonstration of HARINGTON and of HARINGTON and SMITH that small amounts of a strongly fluorescent oil containing small amounts of 3,4-benzpyrene can be eluted with cyclohexane from several sorts of asbestos, has posed the question whether asbestos cancers might not be attributable to a slow release of carcinogenic polycyclic aromatic hydrocarbons from the surfaces of asbestos particles inhaled and retained in the lungs. It was shown that the minute amounts of 3,4-benzpyrene attached to crocidolite can readily be removed from the asbestos by serum. HARINGTON and SMITH demonstrated moreover that 3,4-benzpyrene can be adsorbed by crocidolite, chrysotile and coal dust from which it could readily be eluted subsequently by serum to much the same extent. Only crocidolite, to a lesser degree amosite, but not chrysotile were found to contain an oil with 3,4-benzpyrene, which was present in amounts ranging from 4.9 to 0.2 micrograms per 100 grams of fiber for the various specimens examined. While the absolute amounts of 3,4-benzpyrene adsorbed to asbestos fibers seem to be rather small to be significant carcinogenically, it may be unwise to dismiss these findings as unimportant, because the experiments of SHABAD and of SAFFIOTTI *et al.* with carcinogens adsorbed to carbon particles and iron oxide particles, respectively have demonstrated the carcinogenic effectiveness of such preparations on the lungs of experimental animals. However, if such a combination of asbestos with carcinogenic polycyclic aromatic hydrocarbons should be shown as being a potent combination, such a finding would not exclude a direct carcinogenic effect of asbestos, because chrysotile which lacks, according to HARINGTON, any carcinogenic chemical contamination nevertheless appears to be carcinogenic to man and experimental animals.

Finally, mention must be made of the proposal to regard asbestos carcinogenesis as a manifestation of the formation of cancers by the surface forces of polymer plastics (NOTHDURFT; OPPENHEIMER *et al.*). An application of this hypothesis, mainly based on speculations, to asbestos cancers appears to be unjustified, since asbestos exerts its carcinogenic action as a fine particulate powder, which, according to the proponents of this hypothesis, represents a physical state in which polymerized plastics are carcinogenically inactive.

3. Chromium

Sites of Chromium Cancers: Recognized: Lung, Nasal Cavity
                                 Suspected: Stomach, Larynx
Exposure Stigmata: Dermatitis, Cutaneous "Chrome Holes", Ulcerated and Perforated Nasal
                     Septum, Laryngitis, Tracheitis, Bronchitis, Chronic Fibrosing Pneumonia,
                     Chronic Gastritis, Indolent Intestinal Ulcers
Compounds of Economic Importance (Di-, Tri- and Hexavalent)
     Chromite ore, Chromium metal, Chromium alloys (Iron, Nickel, Cobalt), Chromium oxide, Chromium trioxide, Chromous Chloride, Chromic chloride, Chromyl chloride, Chromic nitrate, Chromium oxychloride, Chromium boride, Chromium carbide, Ammonium chromate,

Sodium chromate, Potassium chromate, Strontium chromate, Calcium chromate, Barium chromate, Lead chromate, Zinc chromate, Sodium dichromate, Potassium dichromate, Chrome sulfate, Chrome alum, Ammonium chrome alum, Potassium chrome alum, Stearate chromium chloride, Chromium acetate, Chromic acid, Ammonium dichromate, Copper chromate, Chrome hydroxide, Chrome-phosphate, Chromite Ore Roast, Chromate Roast Leached Residue, Stearatochromic chloride, Butyl Chromate

Operations and Products with Contact to Chromium for Producers, Processers, Users, Consumers, Residents

Mining, Grinding, Mixing, *Chromate Manufacture*, Electrometallurgical Chrome Production, Stainless Steel Manufacturing and Processing Industries, *Production of Chromium Compounds* for Tanning, Photography, Paint, Ink, Textile, Shingle, Rubber, Plastic, Glass, Petroleum, Pyrotechnical, Pottery, Printing, Wood Preserving Industries; Electroplating plants, Aviation-, Railroad-, Shipbuilding Industries; Dye Manufacturing Industry, Chemical and Pharmaceutical Industries, Explosive Manufacturing Plants, Match Manufactures, Wax and Wax Product Industries; Oil and Fat Industry; Fiberglass Manufactures and Processers; Cement Industry; Blue Print Industry; Metal Wares and Machinery, Electrical Appliances, Anti-corrosive and Antirusting Agent, Polymerization Catalyst, Oil Cracking Catalyst, Anti-corrosive Primer Paint Pigment, Pigment in Paints, Inks, Glass, Plastics, Rubber, Shingles, Linoleum; Glazes, Enamels, etc.; Glass and Pottery Frosting and Etching Agent; Chemical Cleaning Fluid; Textile Mordant; Oxidizing Agent in Dye Production, Bleaching Agent for Fats and Oils; Leather Tannery and Finishing Chemicals; Dry Battery Chemicals; Wood Preservative and Staining Agents; Fiberglass Coupling Agent; Corrosion Retarder in Refrigeration Brines; in Air Washers, in Cooling Water of Diesel Engines, Locomotives, Automobiles, Boilers; Ingredient of Match heads, Explosives, Cements, Water repellent for fabrics, felt hats, glass fiber, drapes, paper

Population Groups with Occupational and Environmental Exposure to Chromium

Occupational Groups: Abrasive Makers, Abrasive Workers and Polishers, Airplane Sprayers; Bleachers, Blue Print Makers, Colored Candle Makers, Cement Manufacturers; Chemical Workers, *Chromate and Chrome Pigment Producers;* Chrome Platers; Chrome-Steel Manufacturers and Processers; Chrome Ore Miners, Loaders, Shippers, Grinders and Mixers, Chrome-Alloy Producers and Processers, Crayon Makers, *Dye Manufacturers,* Dock Workers, Electroplaters, Electrometallurgical Workers, Enamelers, Enamel Makers; Explosive Manufacturers, Fiberglass Producers and Processers, Furniture Polishers, Glass and Pottery Frosters, Ink Makers, Linoleum Workers, Lithographers, Match Producers, Mordanters, Paint Manufacturers, Painters, Metal Cutter and Welders, Oil Refinery Workers, Pyrotechnical Workers, Printers, Paper Dryers, Paper Waterproofers, Photoengravers, Photographic Workers, Pottery Glaze makers, Pottery Glazers, Refractory Brick Makers and Masons, Railroad Engineers, Rubber Workers, Plastic Manufacturers, Soap Makers, Stainless Steel Producers, Processers, Buffers and Polishers, Pyrotechnical Workers, Shingle Manufacturers, Leather Finishers, Tannery Workers, Textile Printers and Mordanters, Textile Waterproofers, Wax Ornament Workers, Welders, Wood Stainers and Preservers, Boiler Scalers, Dry Battery Makers, Colored Glass Producers, Fat Bleachers

Nonoccupational Groups: Residents in vicinity of chromate plants, airplane manufacturing and maintenance establishments, railroad yards, ship building plants, scrap metal smelters, oil refineries; Home users of paints containing chrome pigments and of chromate containing antirusting agents in steam heating plants; Consumers of drinking water polluted with chromates containing industrial wastes and of fats bleached with sodium dichromate.

a) Technologic Aspects

The production and use of chromite ore, chromium metal, chromium alloys and chromium compounds have risen remarkably during the last 50 years as demonstrated by the figures on the world production of chromite ore (Table 39).

The largest increase in the production of chromite ore between 1944 and 1953 (90%) was in the metallurgic manufacture of chromium metal and chromium alloys. The use of chromite ore in the production of chromite cement and refractory brick during this period rose by 70%, while that employed for the manufacture of chromium compounds for chemical uses increased by only 20%. These technologic and commercial observations are of importance in the assessment of the past, present and future scope of occupational and environmental cancer hazards associated with exposures to chromium and chromium compounds. The data indicate that with the rapid recent rise in the production and use of chromium and its compounds and alloys in the human economy (DANKMAN; WALSH) and the thereby conditioned greater occupational and environmental exposure to these agents, there may follow during the next decades a distinct and progressive increase in the number of chromium cancer affecting mainly parts of the respiratory system among members of many special

Table 39. *World Production of Chromite Ore in Short Tons from 1900 to 1958*
P. J. THOMPSON and B. B. MITCHELL

Year	Tons
1900	58,600
1905	158,600
1910	119,500
1915	204,300
1920	189,400
1925	339,000
1930	616,000
1935	865,000
1940	1,605,000
1945	1,170,000
1950	2,655,000
1955	4,020,000
1958	4,050,000

1958 Mineral Yearbook, Vol. I. p. 316, U. S. Government Printing Office, 1959.

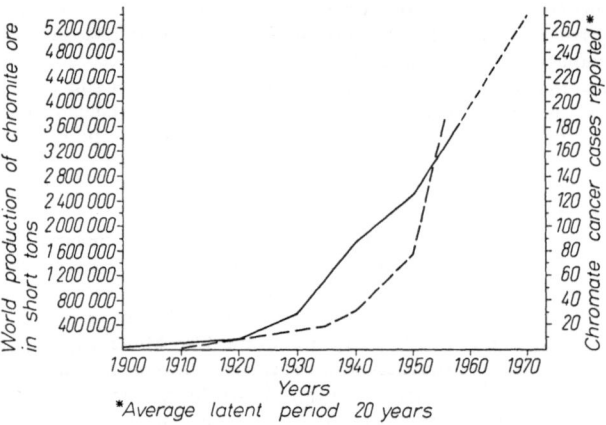

*Average latent period 20 years

Fig. 14. Chromite ore production and chromium cancers of lung

worker groups as well as of the general population (Fig. 14). Cancer hazards to this type may be related to occupational contacts encountered during the production, processing and industrial use of these agents. They may be associated with environmental exposures to chromium-containing industrial effluents contaminating the air, water and soil and after secondarily being transferred to agricultural products and meats, also the human food supply, and they may result from contact with chromium-containing constituents and pollutants of general consumer goods (GRUSHKO; HUEPER). While these industrial developments have been accompanied in many operations by a reduction in the intensity of exposure to chromium-containing dust, fumes and vapors through the introduction of improved production methods and of protective measures, there has not occurred lately any appreciable decrease in the duration of occupational exposure to these agents and, doubtlessly, there has taken place during the same period a remarkable increase in the number of exposed individuals engaged in old and new activities and practices providing contact with, in part, new chromium compounds and alloys. There were employed in the American Navy Shipyards in 1960 about 2,000 zinc chromate spray painters among a total of approximately 60,000 workers. During World War II about 6,000 spray painters worked in the aviation industry in southern California.

b) Epidemiologic Cancer Aspects

The first observation which aroused the suspicion concerning the existence of a cancer hazard to the lung in workers exposed to chromates was made in 1911 and 1912 in two workers engaged in Germany in the production of alizarin which required the use of chromates as oxidizing agents (PFEIL).

Because of the small number of cases and the newness of this finding no serious attention was paid to it, expecially since its significance as an industrial cancer hazard was denied by LEHMANN and KOELSCH. However, 25 years later, ALWENS, BAUKE and JONAS and subsequently GROSS and other German investigators reported the occurrence of lung cancers in a considerable number of workers employed in the manufacture of chromates or having, for other reasons, contact with chromate dust and fumes in such plants and plant areas. It became soon apparent that also the producers of chrome pigments (zinc chromate, barium chromate and lead chromate) exhibited an excessive liability to lung cancer (GROSS and KOELSCH). The entire evidence recorded on the occurrence of these respiratory occupational cancer hazards in Germany up to 1952 was reviewed by SPANNAGEL in 1953, who collected a total of 86 lung cancers and four (4) nasal sinus cancers among German chromate and chrome pigment workers (PFEIL, LEHMANN; TELEKY; KOELSCH; ALWENS and BAUKE; ALWENS, BAUKE and JONAS; ALWENS; GROSS and ALWENS; GROSS; GROSS and KOELSCH; BAADER; RINCK; ASANG; FISCHER-WASSELS; CADOTSCH; LETTERER, NEIDHARDT and KLETT). Among the workers thus affected were not only chromate producers but also workers with intermittent contact to effluents of such operations (GROSS), such as truckers, glaziers, locksmiths, welders, workers employed in buildings located within the fume zone of chromate operations and suffering in part from perforated nasal septa (GROSS) (hydrochloric acid and sulfuric acid workers); chrome pigment producers (GROSS; BAADER; LETTERER et al.; FISCHER-WASELS); a polisher of aluminium casts treated with sodium bichromate (ASANG), and a spray painter (BAADER). A larynx cancer of somewhat doubtful association to an exposure to chromic acid occurred in a galvanizer (CADOTSCH). Recent unpublished observations of HUEPER and of PAYNE and HUEPER established the occurrence of lung cancers in cutters of scrap metal painted with chrome yellow who were employed in a shipyard and in spray painters applying chrome yellow paints as an anticorrosive coating to airplanes. Five cancers of the lung were observed in 1962 in American chrome pigment workers who had been employed in a chromate plant (HUEPER) which formerly had been found free from such occurrences (MACHLE and GREGORIUS).

The first case of lung cancer in a chromate producer in the U.S.A. was recognized in 1946 as the result of a litigation (HUEPER). When subsequently upon suggestion of HUEPER, the American chromate producing industry conducted a survey among workers employed in seven plants, 42 additional cases were discovered (MACHLE and GREGORIUS). These studies and others performed thereafter (BAETJER; MANCUSO and HUEPER; BRINTON, FRASIER and KOVEN; IMPRESCIA; GAFAFER et al.; HUEPER; FISHER and RIECKERT) provided definite proof that workers engaged in the manufacture of chromates exhibited also in American plants a highly excessive attack rate of cancer of the lung. Subsequent similar epidemiologic investigations made in England by BIDSTRUP and by BIDSTRUP and CASE revealed the existence of similar connections for English chromate workers.

These observations came some 60 years after the initial finding by NEWMAN of an adenocarcinoma of the turbinates in a chrome pigment worker in Scotland. During recent years reports on the occurrence of isolated cases of cancers of the lung and nasal septum in chromate producers have been published from other countries (Italy, Czechoslovakia, U.S.S.R.) (VIGLIANI and ZURLO WACKMANN; PORTIGLIATTI-BARBOS; BARBORIK, NANSLIAN, ORAL, SEHNALOVA and HOLUSA; GRUSHKO).

In fact, it has become likely from clinical and experimental findings that the carcinogenic action of chromium may not entirely be limited to the respiratory system, but may extend under special conditions to other tissues such as the skin and bones. Welz recorded the occurrence of a squamous cell carcinoma of the skin of the forearm in a graphic workers suffering from a chronic chrome eczema, while STRUPPLER and McDOUGAL noted the development of bone sarcomas in individuals following the nailing or plating of bone fractures. The occasionally observed development of cancers around bullets and shell fragments embedded in various tissues, including the lung and nasal sinuses, may possibly be attributable to a carcinogenic action of chromium contained in such materials (BLÜMLEIN), since implants of various chromium compounds into rats and mice gave rise to the development of sarcomas of different types (HUEPER; HUEPER and PAYNE; PAYNE). The following table (Table 40) presents a summary of the cases of industrial chromium cancer reported from various countries.

Table 40. *Cancers of the Respiratory System in Industrial Producers, Processers, and Users of Chromates, Chrome Pigments, and Other Chromium Compounds*

Country	No. of Cases	Sites of Cancers				Location in Lung					
		Lung	Larynx	Nares	Nasal Sinuses	Upper Lobe		Lower Lobe		Hilum	
						Right	Left	Right	Left	Right	Left
Germany . . .	93	89	1		3	14	9	16	8	6	4
U.S.A.	77	76			1	12	5	6	3	6	4
England . . .	13	12			1						
Italy	3	2		1							
Czechoslovakia	1	1									
Total	187	180	1	1	5	26	14	22	11	12	8

It should not be assumed that the number of cases listed in this Table represent even approximately the number of cases of chromate cancers which actually occurred among workers employed in plants and operations and inhaling chromium containing air pollutants. While American, German, U.S.S.R., and South-African investigators (GAFAFER et al.; KOELSCH; LUKANIN) noted that chromite ore dust inhaled during the mining and the processing of ore into refractory bricks and cement has not produced a lung cancer hazard, this statement is of uncertain validity because of the absence of acceptable large scale epidemiologic investigations on worker groups thus exposed and the high rate of labor turnover among such workers. The trivalent chromium of finely powdered chromite ore, moreover, is transformed by the action of atmospheric oxygen into a water soluble hexavalent chromium (GROGAN) and thus becomes biologically active. Experiments of HUEPER, moreover, have shown that chromite ore dust inhaled by mice and deposited in their lungs is solubilized, mobilized and demonstrable in the blood.

It appears from observations made in man exposed to chromite ore dust that similar changes apparently take place in the human lung since chromium could be demonstrated in the blood, urine and tissues of individuals thus exposed (MANCUSO and HUEPER).

Apart from the epidemiologic surveys made on rather small worker groups engaged in the manufacture of chromates in Germany, U.S.A. and England, there is a complete lack of similar studies on the many and much larger worker populations who have respiratory contact with hexavalent and trivalent inorganic and organic chromium compounds and with metallic chromium and alloys, such as especially chrome platers, stainless steel makers, welders, metal cutters and spray painters. Even the available epidemiologic studies performed on members of the chromate producing industries in the three countries mentioned yielded only fragmentary information, since they did not include a comprehensive analysis of former workers employed in their plants, who can be expected to have developed at least in part, cancers of the respiratory organs while employed later on in other jobs. The data provided by SPANNAGEL and others on the length of the lag period elapsing between the cessation of exposure and the appearance of the first symptoms of a respiratory cancer illustrate the significance of such epidemiologic relations (Table 41).

Table 41. *Length of Lag Period of Chromate Cancers of the Lung*

Years	1—2	3—5	6—10	11—15	16—20	21—30	Total
Cases	16	8	19	3	1	49	49

In an analysis of HUEPER conducted on 154 former chromate producers employed in a Mid-Atlantic State of the U.S.A. who had been engaged at this work for a minimum of 6 months and who had left the chromate plant at least four years prior to the investigation, it was found that among 20 deaths which had occurred in this group, four (4) were due to cancer of the lung, one (1) to cancer of the maxillary sinus; one (1) to cancer of the colon and one (1) to leukemia. The respiratory cancer death rate in this group which thus accounted for 25 per cent of all deaths, indicates clearly that an excessive liability to cancer of the respiratory system persists for individuals after exposure to chromium has ceased for many years (Fig. 15). It is, therefore, important that SPANNAGEL succeeded in obtaining data on the cause of death in only a part of the former employees of several German chromate plants which had stopped operation many years prior to the time of this investigation. BIDSTRUP and CASE were confronted with similar difficulties in their studies on English chromate producers, since they were unable to ascertain the fate of 217 of 333 former workers of the 723 chromate workers still alive. GAFAFER et al. also emphasized the fact that the number of recorded deaths from respiratory cancer among American chromate producers recorded in their survey was minimal for the following reasons:

1. Deaths of employees who were not members of a sick benefit association were not included.

2. Persons who worked in chromate but left the industry prior to their terminal illness were not included.

3. Members who died over a year after onset of disability due to cancer were not included.

4. Several members who had a clinical course consistent with the presence of cancer of the respiratory tract were not included because cancer was not recorded on their death certificates.

5. Some members whose deaths were not recorded as cancer died without a complete medical examination or biopsy.

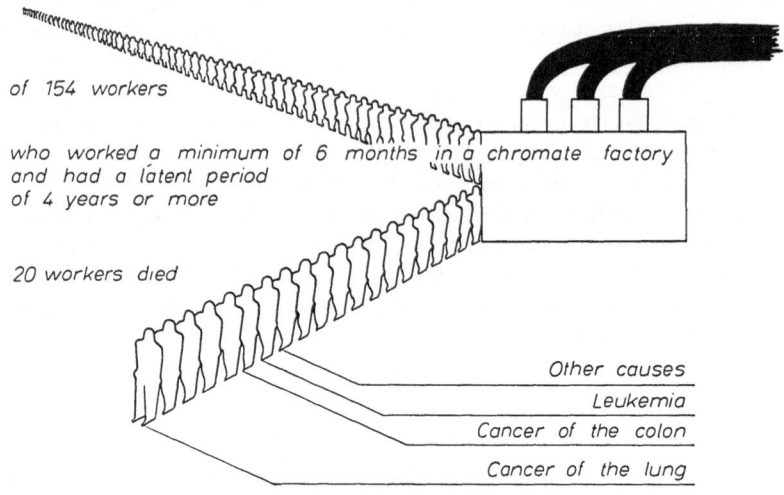

of 154 workers

who worked a minimum of 6 months in a chromate factory and had a latent period of 4 years or more

20 workers died

Other causes
Leukemia
Cancer of the colon
Cancer of the lung

Fig. 15. Environmental cancer

Since work in chromates appears to be objectionable in many respects there is a rather large labor turnover in such plants. Imprescia estimated an annual labor turnover of from 40 to 50% in a chromate plant employing about 400 workers. GAFAFER noted that 38.6 per cent of all workers (37.5 for whites, 41.8 for colored) had worked less than 5 years in chromate operations. In two plants surveyed by them less than 7% of the white workers had been employed there for 20 years or longer. Also BAETJER stated that no information on a delayed occurrence of lung cancer was available in her study of the chromate plant in Baltimore for the many workers who had left over a 15 to 20-year period. The deficiencies in the epidemiologic data produced thereby are bound to lower possibly considerably the lung cancer attack rates calculated from the available information because of the omission of the undetermined number of lung cancers which doubtlessly developed among former chromate workers whose cause of death remained obscure.

Because of these limitations in the available epidemiologic data, the various statements made concerning the incidence and frequency of chrome cancers of the respiratory organs represent at best well considered approximations or are mere educated guesses. All of them are nevertheless definitely indicative of the existence of highly excessive lung cancer rates among chromate producers and chrome pigment makers (Table 42). CAROZZI stated that up to 40 per cent of the employees in chromate plants in Germany developed lung cancers. Estimating that among approximately 2,000 chromate workers who had been employed in German plants between 1880 and 1948, a minimum of 86 lung cancers had occurred, SPANNAGEL noted a morbidity ratio of 43 : 1 for chromate workers. MACHLE and GREGORIUS found that 21.8 per cent of all deaths among American chromate workers were attributable to occupational factors and that the ratio was 16 times the standard one of 1.3%. The range of the ratio for different plants was from 13 times to 31 times. The crude death rates from lung cancer for members of this occupational group stood at from 18 to 50-fold the standard rate *and averaged* 25-fold. MANCUSO and HUEPER estimated a lung cancer rate among American chromate workers to be about 15 times the normal rate, while BAETJER noted that the lung cancer rate in chromate workers was 28 times the standard of the employed male population of Baltimore 18 years and older (34 times for whites, 18 times for colored). GAFAFER *et al.* concluded from the results of their survey that nearly 29 times as many deaths as were expected were found among American chromate workers.

Table 42. *Comparative Frequency Rates of Lung Cancer in Chromate Workers of U.S.A., Germany and England*

Country	Frequency		Lung Cancers per 100,000	
	Expected	Observed	Chromate Workers	General Population
United States .	1.9	31.9	470.8	16.7
Germany . . .	1	43	—	—
England . . .	1.3	7	—	—

They noted, moreover, that a racial comparison of respiratory cancer deaths showed that the ratio of actual to expected number was 40 for whites and 80 for colored. It should not be concluded from this observation that colored individuals possess a racially conditioned higher susceptibility to lung cancer. The difference in lung cancer rates noted by GAFAFER *et al.* for whites and colored individuals employed in chromate operations is attributable to the fact that colored workers are usually employed in the dirtier operations and, therefore, sustain the more severe exposure to the carcinogenic agent. The validity of this reasoning is supported by the observations made by GAFAFER *et al.* on the time of first occurrence and on the frequency of nasal septum perforations among members of the two racial groups (Table 43).

Table 43. *Time of Appearance and Frequency of Nasal Septum Perforations in White and Colored Chromate Producers in U.S.A.*
(GAFAFER *et al.*)

Time of Employment	Number of Workers	Percentage of Perforated Nasal Septa		
		All Workers	Whites	Colored
0—6 months	41	2.4	0	11.1
6 months to 3 years . .	117	39.3	31.5	64.3
3—10 years	370	55.4	44.3	74.8
10 years and over . . .	369	69.6	64.0	93.1
Total	897	56.7	49.3	76.6

Most investigators agreed that the excessive liability to cancer among chromate workers was restricted to cancers of the lung (MACHLE and GREGORIUS; BIDSTRUP and CASE; GAFAFER *et al.*) and did not extend to other organs exposed to chromates (skin, alimentary tract), although chromate workers exhibit frequently inflammatory and ulcerative reactions in these organ systems. TELEKY, on the other hand, has suggested that an occupational cancer hazard in chromate workers might extend to the alimentary system. So far only the occurrence of ulcerative lesions in the stomach and intestine has been reported (BUESS; RIEDL; MOSINGER and FLORENTINI). There is no evidence in support of the view that the development of a cancer of the lung in chromate workers lowers their liability to cancers in any other organ (GAFAFER; BAETJER; MACHLE and GREGORIUS).

c) Special Aspects

The exposure time preceding the development of respiratory cancers in chromate workers exhibited, according to the various assessments, wide variations depending apparently upon differences in exposure conditions as well as upon fluctuations in the individual susceptibility. It was noted, however, that the exposure time of chrome pigment workers developing lung cancer was distinctly shorter than that of the chromate producers (GROSS) (Table 44). This phenomenon may perhaps be due to the

Table 44. *Length of Latent Periods for Cancers of the Lung in Chromate Workers*

Years	3—5	6—10	11—20	21—30	31—40	41 and over	Total	Average length
All cases	2	25	79	45	17	8	176	24 years
Pigment workers	—	1	1	1	—	—	7	15 years
U.S.A. workers	1	11	23	11	1	2	49	17 years

fact that the yellow pigments mainly involved in this respect, particularly zinc chromate, possess higher carcinogenic potency than the chromium compounds encountered in chromate operations (HUEPER and PAYNE).

The entire range of exposure times noted in the 131 cases for which data were available extended from 2 to 47 years with 60% of them falling in the 6- to 20-year range. The existence of marked variations in the length of effective exposure periods is in accord with similar observations recorded for other occupational cancers. Most of the long exposure periods noted are most likely merely incidental because they are identical with the latent periods observed in these cases. Whenever relatively short exposure periods were followed by a longer lag period, it may be assumed that the intensity of exposure may have been quite severe, or the inhaled material was rather water insoluble, therefore was retained in the lungs over long periods of time and was gradually released from its intrapulmonary depots. It is also possible that in a particular exposed individual some special exogenous or constitutional additional factor of local or systemic nature was operative which favored and accentuated the action of the inhaled carcinogen. It is, for instance, conceivable that the irritative respiratory effect of inhaled acid fumes in German acid workers developing chrome cancers of the lung acted in such a capacity (neighborhood cases), since it is likely that the concentration of the carcinogenic air pollutants must have been rather low in the atmosphere of the acid operations.

A similar connotation have the distinct fluctuations in the length of the latent period which varied in the individual cases from a minimum of three (3) years to a maximum of 58 years. About 70 per cent of all cases had a latent period extending from 11 to 30 years.

The relative length of the latent period in the individual cases may be taken as reflecting the intensity of exposure, the carcinogenic potency of the particular chromium compound or compounds to which the individual became exposed, and his reactivity as a host.

d) Histologic Types of Chrome Cancers of the Lung

While four (4) nasal sinus carcinomas observed in chromate workers were all squamous cell carcinomas, those affecting the lung exhibited a degree of variation which roughly corresponded with that seen in "spontaneous" cancers of this organ. This observation offers a good illustration of the fact that there does not exist any definite relationship between any particular carcinogenic agent and any specific histologic type of cancer (Table 45).

Table 45. *Histologic Types of Pulmonary Carcinomas in Chromate Workers*

Types	Squamous Cell Carcinomas	Round, Anaplastic and Undifferentiated Cell Carcinomas	Adeno-carcinomas	Total
No. of cases . . .	46	66	11	123

In two American cases, two different types of carcinomas coexisted in the lungs. Since one of these double cancers affected the pleura (BAETJER) and was of an undifferentiated type, the possibility must be considered that it might have been a meso-

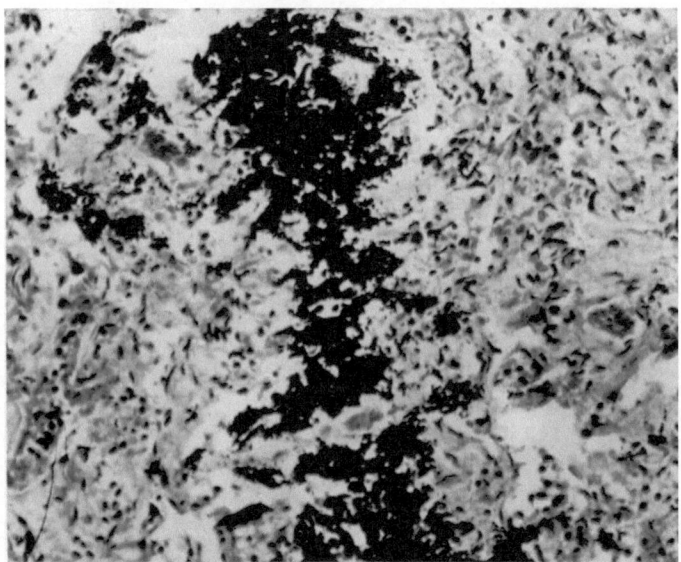

Fig. 16. Massive deposits of black chromite ore dust in the lung of a chromate producer

thelioma of the pleura. There is no sound scientific reason for assuming that the adenocarcinomas are not of occupational origin but result from embryonic malformations (ALWENS). A study of the various histologic intrapulmonary changes preceding the development of lung cancers elicited in man and experimental animals show clearly the multiple potentials of the lung tissue accounting for the development of cancers of the different types which were observed sometimes in the same lung.

Chromate producers exhibit often the manifestations of a chronic sinusitis, chronic ulcerative rhinitis, chronic laryngitis, chronic tracheitis and chronic bronchitis, which

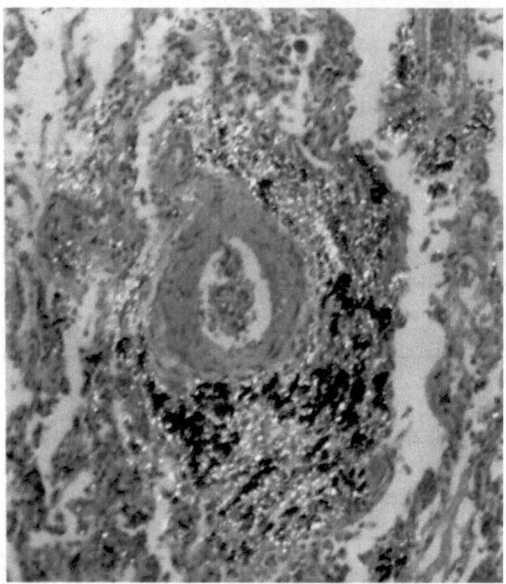

Fig. 17. Numerous fine reflecting particles in the perivascular tissue of the lung of a chromate worker located within a black pigmentary deposit seen under polarized light

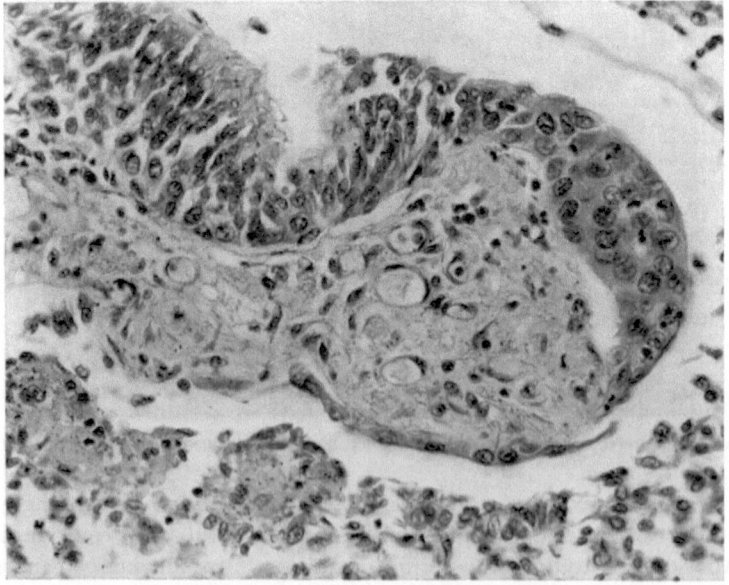

Fig. 18. Large intrabronchial polyp with focal squamous cell metaplasia

at times may assume an ulcerative character (SPANNAGEL; MACHLE and GREGORIUS; MANCUSO). The lungs of chromate producers who are exposed to the inhalation of chromite ore dust show at autopsy often varying degrees of black spotting. These pigmentary deposits which resemble in appearance anthracotic lesions, however, do

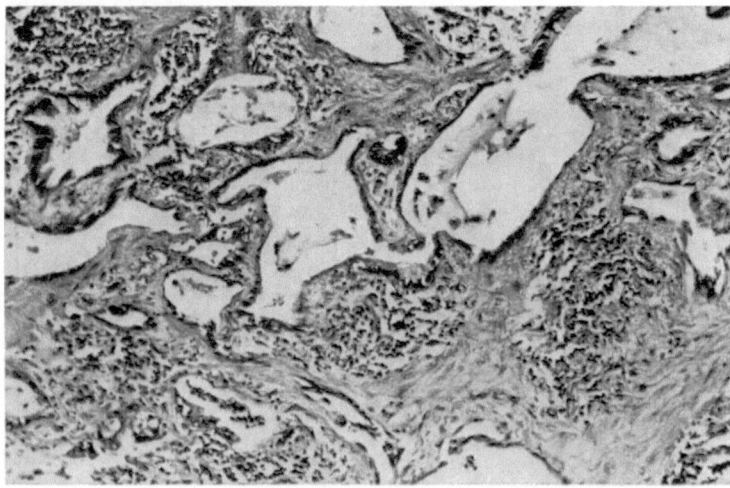

Fig. 19. Fibrosing chronic chemical pneumonitis with adenocystic transformations of bronchioli in a chromate producer

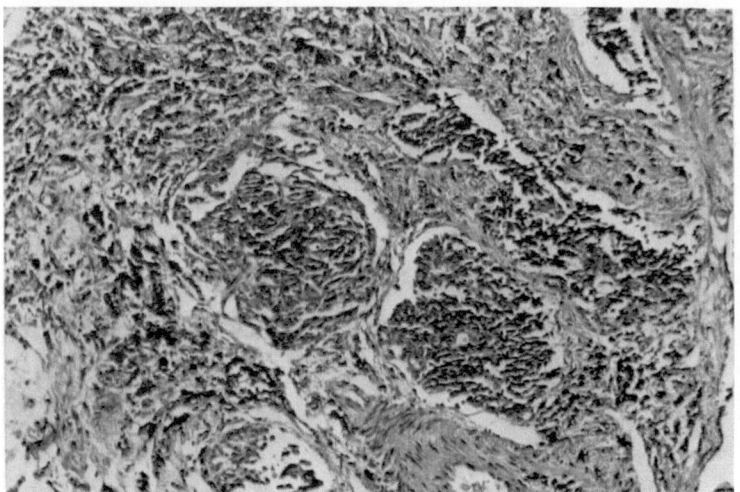

Fig. 20. Miniature, small cell carcinomas in the lung of this worker

not disappear, as anthracotic deposits do, in incinerated sections because of their mineral character. In polarized light they show numerous, small, white reflecting crystalline granules (Figs. 16, 17). The bronchial lumens contain often purulent material, while the bronchial mucosa may form polypous formations covered by a hyperplastic stratified columnar epithelium with localized squamous cell metaplasias (Fig.

5*

18). The retention of toxic chromium-containing dust may give rise to the development of some degree of interstitial fibrosis (chromitosis) (MANCUSO and HUEPER; RINCK; LETTERER; BAADER; LUKANIN; LETTERER, NEIDHARDT and KLETT; ANDRIEVSKAYA and MISLAVSKAYA). In severe conditions of pulmonary chemotoxi-

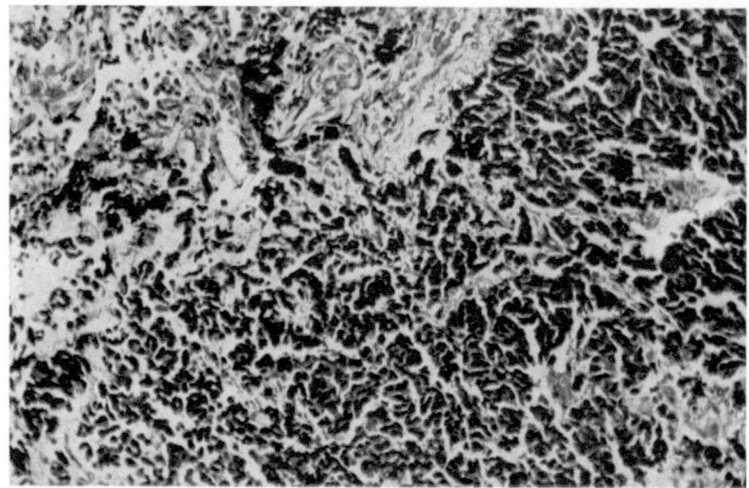

Fig. 21. Small round cell carcinoma of the lung in a chromate worker with black pigment in the fibrous tissue surrounding the tumor mass

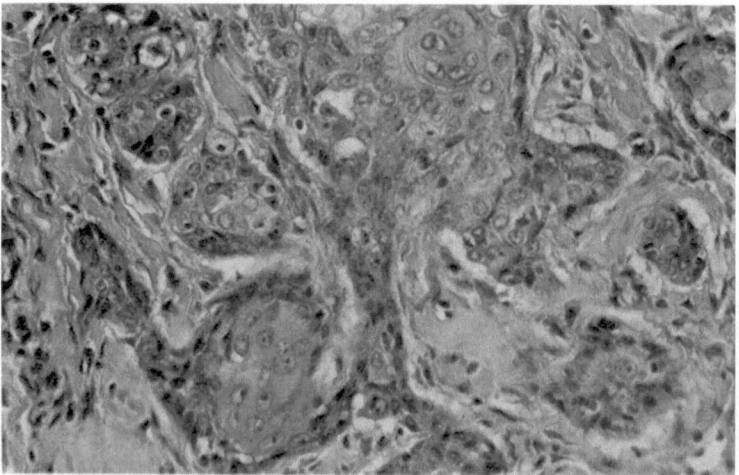

Fig. 22. Squamous cell carcinoma of the lung in a chromate worker

cosis, there occurs a multicystic transformation of the bronchioli. Such lesions at times may be complicated by multifocal proliferations of small hyperchromatic bronchiolar epithelial cells producing the impression of miniature carcinomas (Figs. 19 and 20). Such precancerous lesions of glandular, small cellular and squamous cell nature evidently form the basis for the various histologic types of carcinomas subsequently developing (Figs. 21 and 22) (HUEPER). The irrelevancy of the nature of a pulmonary carcinogen in such matters was clearly shown in a series of experiments in which rats were intrapleurally implanted with various chromium-containing materials (chromite ore roast, chromic chromate, calcium chromate, etc.). The bronchial mucosa responded to the carcinogenic stimulus of chromium with the development of cancers of different histologic types (HUEPER; HUEPER and PAYNE; PAYNE). In some ani-

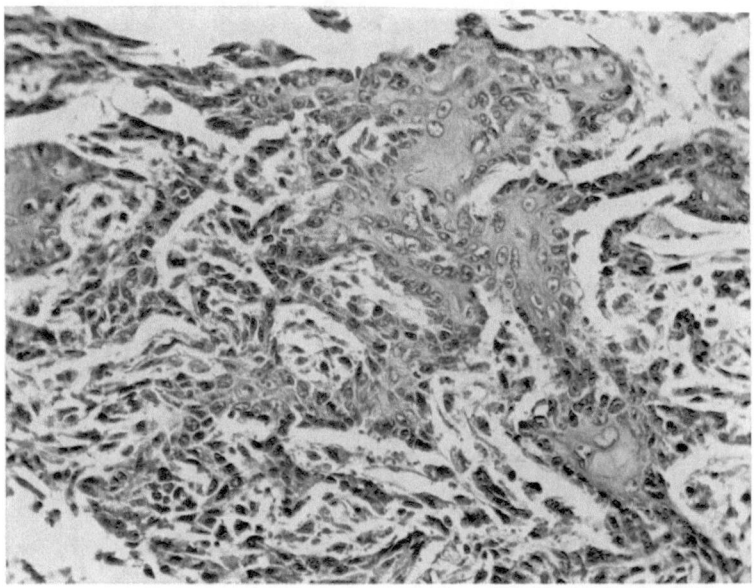

Fig. 23. Squamous cell carcinoma of the lung of a rat following an intrapleural deposition of chromic chromate

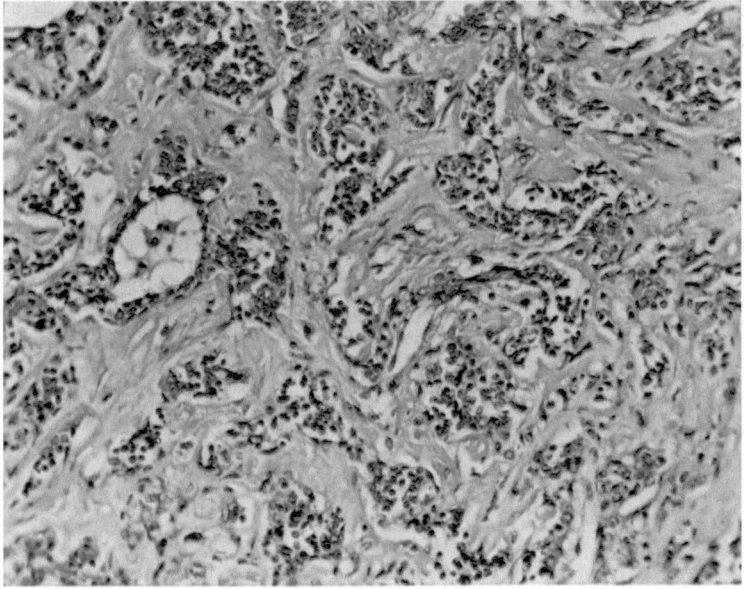

Fig. 24. Adenocarcinoma of the lung of the same rat

mals several cancers of two or three different types coexisted in the same lung (squamous cell carcinoma, adenocarcinoma and sarcoma) (Figs. 23, 24, 25) together with corresponding precancerous lesions.

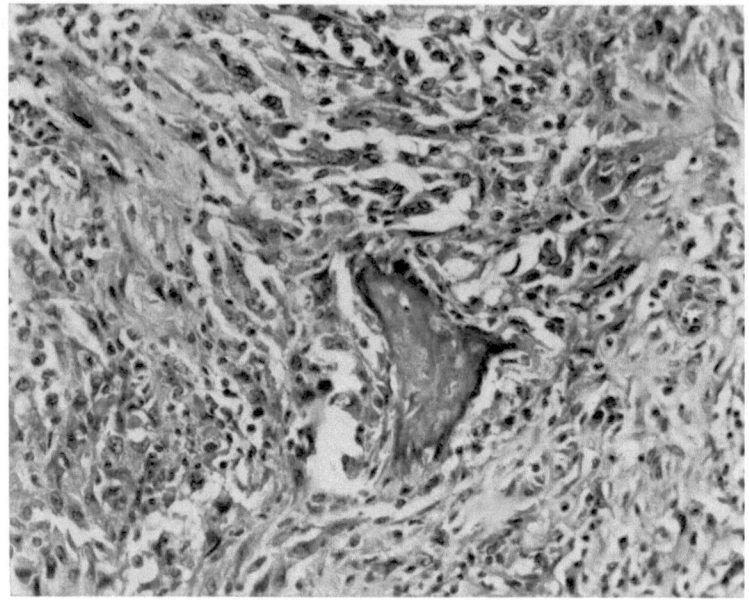

Fig. 25. Osteogenic sarcoma of the lung of the same rat

e) Clinical Aspects

Chrome cancers of the lung in contrast to asbestos cancers, do not exhibit in their location any special preference to any particular part of the lung. Of 93 cases for which some information was available on this point, forty (40) were situated in the upper lobes, 33 in lower lobes and 20 in the region of the hilum.

None of the various symptomatic manifestations observed in chromate workers (perforated nasal septum, chronic bronchitis, unilateral enlarged density of the hilar region and thickening of the peribronchiolar structure in x-ray pictures of the lung, pneumoconiosis, etc.) can be considered as a precancerous lesion characteristic for chrome cancer of the lung. These and other symptoms (chrome holes and chronic eczema of the skin, gastric ulcers, chronic ulcerative colitis and chronic sinusitis) represent merely stigmata of an occupational exposure to irritative chromium compounds. The survival time of the majority of chrome cancer patients did not exceed one year after the discovery of the tumor (SPANNAGEL; GAFAFER et al.; BAETJER), although recently a few cases (3 out of 7) have survived a pneumonectomy for more than six (6) postoperative years (FISHER).

f) Chromium Content of Tissues, Blood and Urine

Since chromium has become an almost ubiquitary element through its widespread use in modern industry and industrial products and the contamination of air, water, and soil with chromium and its subsequent introduction into the human food supply, the blood, urine and tissues of man often contain small amounts of chromium. Considerable quantities of this metal, on the other hand, have been demonstrated in the urine, blood and tissues of chromate producers and other industrial workers processing and using chromium metal and chromium compounds (Tables 46 and 47)

Table 46. *Concentration of Chromium in Body Tissues With and Without Known Exposures to Chromium* (A. BAETJER)

Tissue	Range of Concentrations. Reported in Normal Tissues	Range of Concentrations. Reported in Tissues from Chromate Workers
	Micrograms/100 g Wet Tissue	
Lungs	0—33	130—9,887
Lung tumors	—	0—1,658
Metastatic tumors	—	2— 100
Tracheobronchial lymph nodes	0— 1	12—7,590
Bronchus	—	95— 386
Trachea	—	0— 32
Nasal septum	—	287
Larynx	—	21
Kidney	0— 9.6	0— 211
Liver	1—11	0— 159
Spleen	0—98	0— 91
Abdominal lymph nodes	1	4— 80
Stomach	0— 5	4— 11
Intestines	10	4— 5
Bladder	—	3— 226
Heart	—	0— 20
Muscle	0— 8	0— 19
Pancreas	21	8— 36
Thyroid	43	24— 53
Adrenal	0—41	5— 76
Brain	0— 4	0— 5
Bone	5	0— 292
Cartilage	—	6
Bile	—	1
Hair	—	31
Skin	—	5
Aorta	—	3

(BAETJER; MANCUSO and HUEPER; SPANNAGEL; GAFAFER *et al.* and others) with the analytical methods developed by SPANNAGEL; URONE and ANDERS; CAHNMANN and BISEN. It is of interest that in chromate producers the by far largest amounts of chromium were found in the normal parts of carcinomatous lungs especially their hilar regions, and that the carcinomatous portions contained distinctly smaller concentrations. This is explainable by the fact that chromium containing pollutants cannot be inhaled and be deposited in the newly formed carcinomatous tissue. Chromium can practically get into such parts only when the cancer invades the structures of the lung already containing chromium deposits.

SPANNAGEL commenting on the normally occurring excretion of chromium by the healthy human organism with the urine stated that an increase of the blood chromium level above 20 gamma per 100 cc. should arouse the suspicion of the existence of a bronchial cancer in the individual studied. Since the observations of MANCUSO on exposed, temporarily unexposed and former chromate workers have revealed the occurrence of marked variations in the chromium blood level and a retention of an excessive level many months after cessation of exposure, it is at present perhaps wiser to consider such observations mainly as evidence of a marked and prolonged exposure to chromium containing air pollutants.

Table 47. *Concentration of Chromium in Blood and Urine as Reported in the Literature* (A. Baetjer)

Investigator	Degree of Exposure to Chromium	Blood Concentration of Chromium in Micrograms/100 g of Blood	Urine Concentration of Chromium in Micrograms/Liter of Urine
Gray	No exposure	r.b.c.—20.0 plasma—14	
Grushko	No exposure	3.5—12.0	
Spanngael	No exposure	—	0—16.3
	Occasional exposure	—	Ave 18.2 (Max 76.8)
	Chromate workers	8—580	Ave 78.2 (Range 0) to 832
U.S.P.H.S.	White chromate workers	4.0	43.0
	Colored chromate workers	6.0	71.0
Alwens	No exposure	0—2.02	—
	Chromate workers	trace to 32.7	None
Mancuso	Slight exposure	—	0 — 10.0
	Chromate workers during exposure	0.5—17.0	0 —380.0
	74 days after end of exposure	1.0—16.4	8.0— 54.0
	66 days after reemployment	2.0—13.5	—
	Former chromate workers	0.9—10.0	0 — 20.0
	Chrome platers	—	1.5— 20.0
Urone and Mancuso	Chromate workers	Blood clot 0.6—9.1 Serum 0 —0.8 Cells 0.3—4.7	
	Chromate workers 74 days after cessation of exposure	Defibrinated serum 0.3—4.4 Fibrin 0.3—4.4	
Pascale et al.	Chrome plating industry	—	(0—2,880 micrograms/hr.)

		Cells	Plasma	
Budacz et al.	No exposure	3.7—4.6	2.6—3.9	0
	Chromate worker during exposure	14.0	1.7	51.2
	Chromate worker 5 years after low exposure	3.0	0	3.6
	Chromate worker 23 years after exposure	5.4	2.0	0
	Chromite worker	2.2	0.6	0

g) Atmospheric Neighborhood Pollution

In view of the observation of several intraplant neighborhood cases of chrome cancers of the lung in a German operation attesting to the high carcinogenic potency of certain chromium compounds, it is of importance to note that there exists a carcinogenically perhaps not insignificant pollution of the air in the neighborhood of chromate producing plants and of other chromium using and processing establishments, which involves in part larger urban areas (BOURNE and RUSHIN; BELTH, KAPLAN and COUCHMAN; TABOR and WARREN) (Fig. 26). According to the observations of BELTH *et al.* the concentrations of chromium in the air of Baltimore fluctuated with the activity of a chromate producing plant located in the city. They were highest in the afternoon and lowest in the 2 hours before major operations began in

Table 48. *Concentrations of Chromium in the Urban Air Near Chromate Producing Plants*

Author	Concentration mr/cm³	Distance from Plant
BOURNE and RUSHIN . . .	0.12	100 ft
	0.06	2,000 ft
	0.001	10,000 ft
BELTH et al. . .	0.0001 minimum	
	0.018 maximum	700 ft

Table 49. *Chromium Content of the Atmosphere in Selected American Cities 1953—1957 Sanitary Engineering Center, USPHS*

Cities	Chromium in micrograms per cbm of Air		Industry
	Maximal Value	Minimal Value	
Baltimore	0.290	0.023	Chromate Plant
Pittsburgh, Louisville, East Chicago, Denver	0.100—0.200		Steel Plants, Oil Refineries
Average American City	0.0002—0.040		

Table 50. *Concentrations of Chromium in the Air of Different Areas of Chromate Producing Plants*

Country	Author	Operations	Cr in mg/m³
France	SPANNAGEL	Chromite Ore Crusher	8.0
		Sodium Chromate Barrelling	0.16
Germany		Chromite Ore Crusher	0.44 — 0.60
		Furnace	0.35
U.S.A.	MACHLE and GREGORIUS	Kiln and Mills	0.01 —· 2.8
		Packing	0.20 —21.0
		General Area	0.003— 1.0
	GAFAFER et al.	Mill Room	1.07
		Potash Production	0.17

the plant each morning. Whether such pollutions may give rise to the creation of industry-related environmental cancer hazards for individuals working and living in the dust and fume zones of such establishments is at present unknown and remains to be determined.

The actual existence and the potential degree of such an environmental industry-related lung cancer hazard depends not only on the absolute amounts of chromium polluting the general atmosphere in the vicinity of such plants, but also in the chemical type and biologic availability of the chromium pollutants (MANCUSO and

Table 51. *Comparison of Average Concentrations of Chromium in British and American Chromate Factories* (M. BUCKELL and D. G. HARVEY)

Phase in Process No.	General Description	Details of Sampling Points	British (Concentrations in mg. Cr./cu. m.)						American (Concentrations in mg. Cr./cu.m.)				
			Cr^{+3} Average	Range	Cr^{+6} Average	Range	Total	$Cr^{+3}:Cr^{+6}$	Cr^{+3}	Cr^{+6}	Total	Cr^{+3}	Cr^{+6}
1	Pre-reaction phase: mainly insoluble chromium (chromite) (lime and ash)	Near mixers only	2—14 (3)	3—27 / 0—818	0—005 (3)	0—01 / 0—002	2—145	430:1	1—52 / 1—2	0—03 / 0—1	1—55 / 1—3	6:1	(6)
2	Reaction phase: conversion of insoluble chromite to soluble chromate (roast)	Discharge end of furnace; by frit hopper during discharge by wash tanks during emptying of frit	0—17 (9)	0—660 / 0—0033	0—029 (10)	0—146 / 0—0005	0—199	5—8:1	0—26	0—39	0—65	2:1	(62)
3	Reaction phase continued: extraction (filtering)	By wash tanks before, during and after flooding; digging out of extracted frit; running off monochromate liquor	0—037 (6)	0—214 / 0—0009	0—52 (10)	4—15 / 0—0005	0—557	1:14	0—08	0—12	0—2	2:1	(10)
4	Formation of di-chromate (liquor)	By acidifier tanks	0—014 (7)	0—094 / 0—0002	0—056 (8)	0—175 / 0—005	0—070	1:4	0—09	0—09	0—18	2:1	(12)

HUEPER; HUEPER; GAFAFER *et al.;* HUEPER and PAYNE) which determine their carcinogenic reactivity. The following data on the concentration of chromium found in the urban air near such plants and on the amounts and types of chromium present within various areas of chromate plants may help to place this problem into proper perspective. Consideration must here be given to the fact that the minimal carcinogenically effective concentration of chromium in the air is unknown (BAETJER) (Tables 48 and 49).

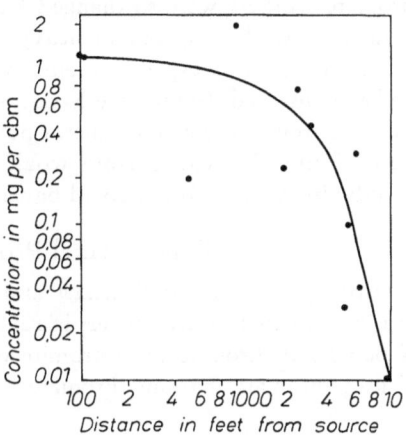

Fig. 26. Chromium content of the air in the environment of a chromate plant (BOURNE and RUSHIN)

h) Atmospheric Intraplant Pollution

The following two tables (Tables 50, 51) present the atmospheric conditions prevailing in British and American chromate producing plants in greater detail and illustrate at the same time the carcinogenically important variations in the types of chromium compounds present in different parts and with different activities of these plans (BUCKELL and HARVEY; GAFAFER *et al.*). The threshold limit value for chromic acid and chromates (as CrO_3) for 1961 has been set at 0.1 mg/cbm. of air (BALL *et al.*). While this value may represent a concentration at which under ordinary circumstances of occupational exposure, toxic health hazards are not encountered among the great mass of workers, they definitely do not constitute a measure by which industrial carcinogenic hazards can be determined, expecially since it is well known that the carcinogenic dose of many chemicals is distinctly lower than their minimal toxic dose.

i) Chromate Carcinogenesis and Smoking Habits

At various occasions doubts have been voiced concerning the real causal role of chromium compounds in the production of cancers of the respiratory organs (LEHMANN; OETTEL). OETTEL in fact only recently alleged that cancers of the lung develop only in those chromate producers who smoke cigarettes and that the carcinogens present in cigarette smoke act specifically and syncarcinogenically on the cellular changes elicited in the bronchial mucosa by the irritative action of the inhaled chromimium compounds. ALWENS in an early publication on the subject of chromate cancers of the lung pointed out that an abuse of tobacco could not be demonstrated in most of his patients. GAFAFER *et al.* recorded that 81.1% of the chromate workers with lung cancers and that 79.4% of the foundry workers used as controls had been smokers. These investigators noted, moreover, that the white chromate workers smoked more heavily than the colored ones and that, on the other hand, the lung cancer liability of the colored workers was considerably higher than that of the white workers. In the brief report of FISHER, mention is made of the fact that among the 38 chromate producers with lung cancer, two (2) were non-smokers, three (3) smoked pipe and/or cigar, three (3) smoked less than one pack of cigarettes per day, nineteen (19) smoked between 1 and 1½ packs per day and five (5) smoked two (2) packs.

This evidence also does not support the dogmatic statement of OETTEL concerning an exclusive role of cigarette smoking as a cause of lung cancer in chromate workers. The most valid analysis on this matter has been provided by BIDSTRUP and CASE who came to the following conclusion: "Thus even if the smoking habits of the chromate workers were so changed from those of the general population that all of them fell into the category of heavy smokers, the increase of carcinoma of the lung that then would be expected would not satisfactorily account for the increase which we have observed. In fact, we have no reason to believe that their smoking habits are different from those of the general population, and an explanation based on a hypothesis of altered smoking habits would need to be supported by satisfactory evidence of such alteration before it could be seriously considered."

k) Experimental Production of Chrome Cancers

Attempts of GROSS; SHIMKIN and LEITER; BAETJER *et al.*; STEFFEE and BAETJER; and HUEPER to produce cancers in rabbits, guinea pigs, rats and mice by the inhalation of powdered chromite ore, chromite ore roast, yellow chromium pigments (mixture of lead chromate, barium chromate and zinc chromate) and green chromium oxide

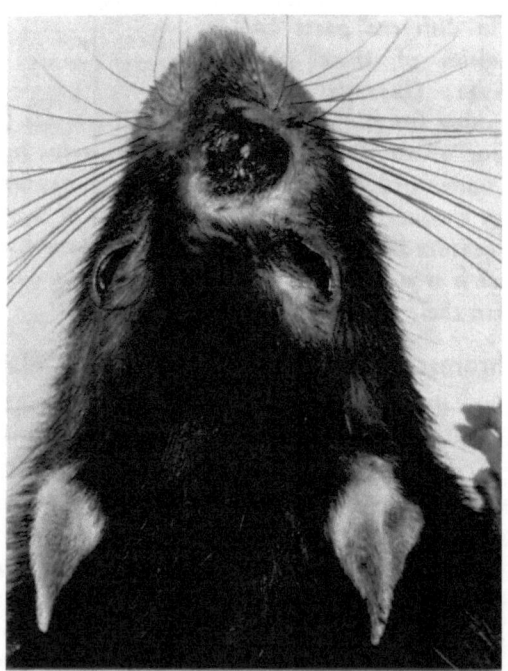

Fig. 27. Ulcerative squamous cell carcinoma of the snout of a rat exposed to chromite ore roast dust

yielded negative results except that rats exposed to chromite ore and with chromite ore roast developed ulcerative squamous cell carcinomas of the skin of the snout (HUEPER and PAYNE) (Fig. 27).

While an intratracheal introduction of basic potassium zinc chromate and of barium chromate into mice proved likewise unsuccessful in eliciting bronchial carcinomas (BAETJER *et al.*), HUEPER and PAYNE using the same procedure on rats which were insufflated with suspensions of strontium chromate, calcium chromate and zinc chromate in gelatin solution, obtained pulmonary sarcomas in two rats out of 79 intratracheally injected with calcium chromate and one (1) rat out of 49 given by this route, strontium chromate. The total tumor yield was nevertheless disappointing in view of the high carcinogenic potency of the chromates employed when introduced into rats by the intrapleural and intramuscular routes (Table 52). PAYNE subsequently

Table 52. *Cancerous Responses at the Sites of Implantation of Several Chromium Compounds in the Tigh Muscle and Pleural Cavity of Rats*

Compound	Route 35 Rats	Number of Cancers at Site	Percent Cancer Yield	Minimal Latent Period
Chromic	IM	30	86	7
Chromate	IPl	34	97	7
Calcium	IM	10	29	7
Chromate	IPl	28	80	7
Sintered Calcium	IM	13	37	—
Chromate	IPl	21	60	6
Strontium	IM	16	46	6
Chromate	IPl	17	50	6
Barium	IM	0	0	—
Chromate	IPl	2	6	14
Lead	IM	3	9	—
Chromate	IPl	3	9	16
Sodium Dichromate	IM	0	0	—
	IPl	2	6	—
Chromite Roast	IM	1	3	19
Residue	IPl	8	23	12
Zinc	IM	16	45	5
Yellow	IPl	22	65	6
Chromium	IM	1	3	16
Acetate	IPl	1	3	—
Sheep	IM	0	—	—
Fat	IPl	0	—	—

demonstrated that also mice subcutaneously injected with calcium chromate and sintered calcium chromate developed cancers, after HUEPER had shown that chromite roast intrapleurally introduced into rats elicited sarcomas and carcinomas of the lungs and of the mediastinal tissues.

A contradictory outcome was recorded when powdered metallic chromium was implanted into the femoral cavity of rats, dogs and rabbits, by HUEPER and by VOLLMANN and by SCHINZ. Whereas rats kept for two (2) years and dogs observed for eight (8) years following such procedures did not develop any tumors at the site of metallic depots, SCHINZ observed in three (3) out of twenty (20) rabbits with intraosseous chromium depots in the femur, the development of sarcomas after a minimal latent period of 4 years. Since these tumors, however, did not involve the sites of the implants but were found remote from them (2 in the chest, one (1) in the bony pelvis), it is uncertain whether they actually represent reaction products to chromium.

The histologic examination of the cancers observed in the thighs and chests of rats and mice receiving implants of the various chromates demonstrated that chromium is a carcinogenic agent capable of eliciting cancers from various tissues and of different types (Fig. 28). Sarcomas apparently derived from fibrous tissue, bony tissue, muscle tissue and myxomatous tissue were observed, as were carcinomas of squamous cell

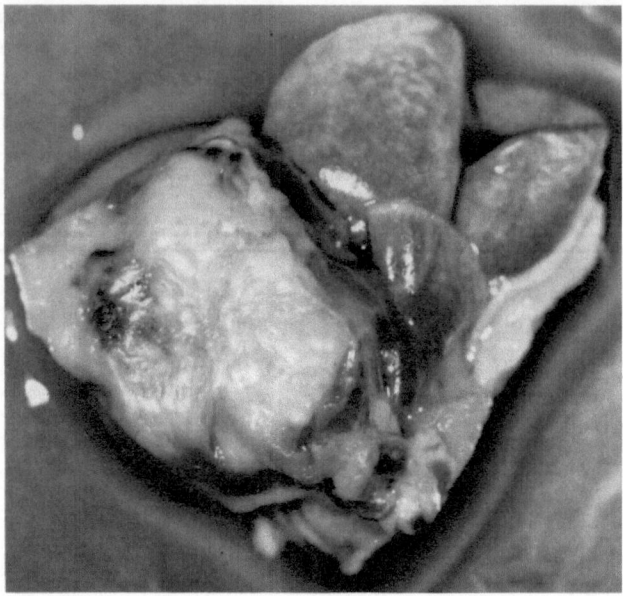

Fig. 28. Cornified squamous cell carcinoma in the lung of a rat intrapleurally implanted with calcium chromate

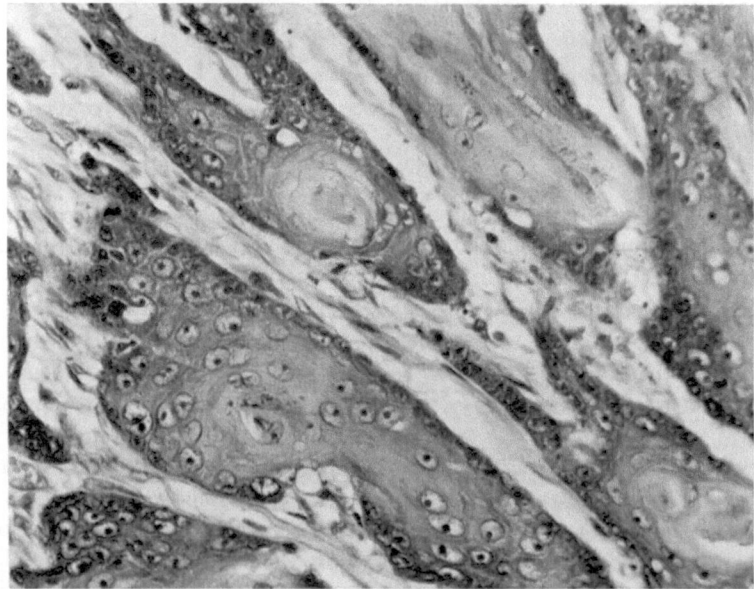

Fig. 29. Cornified squamous cell carcinoma of the lung in a rat with an intrapleural implant of calcium chromate

type, round-cell type and glandular type involving the lung often combined with various adenocystic and metaplastic bronchiolar lesions and at times associated with sarcomatous tumors occurring in the same lung or in the form of carcinosarcomas, such as those occasionally seen also in man (PRIVE *et al.*) (Figs. 28, 29, 30, 31, 32, 33).

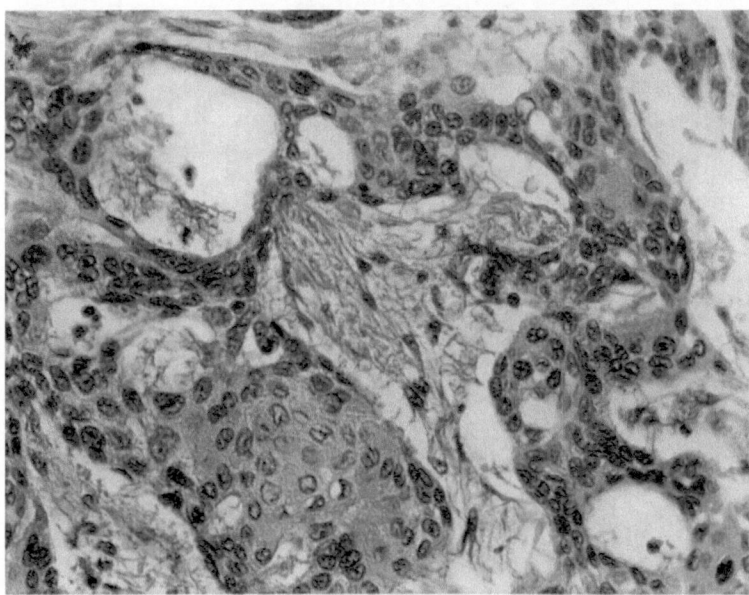

Fig. 30. Adenocarcinoma with squamous cell transformations in the lung of a rat given lead chromate intra-pleurally

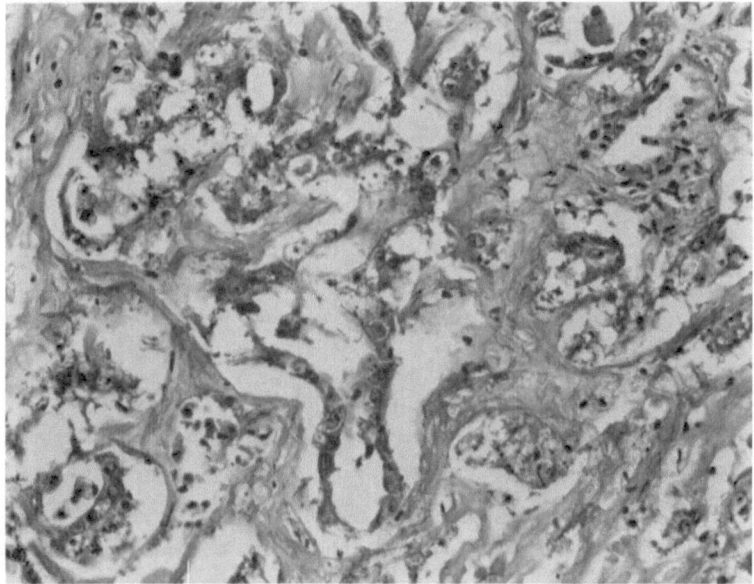

Fig. 31. Adenocarcinoma of the lung in a rat after intrapleural administration of strontium chromate

It is noteworthy, moreover, that the lungs exposed to these chromium compounds and thus involved, showed distinct chronic inflammatory and fibrosing changes which were similar to those reported to occur in rats following a respiratory introduction. of chromic oxide and zinc chromate (MASSMANN and PILGRIM; BISTER *et al.*).

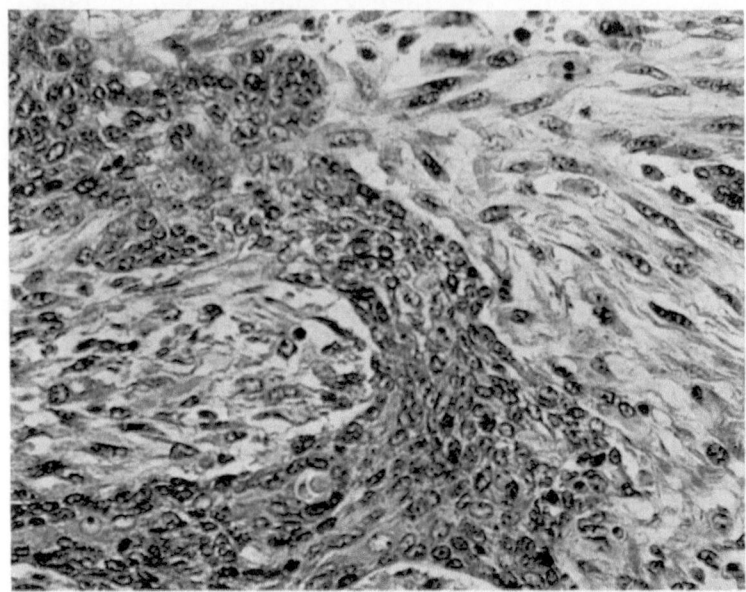

Fig. 32. Carcinosarcoma of the lung in a rat following intrapleural deposition of chromic chromate

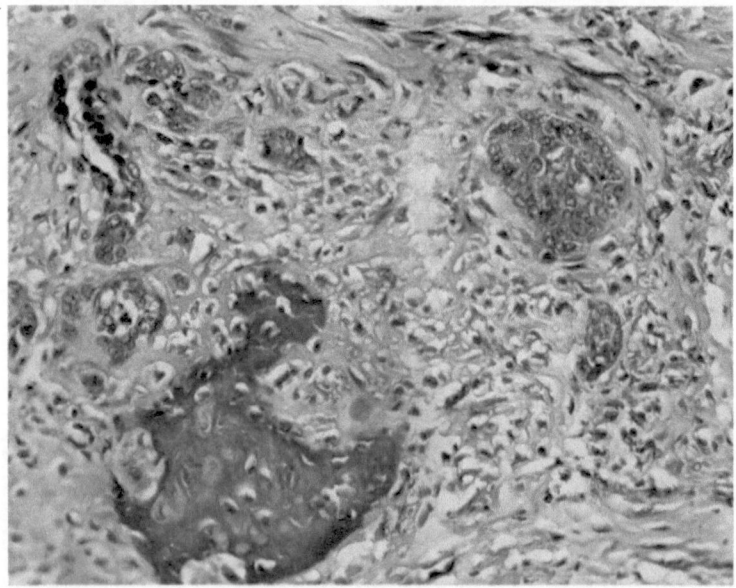

Fig. 33. Osteogenic sarcoma with squamous cell nests in the lung of a rat implanted intrapleurally with chromic chromate

I) Causative Mechanism of Chromium Carcinogenesis

As long as the exact carcinogenic role of chromium in the production of cancers of the respiratory organs of chromate producers and similarly exposed workers remained uncertain, various concepts were advanced concerning the causal agent active in their production, i.e., whether these cancers were elicited by trivalent or hexavalent chromium compounds, by monochromates or dichromates, by water soluble or insoluble derivatives, by chromite ore, intermediary roasting products or chromium metal, or by chromium in all these forms under proper conditions of exposure (GROSS; BAETJER; MACHLE and GREGORIUS; GAFAFER et al.; MANCUSO and HUEPER; HUEPER; HUEPER and PAYNE). Even the possibility was considered that chromium in any form was causally not related to the development of the lung cancers, but was attributable to respiratory contact with other constituents of the chromite ore, such as iron and vanadium, or to exposure to incomplete combustion products of the fuel (coal, fuel oil, gas) extensively used in the roasting process of the ore, and representing the cause of lung cancer occurring among workers inhaling such products for occupational reasons (coke oven workers, gashouse workers).

The two last mentioned possibilities could be dismissed as relevant for the following reasons. Cancer of the lung had been observed among chromium pigment makers who had no respiratory contact with incomplete combustion products of carbonaceous fuel. Investigations of CAHNMANN, moreover, had shown that 3,4-benzpyrene could not be demonstrated in chromite ore roast, where it would be likely to occur as an impurity, if this aromatic polycyclic hydrocarbon would occur or would be stable under the condition present in the roasters. This aspect was subsequently re-investigated by PAYNE who found that the addition of hexavalent chromate phosphate and of chromate roast residue to 3,4-benzpyrene before this chemical was subcutaneously injected into mice, reduced because of their oxidative action on 3,4-benzpyrene, its carcinogenic potency as evidenced by a decrease in the tumor yield and a lengthening of the latent period.

As a by-product of this investigation, PAYNE moreover, demonstrated that the leached roast residue retains some carcinogenic potency for rats, since out of two series of 35 rats each, one implanted intrapleurally with the residue, the other implanted intramuscularly, three developed intrathoracic sarcomas and one (1) an intramuscular sarcoma, respectively. The pollution of the intraplant and extraplant air with roast residue, therefore, may create a cancer hazard for workers and residents of the dust zone.

The experimental observations of HUEPER and PAYNE made on a series of hexavalent and trivalent chromium compounds showed definitely that chromium as such when present in a biologically available form accounts for the carcinogenic potency of chromium derivatives, and that the degree of biologic availability as reflected by their relative degree of water solubility determines the relative potency of a particular compound.

The various findings on the type of chromium compounds and the tissue reactions of degenerative, fibrosing, hyperplastic, metaplastic, precancerous and cancerous nature elicited by them indicate that chromium is capable of producing cancers of the lungs and other tissues without the intervention of any additional factor considered essential for preparing the tissues exposed to chromium compounds for their carcinogenic action as suggested by KUSCHNER and NELSON. It appears also from the experimental evidence available that both trivalent and hexavalent chromium compounds possess carcinogenic properties contrary to the opinion of SPANNAGEL who held that trivalent chromium is noncarcinogenic because it cannot be oxidized in the body into biologically active hexavalent chromium. The studies of HUEPER and GROGAN demonstrated that this concept is not correct inasmuch as trivalent chromium may operate as a depot chromium in the body which is gradually transformed into hexavalent chromium through the oxidative action of biologic processes. It thereby may become of distinct carcinogenic importance since it can exert a prolonged effect on the tissues in the vicinity of such depots. Such an action may extend long after an occupational exposure to chromium has ceased. The relative low carcinogenic effect of sodium chromate upon rats under experimental conditions may not adequately reflect its potency under occupational conditions inasmuch as occupational exposures may involve relatively smaller and, therefore, necrotically little effective doses of sodium chromate. Under such circumstances of contact the carcinogenically important proliferative effect of chromium on tissues may dominate over its necrotizing one and thereby enable the development of a cancer, especially since the corrosive hexavalent chromium ion is reduced finally in the cells into the less active trivalent one (GROGAN; BAETJER et al.).

Because chromium is an eminently allergenic substance giving frequently rise to the development of chromium dermatitis (cement workers, locomotive engineers (anticorrosive in water), metallurgical workers (antirusting agent in cutting oils), leather manufacturers (MORRIS), HUEPER suggested in 1942 as a part of the allergenic theory of carcinogenesis that immunochemical processes related to the formation of chromium-protein complexes might play a significant role in the carcinogenic process initiated by chromium. Similar thoughts were advanced by SCHINZ and UEHLINGER. Subsequent investigations carried out by GROGAN and OPPENHEIMER and by GROGAN in further pursuit of this concept demonstrated the in vitro formation of such complexes by both trivalent and hexavalent chromium compounds with egg albumin and human plasma proteins. BAETJER, DAMRON and BUDACZ also showed that cationic as well as anionic chromium brought in contact with lung tissue is bound in such a way that it became insoluble in saline extractants, while CLARK found in in vitro experiments that both trivalent and hexavalent chromium compounds denature blood plasma albumin. It is likely that such complexes may possess antigenic properties, since ISHIKAWA succeeded in producing chromium specific antibodies in rabbits by the repeated intramuscular injection of potassium bichromate, potassium chromate, chrome alum and chromium carbonate (LOISELEUR and SAUVAGE). Although EDMUNDSON stated that chromate producers suffering from perforated nasal septa and chrome ulcers show negative patch tests for potassium bichromate, some preliminary experiments with antisera produced in rabbits by the repeated intra-abdominal injection of egg albumin-chromate complexes and tested on blood sera of chromate workers with and without lung cancers, gave results which suggested the presence of immunochemical reactions to chromium in some of the workers investigated (HUEPER and PAYNE). More comprehensive and exact studies of this type, therefore, may yield results important for diagnostic and therapeutic reasons.

m) Preventive Measures

The serious nature of the respiratory cancer hazards connected with the production, processing and industrial use of chromium compounds and possibly also of metallic chromium and its alloys provide sufficient reasons for the institution of adequate preventive and prophylactic technologic, industrial-hygiene and medical measures for obtaining the maximal possible protection of the workers employed in such operations as well as of the general population working and residing in the vicinity of such plants.

a) Technologic Measures

The objective of all technologic measures is the maximal reduction of the dissemination of chromium containing dust, fumes and mist in the air of work rooms and of the plant area. Precautionary measures to this end should be applied not only within the buildings and to the production, processing and packaging procedures, but also to the handling of the waste products released into the atmosphere from the stacks and into public waters as well as to the storage and disposal of the finely powdered sludge. The entire operation starting with the unloading of the powdered chromite ore to the packaging of the finished goods should be carried on as far as possible in enclosed machinery preventing the escape of dust, fumes and mist into the plant environment. Whenever such measures are technologically not practical, operations with remaining environmental contaminations should be established in facilities separate from the protected operations, so that the contaminants can be restricted to such areas and can be controlled and removed by other procedures, such as exhaust ventilation, vacuum cleaning and washing of floors, walls and ceilings with water. Chromium-containing matter should be removed from effluents by proper scrubbers and electrostatic precipitators so as to prevent a carcinogenic contamination of the plant environment. The effectiveness of control measures should be ascertained at frequent intervals by determinations of the chromium content of the air. SPANNAGEL stated that the presence of 0.1 mg. of chromium per cbm. of air does not create any toxic hazards, although it still might cause a carcinogenic hazard. A chromium content of 2.5 mg. to 6.5 mg. of chromium/cbm. causes, according to SPANNAGEL, severe reactions in individuals working in such an atmosphere. Good housekeeping for preventing accumulation of spillage and dusts is an essential practice for safe plant operation.

It is advisable to incorporate the following principles and considerations in the control program and practices of chromate producing and processing plants.

a) All operations should be carried on as far as possible in closed systems that can receive routine servicing, lubrication and cleaning without being opened.

b) The filling of leaching and condensation tanks should be controlled by automatic devices preventing any accidental overflow of chromate solutions.

c) Cleaning of floors should be done by washing with water and not by sweeping with broom, so as to prevent the production of dust.

d) All pipes, ducts, rafters, ledges, etc. where dust may accumulate should be grouped in such a way that they can be boxed in, since the dust accumulating under ordinary conditions of construction on these parts cannot be removed without liberating considerable amounts of dust into the air, and removing this dust is technically difficult to accomplish.

e) Walls should be constructed of smooth, washable material, such as glassed brick, so that they can be cleaned easily with water.

f) The spilling of chromates or chromate containing wastes on the floors should be kept at a minimum at all times. This material should be washed away immediately whenever such spillage has occurred.

g) The bagging of chromate should be performed under an exhaust hood which covers both the filling and weighing apparatus and the sewing arrangement so that the small cloud of dust issuing from the bag when it is compressed is removed into the exhaust system. It may be advisable, moreover, to have the bags rest on a movable common grate on which they slide without lifting and through which any spillage drops on a pan continuously rinsed with water.

h) Floors at various levels within large sheds should be constructed of iron grating or of smooth hard concrete or tile.

i) Expecially hazardous operations should be separated from the rest of the operations by placing them in special compartments or even separate buildings.

j) All precautionary measures should be, as far as possible, of technical and mechanical nature, since workers do not seem to be inclined to use individual safety devices. Good housekeeping within the plant and safe disposal of hazardous wastes together with adequate engineering of the production machinery are the keystones to effective control of the cancer hazard.

Workers employed in operations in which a certain pollution of the air and cutaneous and ingestive contact remains unavoidable should be provided with adequate protective devices, such as proper work clothes frequently cleaned, gauntlets, respirators, goggles, etc. which must be inspected for defects and operation at frequent intervals. Since a complete removal of all potential and actual cancer hazards is difficult if not impossible in such operations, only workers at least 35 years of age should be employed there. Through preemployment examinations, all applicants with a history of respiratory diseases, especially chronic bronchitis, chronic sinusitis, tuberculosis, hay fever, etc., gastrointestinal disturbances, liver and kidney ailments and chain smokers should be excluded.

β) Medical Prophylactic Measures

Workers should be kept under close medical surveillance. The following measures are indicated in carrying out such a policy.

1. Periodic x-ray examination in intervals of 4 months for all workers exposed including foremen and supervisors, i.e., of all persons entering hazardous operations routinely or frequently during the course of their occupational activities. Yard workers, repairmen, truckers, clerks working in offices, laboratory personnel and medical dispensary employees, exposed to chromate dust from adjacent operations, also should undergo these examinations.

2. Whenever clinical evidence suggests the presence of a bronchogenic tumor, bronchoscopy should be performed for obtaining a biopsy and, if possible, a sample of bronchial secretion should be collected for cytologic study for the presence of tumor cells and for spectroscopic examination for its chromate content (qualitative and quantitative).

3. In all cases with chronic bronchial "irritation" the sputum should be examined repeatedly for cancer cells with the Papanicolaou method.

4. It may be advisable to check on the presence and degree of exposure to chromates by performing periodic chemical or spectroscopic analyses of the urine and blood of workers employed there for presence and amounts of chromates, as well as cytologic sputum examinations.

Records should be kept over a period of decades on the operating conditions of such plants, on the results and methods of examinations of air and water contamiones and on accident insurance and compensation commission data for future reference and evidence.

For prophylactic and therapeutic purposes an attempt should be made of removing chromium stored in the tissues from the body. Whether the use of chelating agents, such as edathamine, may prove useful in this respect remains to be seen (MALOFF; HATEM).

Cancers of the lung, larynx, nasal cavity and paranasal sinuses occurring in chromate producing and processing workers should be considered as results of occupational exposures and should be considered compensable occupational diseases (MAGER; WORTH and SCHILLER; HOSCHEK). It is of distinct public interest if such cancers, whenever they are suspected or recognized as being due to occupational exposures to chromium and chromium compounds, are made notifiable to governmental health and labor authorities. Such regulations when adequately enforced would provide the proper factual basis for correcting undesirable and harmful plant practices, for establishing sources of preventable environmental contaminations with a potent carcinogenic agent and for instituting adequate precautionary and preventive measures nants, on employment and medical histories of workers including former and retired whenever needed. The system of obligatory notification of chromium cancers could, moreover, be employed for activating proper compensation procedures by compensation boards whenever indicated, for obtaining proper economic protection for victims of occupational chrome cancers.

4. Nickel

a) Technological Aspects

Nickel and nickel compounds are relative newcomers among the metals used in the human economy. It was first isolated as late as the year 1751. The beginning of an industrial production of nickel dates back as little as about 150 years ago. The bulk of the present day nickel ore used for numerous metallurgical and chemical purposes is mined in Sudbury, Ontario, Canada. Smaller amounts are obtained in the U.S.S.R., Cuba, New Caledonia and Norway (DAVIS). Smelting of nickel ores is carried on in many other countries such as the U.S.A., England and Germany, and often entails in the refining process the production of nickel carbonyl (Mond process). Nickel metal is extensively employed in nickel-plating manufacture of stainless steel and Monel metal, in the production of storage batteries, for metal-spraying operations, for submicron nickel powder production and use, and in the production of various alloys. Nickel carbonyl is used in the manufacture of acrylic resins as a carbon monoxide transfer agent, and as a catalyst in various chemical industrial processes, such as the cracking of bitumen and hydrogenation processes of animal and vegetable oil (INTERNATIONAL LABOUR OFFICE; INTERNATIONAL NICKEL COMPANY; ABRAHAM; MILLER et al.; SAPPINGTON). Nickel compounds are employed as pigments in inks, enamels, glazes and paints. The total world production of nickel stood in 1950 at about 150,000 metric tons. An organic nickel compound has recently been introduced as an antiknock agent and is used as such as an additive to gasoline.

b) Epidemiology

Exposure to nickel fumes and nickel dusts and mists of metallic nickel and its compounds or to nickel carbonyl vapors is, therefore, frequent for industrial workers of many types and in many operations. While skin contact to nickel and nickel salts not infrequently results in the development of an apparently allergic type of dermatitis (MARCUSSEN; FISHER and SHAPIRO; SAMITZ and POMERANTZ CHAUMONT and HIMMELSBACH; WILSON), inhalation of the volatile nickel carbonyl has been responsible for an appreciable number of acute and often fatal poisonings. The pulmonary manifestations (congestion, desquamation of alveolar epithelium, fibrinous acellular exudation into alveolar spaces, bronchial mucosal hemorrhages) are apparently attributable to the toxic action of finely dispersed nickel formed from the disintegration of nickel carbonyl upon the pulmonary structures (KRAFFT; SUNDERMANN et al.; WEST and SUNDERMAN; KINCAID and SUNDERMAN; ARMIT; AMOR BAYER; CARMICHAEL). KRAFFT suggested that these reactions are the result of a nickel allergy having the lung as its shock organ. The use of nickel plated cannulas for intravenous infusions has been blamed for the occurrence of anaphylactoid reactions to nickel (STODDART).

While many of these reactions occur as the result of occupational exposures to nickel and nickel compounds, there exist many occasions of contact for purely environmental reasons which also have been incriminated as actual or possible causes of toxic or even carcinogenic reactions. Thus, MITCHELL et al. have called attention to the fact that various alloys containing nickel, and used in dentures are capable when implanted into rats, to induce the development of sarcomas. SUNDERMAN and SUNDERMAN have advanced the hypothesis that the traces of nickel present in cigarette smoke may be involved in the etiology of lung cancer attributed to the smoking of cigarettes. Perhaps even more impressive are the highly excessive values of nickel demonstrated in the atmospheric pollutants of several American cities in which nickel consuming and processing plants are located. The atmospheric nickel level of Waterbury, Connecticut, stood as high as 2.800 µg. against the next maximal highest level of 0.300 µg. in Boston and as compared with values between 0.005 µg. and 0.100 µg. for most other cities studied. These few data may suffice for indicating the scope of these aspects of potential general atmospheric air pollutants and the need for future investigations in such matters. Doubtlessly the concentrations of such carcinogenic chemicals can be expected to be much higher in the immediate neighborhood of the industrial establishments responsible for such atmospheric pollutions. One may likewise justly assume that any lung cancer hazards possibly related to contaminations of the air from such sources will be much more severe for the population living and working in the immediate neighborhood of such plants. Such actual or possible relationships will doubtlessly attract increasing legal and medicolegal attention and thus will become the subject of compensation and damage suits. The use of a nickel compound as a gasoline additive which doubtlessly will cause a contamination of urban air with nickel appears to be especially important from a health and cancer viewpoint.

The first indication that an occupational inhalation of metallic nickel dust or nickel carbonyl vapors might be associated with a cancer hazard to the nasal cavity, paranasal sinuses and lung was contained in the *Annual Report of the Chief Inspector of Factories for the Year 1932*, which was published in 1933, and in brief comments by G. A. STEPHENS which appeared in 1933 in *Medical Press and Circular,* on the occurrence of respiratory cancers affecting the nasal cavity in English nickel refinery workers. Additional observations on respiratory cancers among English nickel workers were recorded subsequently by BRIDGE; MEREWETHER; COOPER; GRENFELL; BAADER; SCHÄR, BIDSTRUP; AMOR; GOLDBLATT; and PELLER. In the *Annual Report of the Chief Inspector of Factories for the Year 1948,* it was noted that between 1923 and 1948 inclusive, a total of 47 cancers of the nose and 82 cancers of the lung were reported from the Mond Nickel Works at Clydach. The situation at Clydach was reviewed again in a series of papers by DOLL; MORGAN; and WILLIAMS published in 1958. There had been between 1948 and 1958, forty eight (48) additional lung cancers and thirteen (13) nasal cancers among the workers employed in the nickel refinery. The main results of the epidemiologic aspects of this occupational cancer hazard are contained in two tables by DOLL (Tables 53 and 54).

Table 53. *Comparison Between Observed and Expected Numbers of Deaths from Cancer of the Lung in Four Occupational Groups in 1938—1947 and 1948—1956*

Period	Number of Deaths	Nickel Workers	Men in Other Selected Occupations	Steel Workers	Colliery Workers
1938—1947	Expected	2.61	0.89	13.12	20.67
	Observed	36	0	22	8
	Observed as per cent of Expected	1,379	—	168	39
1948—1956	Expected	5.86	4.27	37.62	56.89
	Observed	39	5	45	23
	Observed as per cent of Expected	666	117	119	40

Table 54. *Comparison Between Observed and Expected Numbers of Deaths from Cancer of Nose Among Nickel and Non-Nickel Workers*

Population	Number of Deaths from Cancer of Nose		Ratio of Numbers of Observed and Expected
	Observed	Expected	
Nickel Workers			
Four Areas (1948—1956)	13	0.082	159:1
Two Areas (1938—1947)	16	0.066	242:1
All Areas Available (1938—1956)	29	0.148	196:1
Non-Nickel Workers			
Four Areas (1948—1956)	12	8.279	
Two Areas (1938—1947)	4	2.132	
All Areas Available	16	10.411	

DOLL estimated that the total number of nickel cancers affecting the lungs, nares and paranasal sinuses occurring between 1923 and 1958 at the CLYDACH works stood at least 131 lung cancers and 61 nasal and paranasal cancers (MORGAN). It is of interest, according to DOLL, that during the whole period between 1938 and 1956 only one nickel worker died with cancer of the larynx.

By the end of 1948, 46 of the workers with nasal cancer and 72 of those with lung cancer had died. MORGAN claimed that none of the patients with lung cancer had commenced work in the nickel refinery after 1924, when a reconstruction of the plant had been carried out. The average exposure period for the nasal cancer patients was 23 years (range, 3—26 years), and for the lung cancer patients, 25 years (range, 1—33 years) (Table 55)

Table 55. *Exposure Time and Age Distribution of Nickel Cancers*

Site of Neoplasm	Nose	Lung
Average		
Exposure Time to Dust	9.2	6 Years
Range	3—18	1—16
Average		
Age at Death	51	53
Range	36—66	48.66
Average		
Time from First Exposure		
in Plant (Latent Period)	17	20
Range	11—28	9—27

Published evidence on the occurrence of similar cancers among nickel refinery workers elsewhere is restricted to Norway, where LOKEN found three cases of lung cancer among members of this occupational group who had been employed in the roasting process. Unpublished information, however, indicates that about half-a-dozen cases of nasal cancer have been observed among Canadian nickel workers during the last 15 years. It is claimed, on the other hand, that none have been seen so far among workers employed in a German nickel carbonyl operation (CAROZZI; GOLDBLATT and WAGSTAFF; OETTEL), and none also have been placed on record from nickel ore mining and refining plants in the U.S.S.R., although ZNAMENSKII recently noted that several cases of lung cancer have been seen in workers employed in these operations which he believed were of occupational origin. No records on the occurrence of occupational nickel cancers of the respiratory organs exist also from the U.S.A., despite the fact that large amounts of nickel, nickel alloys and nickel compounds have been used for many years in diverse American industries and have been responsible in some of them for the production of various types of nickel poisoning (SUNDERMAN).

Commenting on the changing ratio of lung cancer to nasal cancer among nickel workers observed since 1923, PELLER noted that "whereas in the first 17 years, the number of nose cancers was about equal to that of lung cancers, in the 1940's there were almost three times as many lung as nose cancers. This change implies that in the nickel refineries lung cancer surprisingly has a consistently longer latent period than those of nose cancer". Similar epidemiologic phase phenomena in regard to the sequential appearance of occupational respiratory cancers located in different organs but induced by the same carcinogen, have been made in connection with the occurrence of arsenic cancers of the skin and of the lung, since the appearance of cutaneous cancers among German vintners suffering from chronic arsenicosis preceded by about a decade that of cancers of the lung and of other internal organs (ROTH). Recent observations on the chronologic occurrence of asbestos cancers suggest also that asbestos cancers of the lung known since 1935, seem to have a shorter latent period than those involving the pleura and the peritoneum, since these have come to observation only during the past decade. Several years ago, HUEPER called first attention to this phase phenomenon which is characterized by a successive appearance of chemical cancers affecting several organs in connection with his studies on experimental cancers induced in rats by the parenteral introduction of several macromolecular colloids. The observations on the sequential occurrence of lung cancers and nasal cancers among nickel workers thus adhere to an epidemiologic pattern common to occupational and chemical cancers in general.

It is remarkable that none of the exposed workers developed any cancers of the skin especially in view of the fact that nickel, like chromium, is a frequent cause of chronic dermatitis, developing often on an allergic basis (DOIG; MARCUSSEN; SAMITZ and POMERANTZ). The biologic reasons for the different behavior of the human mucosa of the respiratory tract which is embryologically an invagination of the ectoderm, from that of the epidermis toward the carcinogenic action of nickel and chromium, is a challenging problem since similar observations exist also in regard to the carcinogenic action of asbestos and beryllium on the lung. Skin contact with these agents also merely elicits granulomatous reactions.

c) Pathology

While nasal cancers of unknown etiology most often involve the paranasal sinuses and rarely the nasal septum and almost never the turbinates, nickel cancers of the nose originate often in the middle turbinates and occasionally in the ethmoids. It is fair to conclude from this characteristic topographical distribution of nickel cancers of the nose that the agent as well as its physicochemical state at contact are important factors in this respect.

The majority of the nasal cancers for which histologic data are available were of an undifferentiated cell type (6), some showed a squamous cell character (3), while a columnar cell carcinoma was present in only one (1) case. A similar diversity of the histologic types of cancers was observed in the nickel cancers of the lung. Among eleven (11) cases of nickel cancers of the lung which were analyzed, seven (7) were squamous cell carcinomas, three (3) were of a small pleomorphic cell type and one (1) was an alveolar cell carcinoma (WILLIAMS; LOKEN; AMOR). In addition to these neoplastic reactions, WILLIAMS found that the lungs exhibited also bronchiectatic and adenocystic formations associated with some interstitial fibrosis, resembling those occasionally also seen in lungs with chromium cancers.

d) Etiology

AMOR originally suggested that the causal agent active in the induction of these cancers was not nickel but arsenic present in the nickel ore (2%) and in the sulfuric acid used and carried over into the heated calcined dust (MORGAN). The following facts militate against these allegations. Nickel workers with respiratory cancers have remained, according to available records, free from symptoms of chronic arsenic poisoning and cancers at non-respiratory sites, such as those forming frequent accompaniments of typical arsenic cancers of the lung. WILLIAMS noted that in the chemical analyses of two cases, nickel and copper were present in excess in the lungs, while no arsenic could be detected. Although MORGAN stated that the incidence rate of these cancers among nickel refinery workers has remained within normal limits in all workers entering the operation after arsenic was eliminated as an environmental pollutant after the production methods were reorganized in 1923—1924, WILLIAMS mentioned that two of the four workers with lung cancer whom he studied pathologically had started to work in this particular plant after 1924.

The suggestion that a chronic corrosive irritation of the alkali dust generated during the calcining operation represented the carcinogenic mechanism (MORGAN) can readily be dismissed as valid because no similar observations on a highly excessive incidence of nasal and pulmonary cancers have been made on various worker groups sustaining exposures to alkali dust.

AMOR stated that the refined nickel-copper ores are free from radioactive matter. The respiratory cancers observed among nickel refinery workers thus are not identical in etiology with those seen in miners employed in the radioactive mines of Schneeberg and Joachimsthal.

Workers employed at the roaster, in the nickel carbonyl operation, and in other parts of the plant, on the other hand, become exposed to the inhalation of dust, fumes, or vapors containing nickel. Nickel is the common denominator for all of them.

As the result of such exposures, LOKEN demonstrated in one of his cases the presence of 2.8 mg. of nickel per gm. of dry lung.

The scientific and medicolegal significance of these analytical findings, however, depends on the fact that nickel is a trace element present not only in normal tissues but also in benign and malignant tumors (ARAKI and MURE; TIETZ, HIRSCH and NEYMAN; OLSON, HEGGEN and EDWARDS).

MORGAN reported that the nickel content of the urine in persons employed in a nickel refinery varied somewhat for workers engaged in different departments: 0.008—0.15 ppm for nickel carbonyl workers, 0.01 to 0.043 ppm for furnace workers, 0.005—0.06 ppm for workers engaged in chemical precipitation, and 0.002—0.05 in calcination workers. He cited, moreover, GHIRINGHELLE and DAKLI as having found in nickel carbonyl workers a urinary nickel content of 0.365 ppm, and SORINSON, KORNILOVA and ARTEMEVA as having recorded a value of 0.67 to 1.78 ppm. For people not engaged in work with nickel, GHIRINGHELLE and DAKLI gave a urinary value of nickel ranging from 0.003—0.09 ppm (mean 0.05). SORINSON et al. established this level as between 0.03—0.1 ppm while KINCAID, STANLEY, BECK-WORTH and SUNDERMAN recorded a value of 0.011 ppm as an average for the urine of 69 unexposed persons. MORGAN suggested that this "normal" content of nickel in the urine might be derived from nickel naturally in food and possibly introduced into it by the use of nickel-containing kitchen utensils. A much wider variation in "normal" values of nickel in blood was recently reported by IMBUS, CHOLAK, MILLER and STERLING, who noted among 153 persons studied a median concentration of blood nickel of 3.0 micrograms for 100 gm. covering a range of from 0.9 to 45.5, while the median nickel value in urine for these individuals was 7.6 micrograms per liter. SUNDERMAN and KINCAID have emphasized the practical usefulness of measuring nickel in urine among workers exposed to nickel carbonyl, while TEDESCHI and SUNDERMAN have demonstrated in metabolic experiments on dogs exposed to nickel carbonyl, high concentrations of nickel in the urine. Such data in their opionion showed the great value of such determination for the detection of nickel carbonyl poisoning.

e) Experimental Production of Nickel Cancers

The production of cancers at various sites, including the lung in experimental animals (rats, guinea pigs) given nickel and nickel compounds by various routes, represents additional important, if not conclusive evidence as to the carcinogenic role

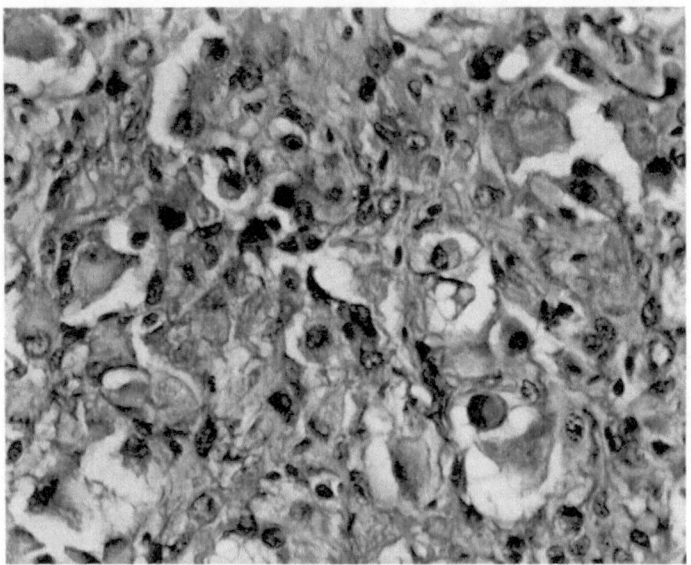

Fig. 34. Rhabdomyosarcoma in the chest wall after intrapleural administration of metallic nickel

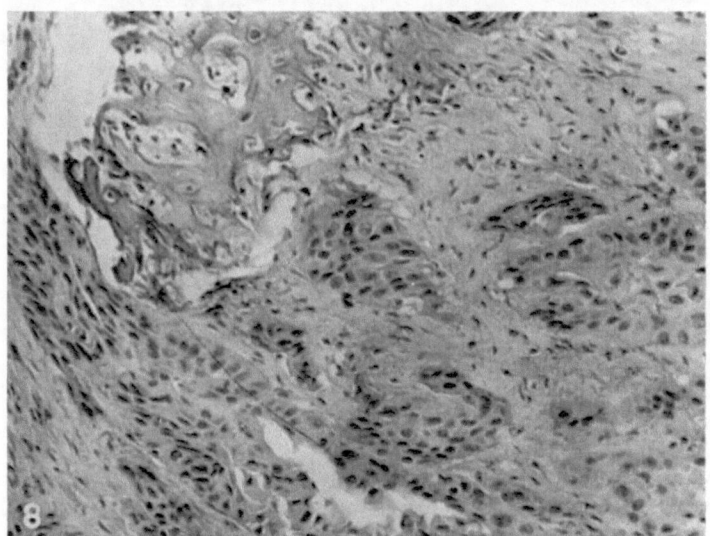

Fig. 35. Squamous cell carcinoma of the skin and osteomyelitic sinus in a rat after implantation of pure metallic nickel powder into the marrow cavity of the femur

which nickel occupies in the induction of cancers of the respiratory organs in nickel refinery workers. HUEPER, and HUEPER and PAYNE succeeded in the production of sarcomas in connective tissue of the subcutis, mediastinum and lung by the parenteral and intrapleural introduction of finely powdered metallic nickel precipitated from nickel carbonyl, and in the induction of adenomatoid and cancerous reaction in the lungs of rats and guinea pigs which inhaled over many months, metallic nickel dust (Figs. 34, 35, 36 and 37). Similar neoplastic responses were obtained in rats subcutaneously implanted with nickel sulfide by GILMAN and HERCHEN; HERCHEN and GILMAN;

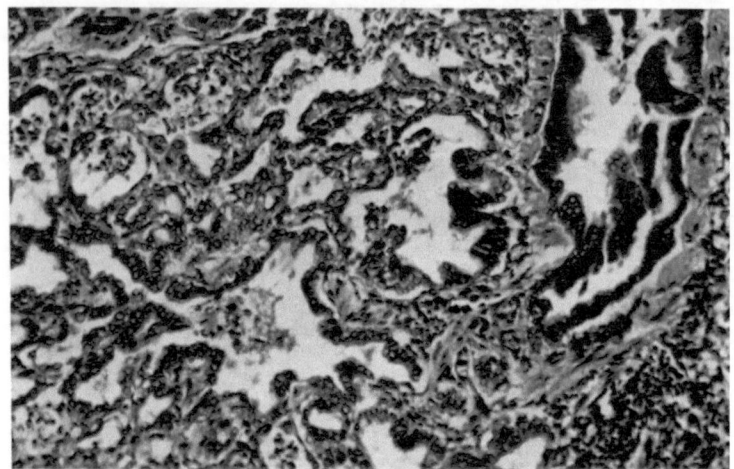

Fig. 36. Adenomatoid proliferations of bronchioli in a rat inhaling powdered metallic nickel

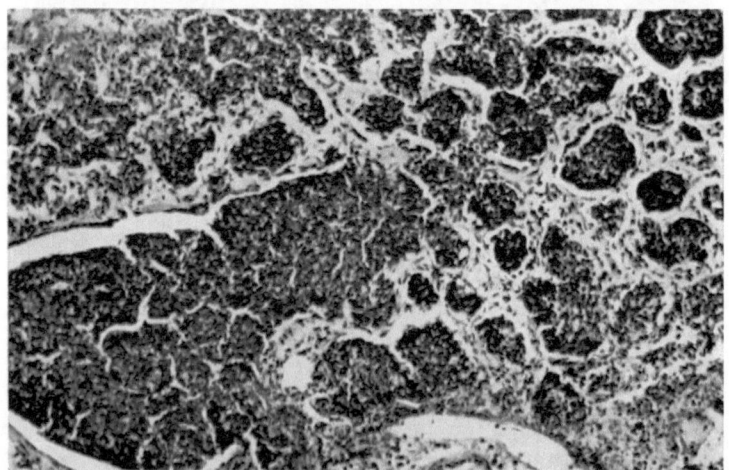

Fig. 37. Small round cell carcinoma of the lung in a guinea pig inhaling powdered metallic nickel

GILMAN and BASRUR; and GILMAN and RUCKENBAUER. The last-mentioned investigators reported sarcoma formation in rats and mice implanted intramuscularly with dust from the flue of a nickel refinery and with nickel oxide. Confirmatory observations on the carcinogenic action of nickel sulfide on the muscle tissue of rats were recorded by JASMIN; and by NOBLE and CAPSTICK. Finally, SUNDERMAN, DONNELLY, WEST and KINCAID found in four rats exposed transitorily to an inhalation of nickel carbonyl, adenomatoid and squamous cell carcinomas of the bronchial epithelium.

f) Carcinogenic Mechanism

The precise role of nickel, like that of any other carcinogenic metals and minerals, in the production of cancer is undetermined. Apart from being an activator of various enzymes and a catalyst of the non-enzymatic decarboxylation of oxalacetic acid, nickel has a high tendency to form complexes with lung proteins (WASE, GOSS and BOYD). Lung protein according to these authors, probably retains nickel. This reaction in turn impairs the catabolic processes involved in the elimination of this element. WEISBURGER, GRANTHAM and WEISBURGER noting the nickel ion complexing properties of various carcinogen metabolites, especially of carcinogenic aromatic amines, commented that it seemed unlikely that this phenomenon played a direct role in the carcinogenic process. HATEM, on the other hand, felt that the formation of nickel-histamine salt complexes in the tissues might explain the appearance of cancers at the site of the nickel action. SUNDERMAN and SUNDERMAN demonstrated that there was an increased nickel binding of RNA isolated from the cells of pulmonary tissue of rats which had inhaled nickel carbonyl. This binding was comparatively firm since nickel was not released from RNA by means of prolonged dialysis. The two investigators noted that these observations on a subcellular localization of nickel and an in vivo interaction between nickel and ribonucleic acid might be related to the carcinogenetic effect of nickel (SUNDERMAN). While such conclusions are interesting and stimulating they are not as yet factual but remain speculative.

g) Prophylaxis of Nickel Cancer Induction

The prophylactic and therapeutic use of chelating agents for mobilizing various carcinogenic metals (lead, arsenic, chromium) has been proposed also for nickel (HATEM; WEST and SUNDERMAN). HATEM claimed that the cancerigenic effect of nickel can be prevented by the administration of EDTA (Edathamil: calcium disodium salt of ethylene diamine tetra acetic acid) because this salt is capable of destroying the nickel-histamine complex. While WEST and SUNDERMAN reported that Edathamil formed stable chelates with nickel, it was ineffective to combat the effects of nickel carbonyl poisoning produced in mice and rabbits. They found that another chelating agent, diethyldithiocarbamate (DITHIOCARB) provided, however, an effective protection against lethal nickel carbonyl poisoning produced in rabbits. Whether such an action of DITHIOCARB would effect also in man exposed to nickel, an adequate denickelization of the tissues, expecially the lung, and would counteract the carcinogenic action of this metal, is at present quite problematical.

While an occupational contact with nickel dust and fumes can be reduced or eliminated in industry by proper technologic preventive and protective measures, such procedures are evidently not applicable to the control of potential respiratory cancer hazards associated with the use of nickel in a gasoline additive.

5. Iron

a) Technological Aspects

Since iron is the by far most extensively used metallic element, occupational and non-occupational exposures of man to metallic iron and its compounds are relatively common. The inhalation of dust of metallic iron, black ferrous oxide ($Fe_3O_4 \cdot H_2O$), red ferric oxide (Fe_2O_3), iron ore (hematite) and various other iron compounds (iron carbonate) is sustained by hematite miners, miners of red and yellow ocher, workers employed in iron and steel plants, foundries, metallurgical factories (welders, buffers, grinders, polishers, lathers, cutters), silver polishers, mirror polishers, watchmakers, knife grinders, boiler scalers and others. Through the common release of large amounts of iron oxide with the fumes and dusty effluents of steel plants also an environmental exposure to iron oxide for the persons living and working in the neighborhood of such factories is created. The iron oxide retained in the lungs of such workers is responsible for the development of a fibrosing pneumoconiosis, known as pulmonary siderosis (SCHNEIDER; GLIBERT; HEIMANN; BRADSHAW, CRITCHLOW and NAGELSCHMIDT; LAMY, SENAULT, SADOUL, HUTTIN and GUILLERM; DUNNER, TODD and RICE; HAMLIN; HARDING, McLAUGHLIN and DOIG; DRASCHE; DOIG; HARDING, TODD and McLAUGHLIN; DREESSEN et al.; STEWART and FAULDS; BARRIE and HARDING; OTTO; EHRHARDT and HEIDEMANN). Hematite miners often develop a siderosilicosis, since hematite contains 10—12% of silica. It is important for medicolegal reasons that a siderosis of the lung may develop also on an endogenous basis as a symptom of an idiopathic hemosiderosis, as a manifestation of hemochromatosis, as a sequela of hemolysis following blood transfusions, as a complication of malnutrition, COOLEY's Mediterranean anemia, etc. (HIGGINSON; ELLIS, SHULMAN and SMITH; BRADLOW, DUNN and HIGGINSON; GILMAN, HATHORN and CANHAM; HIGGINSON, GERRITSEN and WALKER; SPRECACE).

b) Epidemiology

The existence of a causal interrelation between pulmonary siderosis and primary cancer of the lung has been suggested by several casuistic and epidemiologic observations. Metal grinders have an excessive incidence of pulmonary malignancy, according to KENNEWAY and KENNAWAY (1947) (2.25-fold of that of the general population). The same conclusion was reached by TURNER and GRACE as well as CAMPBELL. The three cases of lung cancer discovered by VORWALD and KARR among 15,587 workers roentgenologically examined at the Saranac Laboratory were iron miners, only one having at the same time, silicosis. Their ages were 59, 64, and 68 years, respectively, and the period of occupational exposure to hematite dust was 27, 35, and 43 years, respectively. A case of cancer of the lung in a boy, 19 years old, who had been engaged in sandblasting metal parts in an automobile factory was reported by SIMONS. Two similar cases were recorded by DREYFUSS, involving two members of a family who polished screws with iron oxide polish for 12 and 24 years respectively.

These early data of merely suggestive significance have received rather substantial confirmation from epidemiologic observations on the excessive frequency of lung cancer among hematite miners in England and Lorraine and among boiler scalers in England. FAULDS and STEWART reported that among hematite miners in England, the prevalence of lung cancer at autopsy increased from 4.4% in 1932—47 (4 cases in 92 necropsies) to 14.6, and in 1948—53 (13 in 89 autopsies). The prevalence of lung cancer among males of the same region and same age distribution found at autopsy was 2.0 [45 in 2,221 necropsies (Fig. 38)]. Similar evidence on an excessive prevalence of lung cancer among hematite miners of the Cumberland region in England have been recorded by McLAUGHLIN and HARDING; FAULDS and NAGELSCHMIDT;

FAULDS). While DOLL has doubted that these necropsy observations reflect actual conditions concerning the incidence of lung cancer among hematite miners and suggested in support of this contention, that necropsies were performed for reasons of

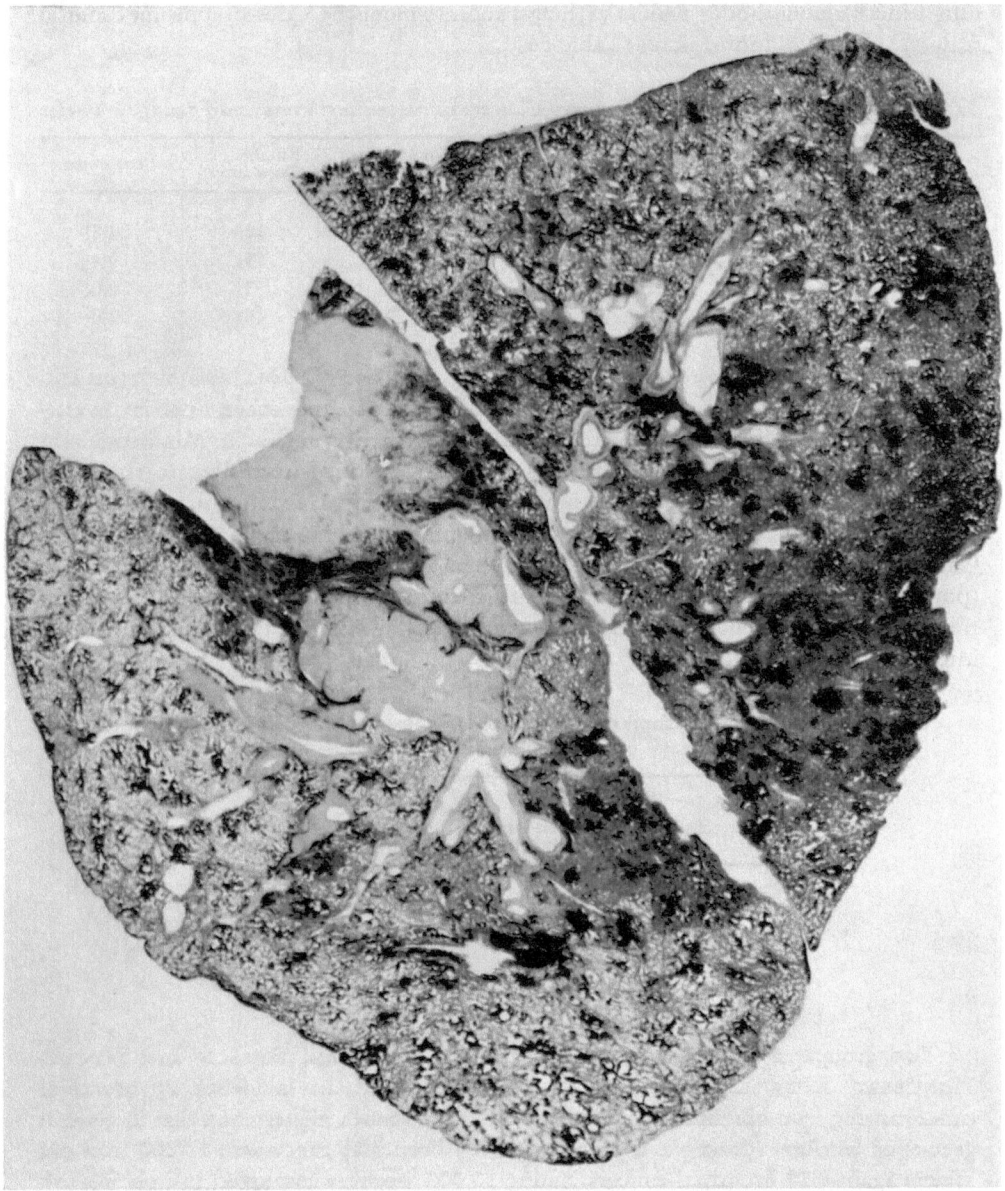

Fig. 38. Lung of an english hematite miner with siderosis and cancer of the lung (courtesy of J. S. FAULDS)

compensation only on miners who showed symptoms indicating the presence of a silicosis, SUTHERLAND alleged that these miners are generally heavy smokers, implying thereby that the lung cancers were attributable to excessive cigarette smoking. It is perhaps important in determining the significance of these speculative allegations by noting that, according to FAULDS, the attack rate of lung cancer among members of this worker group decreased with the degree of silicosis. DUNNER and HICKS as well as DUNNER and HERMON, moreover, reported a similarly high frequency rate of lung cancer among boiler scalers (5 lung cancers among 17 cases of pneumoconiotic scalers) (HARDING and MASSIE) (Table 56).

Table 56. *Siderosis of Lung and Pulmonary Cancers in Hematite Miners and Foundry Workers*

Author	Occupation	Number of Autopsies	Number of Lung Cancers	Percentage
MCLAUGHLIN and HARDING	Foundry Worker	149	16	10.8
FAULDS and STEWARD . . .	Hematite Miner	180	17	9.4
HARDING and MASSIE . . .	Boiler Scaler	12	3	20.0
FAULDS and STEWARD . . .	Controls	2,220	45	2.0

Additional doubts as to the validity of the criticisms of DOLL and SUTHERLAND on the findings of FAULDS; MCLAUGHLIN and HARDING, and other English investigators are provided by observations made on hematite miners in Minnesota and Lorraine, which are of similar nature as those of England. According to statistical data provided by J. W. BROWER, Minnesota State Health Department, on the number of deaths from lung cancer among iron ore miners residing in St. Louis and Ithaca County (total number of miners, 13,313) against that of residents of Minnesota (population base: 2,982,483), there prevails a consistently higher lung cancer death rate for iron ore miners for the five-year period evaluated than that noted for Minnesota residents (Table. 57).

Table 57. *Deaths Due to Cancer of the Lung Among Iron Ore Miners and Residents of Minnesota, 1950—1954*

Year	Number of Deaths		Death Rate per 100,000	
	Minnesota Residents	St. Louis-Ithaca County Miners	Minnesota Residents	St. Louis-Ithaca County Miners
1950	328	5	11.0	37.6
1951	289	4	9.7	30.0
1952	329	12	11.0	90.1
1953	367	8	12.3	60.1
1954	345	6	11.6	60.1

Two groups of French investigators (BRAUN, GUILLERM, PIERSON and SADOUL; MONLIBERT, ROUBILLE and HAYANGE) likewise noted an incidence of bronchial cancer among iron ore miners in Lorraine which was much higher than that in control groups of workers (during a 6-year period, 64 bronchial cancers in 10,000 iron ore miners against 28 bronchial cancers among 10,000 workers employed in iron works). BRAUN et al., like SUTHERLAND, however, called attention to the fact that the French iron ore miners are heavy cigarette smokers.

Mention may also be made of the report of BLAHA on the occurrence of a pachydermia of the larynx which later on became cancerous, in six employees of a workshop where they welded iron parts of tenders and locomotives, and thus became exposed to iron oxide fumes in association with smoke containing 3,4-benzpyrene. A similar combination of agents doubtlessly polluted the air of workshops of English metal moulders and casters and of iron foundry furnace men and labourers, who according to the study of the Registrar General had, during 1930—32, an excessive mortality from cancer of the lung (93% and 88% above standard) (DOLL). In view of these incriminating observations from various sources, it is noteworthy that MÜLLER and EHRHARDT mentioned the absence of lung cancer among 10 German ocher miners who came to autopsy. The absence of any reports on any excessive liability to lung cancer by individuals suffering from endogenous siderosis of the lung also deserves consideration in this connection.

c) Experimental Iron Carcinogenesis

In 1940 CAMPBELL reported that there was an increase of lung tumors in mice inhaling iron oxide dust ($Fe_2O_3 \cdot H_2O$) (32.7% in test mice against 9.6% in controls). CAMPBELL concluded from this observation that the experimental evidence

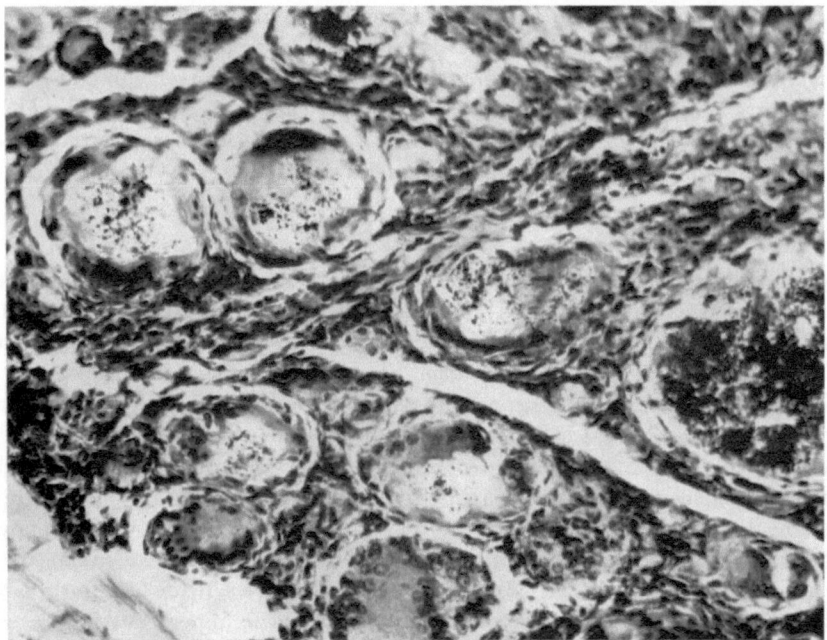

Fig. 39. Sideroma in the thigh muscle of a rat injected with powdered metallic iron

provided support for the high incidence of lung cancers in iron workers, metal grinders, engineers, and foundry workers. SAGAIDAK observed the development of chronic bronchitis and bronchogenic carcinoma in rats intratracheally injected with solutions of radioactive ferrous citrate and suspensions of ferrous oxide in physiologic saline. Mice intraperitoneally injected with FeO_2, on the other hand, did not develop any cancers within five months (MÜLLER and EHRHARDT). MÜLLER and EHRHARDT concluded from this evidence which, however, is inadequate because of the insufficiently long observation period, that iron oxide is not a carcinogen but may possibly exert a syncarcinogenic action. Similarly negative results were reported by HUEPER and PAYNE on rats which were intramuscularly and intrapleurally implanted with pellets containing 25 mg. of finely powdered metallic iron obtained by degradation of iron carbonyl and suspended in 50 mg. of wool fat. The rats developed only granulomas containing large amounts of extra- and intracellularly located iron oxide (sideromas) (Fig. 39) and showing no tendency toward a malignant change. SAFFIOTTI, CEFIS, KOLB and GROTE succeeded in inducing bronchogenic carcinomas in hamsters when suspensions of iron oxide ground together with 3,4-benzpyrene and 7,12-dimethylbenz(a)-anthracene were instilled into their trachea.

The successful production of sarcomas in the subcutaneous tissue of mice, rats, hamsters, and rabbits, but not in dogs, injected repeatedly with large amounts of iron-carbohydrate complexes (dextran; polymaltose; dextrin) (RICHMOND; FIELDING; ZOLLINGER; HADDOW and HORNING; LUNDIN) has been ascribed by HADDOW and HORNING as a specific carcinogenic effect of iron related to its chelating effect since dextran injected alone did not produce sarcomas. This interpretation, however, is open to question since other investigators have shown that certain dextrans, like other water-soluble carbon polymers when injected repeatedly in large amounts, induce sarcoma formation at the site of deposition (HUEPER; LUSKY and NELSON). These observations, therefore, are at present of doubtful value as evidence showing a carcinogenic action of iron. They strongly support, however, the view that iron-dextran, iron-dextrin and iron polymaltose preparations are carcinogenic to various species, including possibly man, although this is denied by GOLDBERG.

d) Etiology

Since iron is an element of distinct physiologic importance which is present in appreciable amounts in the animal and human organism, this consideration alone militates against the conclusion that iron or its compounds are carcinogenic under ordinary circumstances. It is, on the other hand, conceivable that iron ore or iron oxide dust may play nevertheless, under the special conditions prevailing often in industry, an important role as a carrier of carcinogenic materials, such as carcinogenic hydrocarbons present in soot. The experimental observations of SAFFIOTTI and his associates suggest such a role of iron oxide. Iron oxide would prolong, under such conditions, the length of exposure time of the bronchial mucosa to the carcinogenic chemicals adsorbed to the surfaces of the dust particles and would accentuate thereby their carcinogenic effectiveness (HUEPER). Special inquiries made on this point in regard to exposure conditions sustained by English hematite miners, have divulged the fact that diesel engines have been used since 1950 and in part are still used in the English iron ore mines (FAULDS). The high content of 3,4-benzyrene in the environmental air of foundries, steel works and similar establishments with iron oxide pollutants of the atmosphere is well established. This explanation is in general agreement with the observation on the high lung cancer incidence among English metal workers and on the occurrence of larynx cancer in CZECH welders (BLAHA).

Since FAULDS failed to demonstrate any radioactivity in the lung tissue of the English iron ore miners upon autoradiographic examination of large lung sections, any contributory radioactive factor in the causation of lung cancers appears to be most unlikely.

The size of the iron mining industry and of the steel and iron metal industries with their many thousands of workers exposed to iron oxide as well as the prevailing exposure to iron oxide fumes and dust for residents of the vicinity of modern steel plants provide a weighty reason for conducting competent and trustworthy epidemiologic surveys for demonstrating conclusively whether or not occupational and environmental siderosis of the lung creates an excessive liability to cancer of the lung and, if so, under what type of exposure conditions.

6. Beryllium

a) Technological Aspects

Although beryllium has been known since 1797, it has found significant industrial use only since about 1920, particularly in Europe. Its large-scale and rapidly growing industrial use in the United States started with World War II. Beryllium metal and its compounds are being employed in a great variety of processes and products (beryllium alloys with copper, aluminium, and nickel; phosphors in fluorescent and Neon tubes, ceramics, refractory crucibles, x-ray tube windows, vitreous enamel, radio tubes, textile fibers, gas mantles, atomic energy reactors, guidance systems, space vehicles, rocket motors). Beryl, the ore from which beryllium is refined, is mined in the U.S.A., Argentina, Brazil, India and Madagascar. The data listed in Table 58

Table 58. *Industrial Manufacturing Processes and Products and Types of Beryllium Compounds*

Source	Probable Compound
Processing Be from ore	BeO
Fluorescent powder manufacture	BeO, $ZnBeSiO_2$
Machining Be	BeO
Fluorescent lamp works	$ZnBeSiO_2(BeO)$
Alloying Be	BeO
Laboratory work	BeO
Sign tube manufacture	$ZnBeSiO_2(BeO)$
Ceramics	BeO
Crystal manufacture	BeO
Fluorescent lamp salvage	$ZnBeSiO_2$

provide some information on the type of beryllium compounds which are used in different industrial operations and products, and to which workers in such establishments may become exposed (MINERAL YEAR BOOKS; HARDY; BRESLIN; CAMPBELL; REYNOLDS; SANDER; FENN; HASTERLINK; METZNER and LIEBEN).

b) Epidemiology

Disease related to inhalation of beryllium metal and beryllium compounds was documented in Europe in the early 1930's and in the USA in the early 1940's. The manifestations related to occupational contact with these agents were of acute, subacute and chronic character and affected the lung, skin and occasionally other organs

(HARDY; AUB and GRIER; STERNER and EISENBUD; CONFERENCE; SCHEPERS; DE-NARDI, VAN ORDSTRAND, CURTIS and ZIELINSKI; DUTRA). The pulmonary reactions assuming the symptomatic and morphologic characteristics (acute and chronic chemical pneumonitis) are known under the term of berylliosis and in their chronic form represent a sarcoidosis symptomatologically and histologically similer to that present in BOECK's sarcoid. It has been claimed that beryl mining does not entail such a hazard.

The appearance of such reactions among persons living in the vicinity of beryllium plants and rocket motor testing grounds, demonstrated soon that such hazards are not restricted to workers employed in such establishments but extend to residents of their environment (EISENBUD, WANTA, DUSTAN et al.; EISENBUD, BERGHOUT and STEADMAN; CHESNER; MACHLE; PERRY; METZNER and LIEBEN; CAMPBELL) because of a pollution of the environmental atmosphere with beryllium-containing effluents (neighborhood cases of berylliosis). Recent studies showed, moreover, that beryllium hazards may be transferred into the environment when contaminated work garments are laundered in commercial laundries (COHEN). While the primary environmental beryllium hazard related to the use of beryllium phosphors from broken fluorescent tubes has largely disappeared with the discontinuation of such phosphors for this particular purpose, hazards from other sources have taken its place. Because of the seriousness of the prognosis of berylliosis and the rather minute amounts of atmospheric beryllium which may induce in some persons the development of a berylliosis, LISCO advised to treat beryllium like radioactive chemicals in the design of protective technologic measures. Indeed elaborate technologic control procedures have been introduced during the past decade into the various industrial operations for eliminating or reducing beryllium hazards (MITCHELL and HYATT; SILSON, BENJAMIN and WILSON; BRESLIN; LINDEKEN and MEADORS; HEUSTIS; BRESLIN and HARRIS). Such precautionary procedures include determination of the beryllium content of the air and on protective garments (WALKLEY; COHEN; CHOLAK and HUBBARD; VAN ORDSTRAND) as well as of the urine and in lung tissue of workers employed in such operations (CHOLAK and HUBBARD; DUTRA, CHOLAK and HUBBARD; LIEBEN and METZNER; KLEMPERER, MARTIN and VAN RIPER). The widespread nature of contact with beryllium is indicated by the fact that a large sector of the general population harbors significant amounts of beryllium in their pulmonary tissues (TIETZ et al.).

The pulmonary reactions may become manifest years after cessation of exposure to beryllium (24%) (HARDY). Since the clinical complaints are not infrequently nonspecific in nature and since their onset may be delayed and mimicries other pulmonary diseases (BOECK's sarcoid, miliary pulmonary tuberculosis), berylliosis is hard to diagnose reliably, and therefore may escape correct recognition. The scope of the occupational type of berylliosis is suggested by the fact that HARDY could collect in 1962, 650 reasonably well documented cases of beryllium poisoning occurring in 70 companies and in 12 different operations.

In addition to such acute and chronic inflammatory and granulomatous responses to the introduction of beryllium and its compounds into the lung (WILLIAMS; etc.), there were observed an appreciable number of cases of beryllium granulomas of the skin and other superficial tissues often developing at the site of injury with beryllium-containing materials (GRIER, NASH and FREIMANN; DUTRA; LEDERER and SAVAGE;

RIZZUTI; HELWIG; etc.). None of these lesions, like those elicited by asbestos in the skin (asbestos warts), has ever displayed a tendency to become cancerous.

c) Beryllium Cancers

The first suggestion that beryllium might be another chemical carcinogen which was added recently by man to his environment, was provided by the experimental production of osteogenic sarcomas in rabbits which were intravenously injected, or inhaled various beryllium compounds, or powdered beryllium metal (beryllium oxide, beryllium silicate, zinc beryllium silicate, beryllium phosphate) (GARDNER and HESLINGTON PRICE; DUTRA and LARGENT; SISSONS; DUTRA, LARGENT and ROTH: NASH; GARDNER; BARNES, DENZ and SISSONS; YAMAGUCHI; HOAGLAND, GRIER and HOOD; VIGLIANI; ARAKI, OKADA and FUJITA). This suspicion was intensified when VORWALD and later SCHEPERS succeeded in producing pulmonary carcinomas in rats and subsequently in monkeys which inhaled for many months beryllium sulfate or beryllium oxide (TEPPER, HARDY and CHAMBERLIN; SCHEPERS; DURKAN, DELAHANT and CREEDON; VORWALD). Some of the pulmonary neoplasms induced thereby were adenocarcinomas, others were squamous cell carcinomas. Various beryllium salts thus proved to be potent respiratory carcinogens active in rats as well as in monkeys (VORWALD; SCHEPERS).

The earliest clue concerning a similar carcinogenic effect of inhaled beryllium on the human lung was given by KAHLAU who reported the coexistence of berylliosis and carcinoma in the lung of a man examined at autopsy. During recent years, three additional such combinations have been recorded with the National Beryllium Case Registry, according to HARDY (1962) and three other cases of this type have recently been described by NIEMÖLLER. These lung cancers made a delayed appearance some 15—20 years after a previous occupational exposure to beryllium dust, fumes or gas. NIEMÖLLER noted that such lung cancers may develop in lungs lacking the typical radiographic changes of a berylliosis, yet containing beryllium upon spectrographic analysis. Sutherland, commenting on this report, suggested that traces of beryllium present in cigarette tobacco and inhaled with the smoke (WILLIAMS and GARMON) might have played a contributory role in eliciting these cancerous reactions. The true scientific merits of such unfounded allegations are perhaps best indicated by the fact that similar claims have been advanced in connection with the causation of occupational cancers of the respiratory system resulting from exposures to chromates, nickel, arsenic, and radioactive chemicals (polonium). The main effect of such unwarranted speculations is added undesirable confusion of the ill-informed on the relative significance of the multiple causal agents involved in the production of cancer of the lung in man, impediment of badly needed epidemiologic, clinical and experimental research into the numerous actual and potential environmental causes of cancers of the respiratory tract (HUEPER), on which rational control measures may be based, and obstruction of justified compensation claims for cancers of the respiratory organs contracted by occupational exposure to recognized respiratory carcinogens, by misleading courts and compensation commissions through a reckless and irresponsible promotion of exaggerated claims on the role of cigarette smoking.

While the preparatory period of beryllium cancers in animals is between 11 and 24 months, that of beryllium cancers of the lung in man is between 20 and 30 years and is often associated with a lag period of many years.

d) Etiology

It is noteworthy that beryllium apparently once inhaled is retained over a long period of time in the human body, since beryllium has been detected in the urine up to 10 years after cessation of exposure (KLEMPERER, MARTIN, and VAN RIPER) and has been demonstrated in the lungs of rats 1 year after the inhalation of beryllium oxide (DUTRA; LARGENT, CHOLAK, HUBBARD and ROTH) as well as in their bones (STOKINGER, STEADMAN and ROOT; BARNES), where it may replace calcium. The skeleton retains the bulk of the beryllium in the body (50—80 per cent) if the inhaled aerosols are soluble compounds, such as beryllium sulfate and beryllium fluoride; the lungs retain the bulk of beryllium if the compounds are insoluble, such as beryllium oxide. However, there occur marked fluctuations in the beryllium content of the lung of individuals which had varying degrees of exposure to beryllium. LIEBEN, DATTOLI and VOUGHT concluded from their quantitative studies for beryllium in post mortem lungs, that the findings of beryllium in the lungs does not necessarily mean a person has anatomically and symptomatically berylliosis. The amount of beryllium in the lung demonstrated is, in their experience, also not necessarily related to the severity or even to the presence of berylliosis. It is, moreover, important that the relative amounts of beryllium in different parts of the same lung may vary as much as ten times, and that at times a single test may be negative in a person with substantial quantities of beryllium in other parts of the lungs. The retention of beryllium in lungs with berylliosis was reported also by DE NARDI, VAN ORDSTRAND, CURTIS and ZIELINSKI.

These investigators, moreover, proposed that beryllium is probably deposited in the reticuloendothelial tissues of the lungs from which Be ions are released to form a Be-protein complex. In some persons, the Be-protein complex becomes antigenic, thus producing antibodies and hypersensitivity reactions. This concept received some support from the experiments of ALDRIDGE, BARNES and DENZ who showed that beryllium ions react rapidly with certain tissue proteins and form complexes with plasma proteins when introduced into the blood. These complexes protect the beryllium from being precipitated by phosphate ions.

Subsequent studies of VORWALD and REEVES demonstrated that the formation of Be-protein complexes apparently takes place in the cells of lung tissue and that Be combines mainly with the proteinic constitutents of the nuclei. It is postulated by VORWALD and REEVES, and REEVES and VORWALD, that a disturbance of cytoplasmic protein synthesis resulting from the introduction of Be into the cells and causing changes in the kinetics of certain key enzymes might be a factor in beryllium-induced pulmonary carcinogenesis.

The studies on the toxicity and carcinogenicity of beryllium compounds indicate that the toxic and cancerous manifestations are to be considered as responses to the action of beryllium itself and not as the result of the associated anions of its acidic salts (STOKINGER, SPRAGUE, and HALL). In considering possible future carcinomatous developments in persons with previous exposure to beryllium, some consideration also may be given to the toxic effect exerted by beryllium on the liver leading to the development of cirrhosis and to an impairment of the metabolic and detoxicating function of this organ (ALDRIDGE, BARNES, and DENZ; HOAGLAND, GRIER, and HOOD).

It appears to be wise to study in the future, individuals with cancers of the lung and sarcomas of the bones for previous occupational and environmental exposure to beryllium metal, alloys and compounds.

7. Mustard Gas — Yperite-Lost — Beta, beta'-dichlorodiethyl sulfide — Bis(beta-chloroethyl)Sulfide

a) Technological Aspects

Mustard Gas is a vesicant, irritative gas which was extensively used during World War I as a warfare agent and which, in this role, has caused many thousand cases of fatal and non-fatal war gas poisoning (MACY, JARMAN, MORRISON and REID; LINDQUIST). While this gas has not been employed officially during World War II, it nevertheless was produced in large quantities for the manufacture of gas ammunition. Workers engaged in such activities in Japan and in the United States have sustained poisonous exposures and as the result of them have suffered from acute and chronic mustard gas poisoning. These, in their acute form, elicited mainly inflammatory reactions in the skin and lung and in their chronic responses not infrequently led to the development of a chronic bronchitis, chronic chemical pneumonia, bronchiectases and emphysema. Such pulmonary manifestations continued to exist in some cases for many years after such events (FUJITO; SARTORELLI, GIUBILEO and BARTALINI; SECRETARY OF HEW). In addition to such direct occupational and military poisonings observed in the production and application of mustard gas, there have occurred also accidental ones among the civilian population (MONGELI-SCIANNAMEO; ROCHE, GRUNWALD and ROUANET). In more recent years this sulfur mustard as well as chemically related nitrogen mustards, have widely been employed in the treatment of cancers, expecially leukemias as well as mucosis fungoides, and thereby have furnished an additional source of therapeutic and accidental poisonings (WOLFSON and OLNEY; VISSER and TEN SELDAM; GILMAN and PHILIPS; BROCK; PREUSSMANN; RHOADS; WINTROBE and HUGULEY; BOYLAND; PHILPOTT, WOODBURNE and WALDRIFF; OSBORNE, JORDON, HOAK and PSCHIERER). The toxic action of such therapeutically used mustards was exerted especially upon the blood-forming tissues and the liver (URAM, FISHER and FISHER; SHULLENBERGER, WATKINS and KIERLAND; SPITZ). Similar pathologic responses have been induced with these mustards in experimental animals (GRAEF, KARNOFSKY, JAGER, KRICHESKY and SMITH; KINDRED; AXELROD and HAMILTON; KARNOFSKY, GRAEF and SMITH).

b) Epidemiology

The alleged carcinogenic action of war gas poisoning figured prominently in the speculations as to the cause of the increase in lung cancers observed during the early 1920's (KIKUTH; BROCKBANK; KLOTZ; DERISCHANOFF; HÜNERMANN; REICHE). Residuals of warfare gassing were noted by MATZ in ten (10) out of 138 cases of pulmonary cancer among American World War I veterans. Four out of 64 cases of lung cancer, recorded by BROCKBANK, were gassed badly during this war. MACKLIN noted that war gas poisoning occurred in 5 per cent of 164 cases of lung cancer among males, while it was present in only 2 per cent of soldiers without this disease. KOELSCH conceded that a few cases of lung cancer exhibited a doubtful etiological relation to war gas injury, which was claimed to have caused also two cancers of the larynx (SPAMER; TILLEY). No distinction was made at that time as to the particular chemical nature of the various gases used during World War I.

The actual human evidence incriminating mustard gas as a human respiratory carcinogen remained at that time restricted to a modest number of isolated cases or small groups of cases of cancers of the lung and larynx occurring in veterans of World War I who had sustained some form of war gas poisoning. It was in 1955 when CASE published a study on a possible relation between mustard gas poisoning in veterans of World War I and the subsequent development of lung cancers, that the first evidence of a statistically significant excessive liability to lung cancer for gassed British veterans was obtained. A similar conclusion was reached by BEEBE (1960), when analyzing American veterans of the first World War who had suffered non-fatal attacks of war gas poisoning.

The up-to-then suspected etiologic relations between exposures to mustard gas and the development of respiratory cancer have recently been placed on much firmer factual grounds by the investigations on former employees of a war gas factory located on the island of Okuno near Hiroshima (KOBAYASHI et al.; YAMADA; NAKAMURA; WADA; WATANABE; YOKORO et al.; YAMADA et al.; WADA et al.). These were started in 1952 by WADA and WATANABE with the discovery of a bronchogenic carcinoma in a 30-year old former war gas worker who had been exposed to mustard gas for about two (2) years. In the most recent publication by WADA et al. (1962), an analysis of 175 death certificates of former war gas workers revealed a total of 49 cancers of which 29 were situated in the respiratory tract, 19 in the gastrointestinal system, and two (2) in the skin. The ratio of deaths from respiratory cancers in this occupational group stood at 16%, while it was 0.3 to 0.5% in larger non-exposed population groups of the same region. In 11 of the 19 cases of lung cancer, a squamous cell carcinoma was found while in the remaining eight (8) cases an undifferentiated carcinoma was present. The age distribution was as follows:

30—40 years: — 1 case   51—60 years: — 9 cases
41—50 years: — 3 cases   61—70 years: — 6 cases

The latent period was over 10 years and in fact for 13 cases, over 20 years. The site distribution of 28 cancers found in members of this group and affecting the respiratory system and upper alimentary tract was as follows:

Bronchi   14 cases   50.0%   Pharynx   3 cases   10 %
Trachea   1 case   3 %   Tongue   1 case   3 %
Larynx   6 cases   21.4%   Mediastinum   2 cases   6 %
Nasal Sinus   1 case   3 %

Cancers of the respiratory organs represented cause of death in 16% of deceased former mustard gas producers (Table 59), while there were only between 0.3 and

Table 59. *Respiratory Cancers in Mustard Gas Producers* (WADA et al.)

Mustard Gas Producers	Bronchi	Trachea	Larynx	Nasal Sinus	Pharynx	Tongue	Media-stinum	Total
Cases	14	1	6	1	3	1	2	28

0.5% of deaths in the general population during the same period (1937—1960) in the neighborhood cities. The observations made in Japanese war gas producers thus confirmed the epidemiologic data on the frequency of lung cancer among English and American veterans of World War I who suffered from war gas poisoning (BEEBE; CASE and LEA).

In addition to cancers of the respiratory tract, individuals occupationally exposed to mustard gas in Germany have shown, according to Baader, an excessive liability to lymphosarcoma (HUEPER).

c) Experimental Mustard Cancers

Experimental studies on animals have established the mutagenic and carcinogenic potency of mustard gas (sulfur mustard) as well as its nitrogen analogue, nitrogen mustard (BOYLAND and HORNING; HESTON; ROGERS; KELLNER and NEMETH; GRIFFIN et al.). The tumors produced by these mustards in mice involved several tissues: lung adenomas and carcinomas, lymphosarcomas, fibrosarcomas at site of subcutaneous injection.

Because of the epidemiologic evidence on a carcinogenic action of mustards in man and in view of the available confirmatory observations made in experimental animals, the following additional epidemiologic studies are indicated for ascertaining the actual scope of past human mustard cancer hazards.

1. Inquiries are in order in all countries where in former years a large-scale production of mustard gas and manufacture of war gas ammunition was carried on, for obtaining evidence whether similar occupational cancers occurred in individuals employed or formerly employed in such works. Such epidemiologic studies on carcinogenic effects of mustard gas and related chemicals should apply not only to cancers of the respiratory system, but also to those of the digestive tract, the hematopoietic organs and the skin. Besides the scientific importance of any data yielded by such surveys, their results would be of direct medicolegal importance to former workers employed in such operations during both wars and to veterans of World War I who sustained war gas poisoning and later became affected by cancers.

2. Patients with long survival periods whose cancers and related disorders were controlled by the administration of mustards should be reinvestigated for evidence of cancers attributable to a carcinogenic action of the mustards given.

d) Etiology

A carcinogenic action of mustard gas upon the bronchial mucosa of man may be related to its cross-linking and radiomimetic effect (SCHRECK; HADDOW and TIMMIS; BOYLAND). Mustards react with a wide variety of aminoacids and enzymes. However, the supposition that the mustards react with sulfhydryl enzymes, in general, is invalid according to BRANDT and GRIFFIN, owing to the number of known sulfhydryl enzymes that are not affected. Mustards display both anticarcinogenic and carcinogenic effects, and thereby exhibit ambivalent properties frequently observed in other carcinostatic agents used in medicine for the control of cancers.

8. Isopropyl Oil

a) Technological Aspects

Isopropyl oil, the crude, slightly turbid liquor from which isopropyl alcohol is distilled and which is obtained by an interaction of sulfuric acid with butylene and propylene in a low temperature reaction, contains, in addition to isopropanol, isopropyl ether, isopropyl sulfate, acetone, polyaromatic ring compounds, alkyl benzenes, and polypropylenes. The latter compounds account for the viscosity of the product and for its tendency to form upon contact with air through progressive polymerization, a brownish-tarry matter.

The isopropyl alcohol (isopropanol) is widely used in various industries as well as in cosmetic and medicinal preparations (KEESER; FOWLER). It is more toxic than ethyl alcohol and, therefore, subjected to regulations limiting its use in the human economy (LEHMAN and CHASE).

b) Epidemiology

Workers employed in isopropanol manufacture have been exposed to the inhalation of vapors, mist, and dust of isopropyl oil escaping from leaky pipe connections, defective pumps, and gaskets, or spilled on the floor at the occurrence of breaks in pipelines and during repairs on pipes, pumps, and stills.

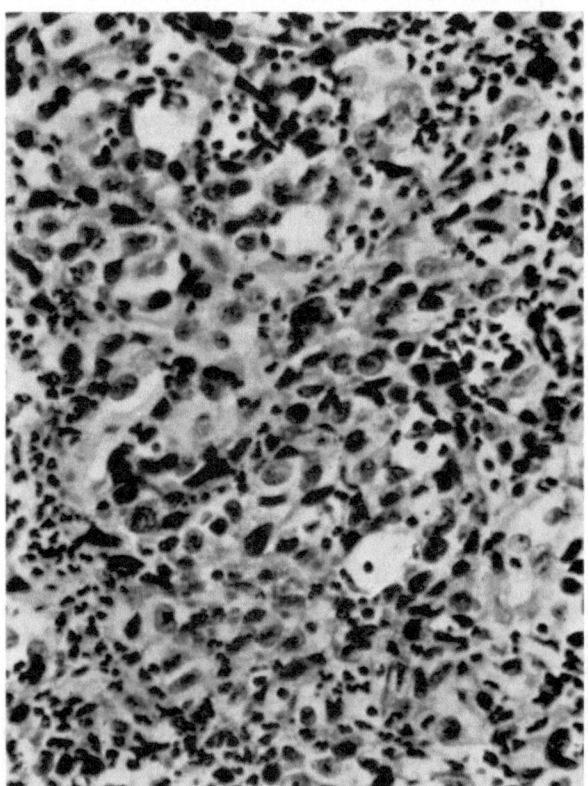

Fig. 40. Lymphoepithelioma of a paranasal sinus in an isopropanol producer

During 1937 to 1946, six cancers of the respiratory system (4 nasal sinuses, 1 lung, 1 larynx) were observed among about 75 workers employed in an isopropyl alcohol plant in the U.S.A. which was in operation since 1928 (NALE and HUEPER; HUEPER) (Fig. 40). Another American manufacturer of this alcohol subsequently observed two (2) cases of sinus cancers and two (2) of the larynx, occurring in a total of 11 cancers among 779 workers employed at varying periods of time in an identical operation active since 1927. From the data available, it was calculated that the incidence of cancer of the nasal sinuses and of the intrinsic larynx among men working in such operations for more than nine years, exceeds the expected incidence of cancer of these organs in males of the general population of ages 45 to 54 by 21 times (ECKARDT) (Table 60). It was calculated that the incidence rate of cancer of the nasal sinuses and

Table 60. *Respiratory Cancers in Isopropyl Alcohol Producers*

Source	Topographic Distribution of Cancer				
	Nasal Sinus	Larynx	Lung	Total	Morbidity Rate
Manufacturer I	4	1	1	6	
Manufacturer II	2	2		4	21 times mormal

larynx for the second group was 134.5 per 100,000, against a normal rate of 6.3. The minimal latent period of these cancers was about 10 years.

Attempts to produce cancers of the skin in mice, of the lung in mice, and of the lung and nasal sinus in dogs with various constituents of the isopropyl oil, were essentially negative (WEIL, SMYTH and NALE). While a definite decision as to the nature of the carcinogenic agent responsible for these occupational cancers in man is outstanding, there is a certain likelihood that polypropylenes may be involved in their causation which reach the respiratory organs in a low polymerized form and which subsequently undergo increasing polymerization.

Published observations on this occupational cancer hazard have remained restricted so far to the United States (BAADER; DOLL). Similar findings, according to KEESER, have not been made in a large German isopropyl alcohol manufacturing plant using a production method differing from that employed in U.S.A.

Because of the relatively high attack rate of isopropyl oil cancers, indicating the action of a rather potent chemical carcinogen, it would be wise to survey similar operations existing in the U.S.A. as well as in other countries for the existence of similar experiences.

Although this industrial cancer problem has remained so far entirely within the occupational sphere and is of rather small proportions, the recently developed production of polypropylene plastics may furnish additional opportunities for occupational cancer hazards of this type which may be worthwhile to include into future epidemiologic observations on "polypropylene polymer cancers".

Additional experimental investigations are, moreover, indicated for ascertaining the exact nature of the carcinogenic chemical responsible for the causation of these cancers. It may be necessary for this purpose to expose animals to the vapors and mists of freshly prepared isopropyl oil generated in a small pilot operation since the carcinogenic agents may perhaps be rather unstable and may pass rather rapidly from through progressive polymerization.

9. Coal Tar, Tar Oils, Soot, and Other Combustion Products of Coal

a) Technologic Aspects

The onset and development of modern industrialism have been associated for many decades with a large-scale use of coal as the principal source of fuel for the production heat and energy. Coal has also furnished a major source of raw materials (tar, coke, pitch, soot, paraffin, tar oils, kerosene, etc.) for the phenomenal growth of the chemical industry and various related industries. In fact, modern industry was built upon a coal economy which only in more recent decades has been complemented by an oil economy. It is likely that these two types of carbon economies may be supplanted in the near future to some extent by the advent of a uranium economy. Components and by-products of these three agents employed for the production of energy and heat share with the fourth source, solar radiation, the distinction that they possess carcinogenic properties. Distillation and hydrogenation products of carbon or coal when exposed to proper temperatures contain, like any other carbonaceous material subjected to similar conditions, a large variety of polycyclic, aromatic hydrocarbons, some of which have been shown to induce cancers in exposed tissues of man and experimental animals (HUEPER; HENRY; KENNAWAY; ITCHIKAWA and YAMAGIWA; TEUTSCHLAENDER; HELLER, etc.). These chemicals usually belong to the classes of benzpyrenes and benzanthracenes (HUEPER and CONWAY), although some experimental evidence indicates that also certain aliphatic hydrocarbons, such as epoxides, may contribute in conveying carcinogenic properties especially to lower boiling fractions of coal tar and petroleum derivatives (HUEPER).

The carcinogenic chemicals contained in coal tar and related derivatives are of particular importance to the present day knowledge of the etiologic factors responsible for human cancers, since their presence in coal soot and their role in the production of cancers of the scrotal skin in English chimney sweeps is associated with the first demonstration of an occupational cancer (POTT, 1779) as well as with that of an environmental, man-made occupational chemical carcinogen. Since that time, occupational cancers of the skin produced by coal tar, pitch, and derivatives, have been reported from many countries (HUEPER) and represent in fact the largest group of occupational chemical cancers placed on record. There is thus undeniable and definite epidemiologic, clinical, pathologic and experimental evidence available by which the carcinogenicity of incomplete combustion and distillation products of coal, i.e., tar, pitch, asphalt, soot, tar oils, creosote, anthracene oil, methylated naphthalenes, waxes, etc., has been established. In view of the widely promoted allegation that cigarette smoking is the predominant cause of lung cancer, although cigarette tar does not seem to induce cancer of the fingers stained with it, it is noteworthy that coal tar workers develop cancer at such sites (LINK; OPPENHEIM; EPSTEIN).

b) Epidemiology

In contrast to the early recognition of skin cancer hazards related to occupational contact with coal tar and related products, well over one hundred years elapsed before any thought and interest was extended to a possible existence between such exposures and the development of cancers of the respiratory system.

KENNAWAY and KENNAWAY first maintained that "coal tar in the atmosphere, whether derived from roads, domestic chimneys, or any other source, does not cause an exceptionally higher incidence of cancer of the lung". A similar claim was advanced by HUGOUNENQ and by HUSTED and BIILMANN in regard to the liability of cancer of the lung for workers employed in the tar industry and in the construction and maintenance of tarred roads.

Similarly negative statements were made by DOIG; FISCHER-WASELS; MENZ; and HARDING. It was only recently that FALK ventured the opinion from a "critical" analysis of the reported evidence on the carcinogenic action of polycyclic aromatic hydrocarbons contained in tar, pitch, asphalt, mineral and similar products on the respiratory system, that these chemicals apparently exerted only a relatively weak effect upon these tissues to judge from the rather small number of recorded cases of lung cancer among members of exposed worker groups. In the face of the available evidence on occupational respiratory cancers and in view of the highly fragmentary information published on this subject by industry, such a statement must be considered to be unfortunate at this time and in fact, misleading.

The epidemiologic evidence on the relative liability to cancer of the lung for certain worker groups exposed occupationally to respiratory contact with coal tar fumes and pitch dust which has been published during the past forty (40) years, has demonstrated beyond any doubt that the inhalation of incomplete combustion and distillation products of coal is a direct cause of cancer of the lung.

In an analysis of lung cancer deaths among members of different occupations for the years 1933 to 1938, KENNAWAY and KENNAWAY (1947) noted that an above-average (100) lung cancer frequency existed for members of the following occupations sustaining such exposures: gashouse workers, 129; gas stokers, 284; gas producers, 202; gasworks crane operators, 138; gasworks superintendents, 136; printers, 119; chimney sweeps, 119; asphalt workers, 164; street cleaners, 169; and automobile drivers, 149. MORRISON, reporting on lung cancer rates among SCOTTISH workers, listed moulders as having an above-standard mortality rate of 162, and foundry workers as having one of 161. Such workers become exposed during the metal casting process, to pitch dust and fumes from heated pitch and mineral or tar oil grease lining the moulds. In an analysis of the lung cancer rates of eight large industrial worker groups of Ohio, MANCUSO listed steel workers, including coke oven and coke oven by-product workers, as having a death rate of 2.18, while agricultural laborers were listed as having one of 0.81. In an exploratory study on occupational lung cancers, BRESLOW noted 11 cases in firemen and boiler attendants instead of the expected number of one.

KAWAHATA and KURODA reported in 1936 the occurrence of 61 cases of lung cancer among 18,000 workers of the Yahata Steel Works in Kyushu within five years. While the lung cancer mortality among the general plant population inhaling a heavily polluted atmosphere was $1^0/o$, it was $6.69^0/o$ among the particularly severely exposed gas generator workers, and $3.36^0/o$ among engine drivers. One-third of the workers with lung cancer were less than 40 years of age. This shift of the age distribution into younger age groups provided additional evidence of the severity of exposure to the carcinogenic tar fumes.

In a follow-up study of the same workers groups for the years 1946 to 1960 by KAWAI, MATSUYAMA and AMAMOTO, ten (10) additional lung cancers were found, making a mortality rate of 202. Similer observations were recently recorded for Canadian gashouse workers (DOLL). Of fourteen (14) cases of cancer among retort house workers, six (6) were due to cancer of the lung, one (1) to cancer of the ethmoid sinus, and one (1) to cancer of the larynx ($57^0/o$ of the total number in the respiratory tract).

Similar occupational evidence incriminating respiratory contact with coal tar fumes in the production of lung cancer among Norwegian gashouse workers was recently supplied by BRUUSGARD (1959). Among a total of 125 deaths from all causes in this group, 41 were due to cancers of various types. Five (5) of them involved the lung, two (2) the larynx, two (2) the nasal sinuses, three (3) the naso-pharynx and hypopharynx, five (5) the bladder, and three (3) the esophagus (Table 61).

Table 61. *Respiratory Cancer Mortality Rates in Coke Oven and Gas Retort Workers*

Author	Country	No. of Cases	Mortality Rate	Year
KAWAHATA	Japan	21	500	1933—1937
KAWAI *et al.*	Japan	10		1946—1960
DOLL	England	97	284 Stokers 202 Retort Workers	1946—1960
CHRISTIAN	U.S.A.	23 12 11 27	149 Gas Plant Workers 784 Coke Oven Workers 87 General Workers 433 Substation Operators	1946—1960
DOLL	Canada	14	Gas Retort Workers (57% of all cancers affected respiratory organs)	
BRUUSGAARD	Norway	12	Gashouse Workers	1959 (among 41 deaths from cancer)

When in 1952 DOLL reinvestigated the lung cancer death rates among English gas workers, he found among 831 deaths of all causes, 25 deaths due to lung cancer instead of the expected 13.8 cases, i.e., the observed rate was about double the expected rate for a standard male population residing in London, where the lung cancer death rate as well as the pollution of the air with carbon soot are notoriously the highest in the world. When in 1956, REID and BUCK again investigated the lung cancer rates among English coke oven workers, they failed to find any significant difference from the standard mortality rate. In exploring the possible causes for the apparent difference between their findings and those of DOLL and of KENNAWAY and KENNAWAY, they proposed that some part of the difference might be due to improved operating procedures introduced into coking plants during recent years. However, of greater importance in their opinion, was the great change in the prevalence of cancer

Table 62. *Age Distribution at Death of Gas Plant and Gas Retort Workers with Lung Cancers*

Author	Type of Worker	Age at Death in Years					Lag Period	Exposure Time
		31—40	41—50	51—60	61—70	71 and over		
DOLL	Pensioners Gas Plant				14	11	0—16	
KAWAHATA	Gas Retort Workers	7	12	2	1			9—23 (16.6 average)

of the lung in the general population during the intervening years when the crude death rate in males increased five-fold in 20 years, i.e., the degree of exposure of the general population to carcinogenic constituents in the occupational and general atmospheres during this period has apparently risen in England to a level equalling that present for coke oven workers during several decades (Table 62).

Although physicians working in the field of compensation medicine in the United States have been aware for some time of the excessive frequency of lung cancers among American coke oven workers, it was only in 1962 that CHRISTIAN provided published evidence supporting these impressions. Analyzing lung cancer rates for the period 1946—1961 among employees of a public power plant (Consolidated Edison Company, New York) which uses coal as source of fuel, he found considerable differences in the rates per 100,000 per year for the 125 lung cancers observed in the different occupational groups. The rate distribution clearly demonstrated highly excessive lung cancer rates for the various workers occupationally exposed to coal tar fumes (Table 63). It is interesting to note that the highly excessive lung cancer rate

Table 63. *Consolidated Edison. Job Distribution of 125 Cases of Carcinoma of the Lung — 1946—1960* (H. A. CHRISTIAN)

Job Title	Number of Employees	Number of Lung Cancer Cases in 15 Yrs.	Rate per 100,000 per Yr.	Percent Employer Group
Substation Operators, elec.	416	27	432.7	6.5
Clerical	4,466	25*	37.3	0.55
Gas Plant Workers	1,031 total	23	147.7	2.2
Coke Oven Workers	102	12	784	11.7
General Workers	929	11	78	1.2
Field Representatives	508	8	107	1.8
Auto Mechanics	186	6	215.0	3.2
Chauffeurs	140	5	238.1	3.6
Attendants	359	4	74.2	1.1
Meter Testers	515	3	38.8	0.58
Gen. Gas and Elec. Appliance Repair Men	759	3	26.3	0.33
Splicers	274	3	73	1.9
Construction Workers	2,075	3	19.2	0.14
Mechanics "B"	2,489	6	16	0.24
Collectors	448	2	29.7	0.44
Stockmen	449	2	29.7	0.44
Meter Readers	354	1	18.8	0.29
Pharmacists	6	1	1,111.1	16.6
Resuscitator Instructor	1	1	6,666.6	100.0
Linemen	126	1	44.9	0.79
Other Miscellaneous	8,969	0	0	0
Totals	23,564	125	35.4	0.53

* One female.

of 432.7 for substation operators was regarded by CHRISTIAN as not being attributable to any occupational factor. Litigation cases on occupational lung cancer placed before American courts and Compensation Boards in recent years and chemical analyses of atmospheric pollutants from coal tar and pitch connected with such claims and presented at court, provide additional evidence that occupational lung cancer hazards from exposure to coal tar fumes and soot are not restricted to coke oven and gas retort workers (waterproofing, roofing, paving, oil and gas pipe tarring).

The exceptionally high exposures to benzpyrene which workers employed in such operations may sustain are clearly demonstrated also by recent studies of SAWICKI *et al.*, the results of which are summarized in the following Table (Table 64).

Similar observations on the considerable amounts of 3,4-benzpyrene which tar workers inhale with the vapors emitted from heated and melted tar used for the manufacture of cork stones were reported by BONNET, who found that some of the workmen engaged in such activities would inhale as much as 0.32 mg. of 3,4-benzpyrene per hour.

Table 64. *Benzpyrene Content of the Air Polluted with Coal Tar Fumes* (SAWICKI *et al.*)

Source of Outdoor Sample	Benzpyrene Content in Micrograms per 1000 cbm of Air
Industry I	4.8
I	0.52
II	1.3
II	0.73
II	1.5
Sidewalk Tarring Operation	110
Same	52
Same	78,000
Roof Tarring Operation	14,000
Same	870
Same	90

The literature contains a number of isolated observations on the occurrence of lung cancer in workers exposed to tar and pitch dust and fumes and exhibiting additional evidence of such carcinogenic exposures by showing tar dermatitis and cutaneous cancers (PATCH; RÖSCH; MÜLLSCHITZKY; KOELSCH; HUEPER; LANCET; BINI). (The occupations in involved in these cases were production of paraffin from retorting of bituminous coal, tar distillation, soot burning, smithy, waterproofing of masonry with liquid pitch; coke oven operation). BLÜMLEIN, moreover, noted that cancer of the larynx in his clinical material a causal relation to certain occupations involving an exposure to coal tar fumes (stokers, blacksmiths, locomotive engineers, tar and asphalt cookers, bakers, glass blowers and iron foundry workers). While KOLO-MAZNIK, ZDRAZIL and PICHA also recorded a frequent occurrence of laryngeal cancer and of pachydermas and leukoplakias of the larynx among foundry workers and pointed to an etiologic role of 3,4-benzpyrene in the dust and air of the two foundries studied, McLAUGHLIN mentioned the presence of cancer of the lung in three of 64 foundry workers examined autoptically. These observations are remarkable since no similar evidence has ever been mentioned in reports made in the United States on the health hazards existing in iron foundries, although such workers become exposed not only to pitch and tar dust while making cores but also to considerable amounts of fumes from such materials which are generated when the hot metal is being poured into the forms (HEUSTIS). Clinical and experimental observations demonstrated the carcinogenic property of pitch and tar used in several Silesian foundries (GORSKI).

It is likewise remarkable that no reports exist in this country on the frequency of lung cancer among coke oven operators of the steel industry, of the large coal tar distillation and fractionation industry and of the various industries in which carcinogenic tar products are used, such as for instance the manufactures of paper pulp conduits. The possibility of pulmonary cancer has not been considered in such operations according to a statement made rather recently by a representative of a Division of Industrial Hygiene of one of our leading States, although workers engaged in such production have not only developed cancers of the skin, but become also exposed to the inhalation of pitch fumes generated from the huge kettles containing liquid pitch used for coating the paper conduits which caused loss of smell and taste.

A similar situation seems to exist in regard to respiratory cancer hazards related to the inhalation of pitch and tar dust and fumes to which workers employed in electrometallurgical plants become exposed, although some of these workers have not only developed skin warts but also a fibrosing type of "pneumoconiosis" (WATSON, BLACK, DOIG and NAGELSCHMIDT; LOCKHART; MALY and MADER; MADER) having a certain similarity to that reported in commercial soot (lamp black) producers (GÄRTNER and BRAUSS; TÖPPNER).

These observations acquire a definite significance because ASK-UPMARK reported an excessive frequency of lung cancer among Swedish printers inhaling particles of carbon black containing ink in addition to mineral oil mist dispersed from rotary presses in workrooms. It is likely that the occurrence of a carcinoma of STENSEN's duct in a chemist who worked with various types of carbon black also belongs to this type of cancer hazard from contact with coal tar derivatives (MAISEL, PEARCE, CONNOLLY and PEARCE).

Since rubber workers also have exhibited evidence of a carbon black pneumoconiosis (MILLER and RAMSDEN), it is pertinent to note that also carbon black prepared from natural gas and carcinogenic bunker C fuel residual oil of petroleum distillation contains known carcinogenic polycyclic aromatic hydrocarbons which when eluted into benzol extracts, are capable of producing cancers in experimental animals (STEINER; FALK and STEINER; VON HAAM, CAPLAN and SHINOWARA; VON HAAM, TITUS, CAPLAN and SHINOWARA; VON HAAM and MALLETTE; NAU et al.; NEAL, THORNTON and NAU). Commercial carbon blacks or soots thus resemble in this respect ordinary soot (STEINBRÜCK; PASSEY). Because of these chemical and biologic qualities of carbon black, it is remarkable, if not surprising, that INGALLS has not been able to demonstrate any unusual liability of American carbon black workers to cancers of any kind, including cancers of skin and lung, although they have intense cutaneous, respiratory and ingestive contact with an obviously carcinogenic product subject to the influence of natural eluting agents when in contact with human tissues. Carbon black producing and consuming industries, like the coal tar and pitch industries, therefore, seem to represent a profitable field for competent and constructive future epidemiological studies on the frequency of cancers of all sites and especially of those of the respiratory tract among their employees.

Such data should prove to be of definite value in assessing and controlling industrial cancer hazards within such establishments, in providing reliable and significant evidence in connection with litigations for cancers contracted by exposure to occupationally active carcinogenic agents, particularly those related to coal tar, pitch and carbon black, and in determining the relative role which industrially produced and industry-related combustion and distillation products of coal play in the causation of respiratory cancers among members of the general population through their pollution of the environmental atmosphere. The presumptive importance of such atmospheric contaminations of urban and industrial areas is strongly supported by two types of epidemiologic observations made in various countries: 1) It has been shown that lung cancer rates are practically always distinctly higher in urban populations and are especially so whenever a high density population lives in a highly industrialized zone (STOCKS; CURWEN, KENNAWAY and KENNAWAY; SHABAD; DIKUN, SHABAD and NORKIN; SARUTA et al.; GORHAM; POCHE, MITTMANN and KNELLER; HAENSZEL; MAN-

CUSO, MacFARLANE and PORTERFIELD; KOTIN; HUEPER; HUEPER et al.; WILDER; MILLS); 2) The lung cancer rates increase with the decrease in the socioeconomic status, i.e., with residence in heavily polluted parts of communities (CURWEN, KENNAWAY and KENNAWAY; STOCKS; COHART; MANCUSO and COULTER; GRAHAM, LEVIN and LILIENFELD). It can be considered as an established fact that the principal pollution of the air of urban communities with industrial and industry-related carcinogens is of the polycyclic aromatic hydrocarbon type (Table 65).

Table 65. *Reported Values of 3,4-Benzpyrene Concentrations in the Atmosphere*
(Micrograms per 1,000 cbm of Air)
(G. WYNNE GRIFFITH)

Country	Place	Concentration	Season	Source
Wales	Countryside	Annual Average	0.9	STOCKS (1960)
England	Industrial City	Annual Average	108.0	STOCKS (1960)
Wales	Small Market Town	Summer	2.0	STOCKS et al. (1961)
England	Center of Large City	Winter	166.0	STOCKS et al. (1961)
U.S.A.	94 Urban Sites	Range of Annual Averages	0.11 to 61.0	SAWICKI et al. (1960)
	28 Rural Sites	Range of Annual Averages	0.01 to 1.9	SAWICKI et al. (1960)
	9 Cities	Summer	Lowest Value 0.25	SAWICKI et al. (1960)
		Winter	Highest Value 74.0	SAWICKI et al. (1960)
Denmark	Copenhagen	Average	10	DOLL (1958)
Norway	Oslo	Average	6	DOLL (1958)
Iceland	Reykjavik	Summer	2.5	DOLL (1958)

c) Experimental Respiratory Carcinogenesis

In early attempts to demonstrate the carcinogenic action of occupational and environmental air pollutants derived from the combustion and distillation of coal, coal tar was applied to the skin of mice (Fig. 41). This procedure usually resulted in an increase of the number of pulmonary tumors (adenomas and carcinomas) which were formed also spontaneously without such an intervention in the lungs of the particular mouse strains used (MURPHY and STURM; SANSSONOW; SCHABAD). Similar pulmonary neoplastic reactions were obtained with this method in rats (MOLLER). While such a procedure provides adequate evidence of the carcinogenic property of the agent used, it does not actually prove that the effect would be identical if the air pollutant would be inhaled by man.

Of similar connotation are the various experiments in which the tarry fraction of air pollutants collected from cities with an industrial coal economy were subcutaneously injected into mice where they induced the formation of sarcomas (LEITER, SHIMKIN and SHEAR; HUEPER et al.). An intravenous introduction of tar into rabbits merely resulted in the development of inflammatory pulmonary responses and of atypical epithelial bronchiolar proliferations (TEDESCHI; SIMONDS and CURTIS). Similar reactions were elicited in the lungs of rats when tarry constituents of air pollutants were intrapleurally implanted into rats and mice (Fig. 42) (HUEPER), or when coal tar was directly injected into the lungs of rabbits (GARSCHIN and PIGALEW).

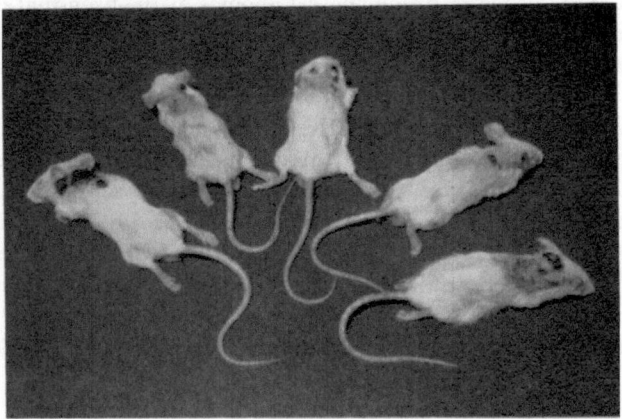

Fig. 41. Carcinomas of the skin of mice painted with carcinogenic Bergius oil tar

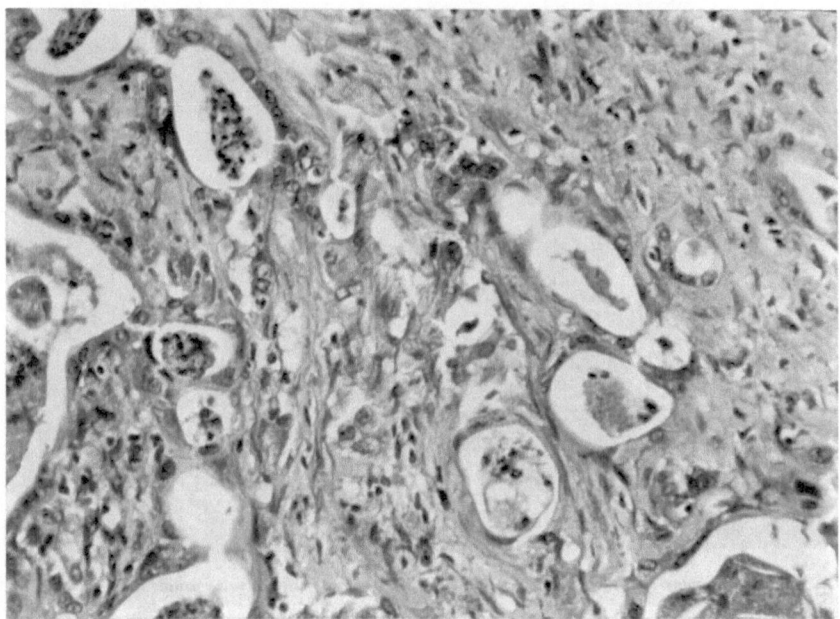

Fig. 42. Atypical proliferations of the bronchiolar epithelium in the lungs of a mouse following repeated intrapleural injections of the tarry fraction of urban air pollutants

It seems that also a direct intratracheal insufflation of coal tar into mice and rabbits elicited merely atypical proliferations of the bronchiolar epithelium but not bona fide carcinomas (SCHABAD), although MINURA made such a claim for a lesion induced in a rabbit thus exposed because a reliable distinction between atypical glandular proliferations and adenocarcinoma may at times be difficult. Of distinctly more definite character as to the production of cancers of different histologic types in the lungs of rats are the observations recently reported by SHABAD and by OSHIMA. These investigators succeeded in producing carcinomas of the bronchial epithelium by introducing into the trachea of rats carbon particles to the surfaces of which known polycyclic aromatic hydrocarbons (3,4-benzpyrene; 7,12-dimethyl benz(a)anthracene) were adsorbed. Through this manipulation a prolonged action of the carcinogen on the bronchial mucosa was obtained, since the carcinogen was only gradually released from its binding to the carbon particles. It may be mentioned that probably a greater part of the carcinogenic polycyclic aromatic hydrocarbons present in polluted air of coal tar operations as well as in urban areas, exists in this type of binding and does not consist of free molecules, as this has been assumed for aromatic carcinogens in cigarette smoke. The experimental evidence cited indeed suggests that carcinogens in free molecular form in the inhaled air are apparently carcinogenically less effective than those attached to the surfaces of particulate matter, such as carbon or iron oxide.

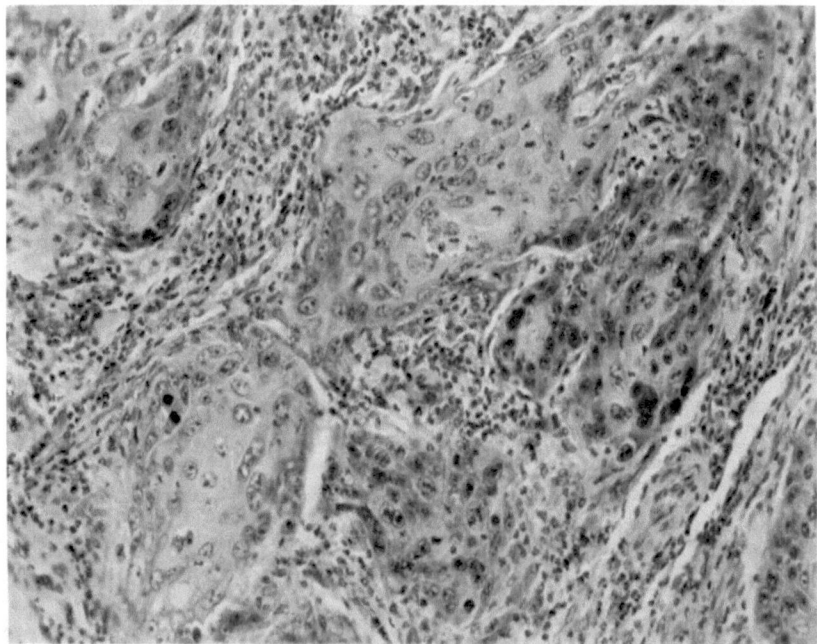

Fig. 43. Cornified squamous-cell carcinoma of the skin of a mouse painted with condensate of coal tar fumes

The inhalation of tarry matter present in the dust obtained from tarred roads (CAMPBELL), or produced by the burning of bituminous coal and used as bedding material (SEELIG and BENIGNUS), caused an increase in the number of pulmonary tumors occurring also spontaneously in mice. No such effect, however, was elicited when mice inhaled directly the smoke from burning bituminous coal (SCHNURER and HAYTHORNE) or when lamp black was employed as bedding material (SEELIG and BENIGNUS) or when they inhaled the heavily polluted air of central Glasgow (PEAcock), or when they became exposed to the fumes given off by heated coal tar (Mestitzova and Kossey; Hueper and Payne). Similarly equivocal results were observed when rats, and guinea pigs inhaled for up to two years, coal tar fumes or soot obtained from smokestacks of coffee roasting plants although condensed coal tar fumes as well as coffee soot displayed definite carcinogenic properties when subcutaneously or intramuscularly injected into rats and mice (Hueper and Payne) (Tables 66 and 67), (Fig. 43).

Table 66. *Neoplastic Reactions in Rats, Guinea Pigs, and Hamsters Inhaling Maximal Tolerated Doses of Fumes from Heated Coal Tar and Petroleum Asphalt, Cutting Oil Fog, Coffee Roast Soot for Up to 24 Months*

Substance	Species	No.	Tumors of Lung		Neoplastic Reactions at Other Sites				
			Adenoma	Carci-noma	Bladder	Liver	Lymph Node	Uterus	Others
Coal Tar Fumes	Rat	75	0	0		6	2		
	Guinea Pig	42	0	0					
Petroleum Roofing Asphalt Fumes	Rat	65	0	0		3	2	1	
Cutting Oil Mist	Rat	105		1		1			
	Guinea Pig	65	0	0					
Coffee Soot Dust	Rat	60	3	0		10		1	6
	Guinea Pig	25	2	0	3				

Table 67. *Cancer of the Skin and Muscular and Subcutaneous Tissues of Mice and Rats Produced by the Administration of Condensates of Fumes of Heated Coal Tar and Petroleum Asphalts, of Paraffinic Cutting Oil, and of Acetone Extract of Coffee Roast Soot*

Substance	Species	No.	Route of Administration	Cancers at Site of Administration	Cancers Remote From Site of Administration
Coal Tar Fume Condensate Petroleum	Mouse	50	Skin	22	
Roofing	Mouse	50	Skin	1 (?)	
Asphalt Cutting Oil	Mouse	50	Skin	1	2
		100	Muscle		4
Coffee Roast	Mouse	100	Muscle		2
Soot Extract		100	Muscle	1	2
	Rat	60	Skin	1	4
Coffee Roast Soot	Rat	30	Muscle		3
4 Petroleum Road	Mouse	250	Skin	2	7
Asphalts		200	Muscle	3	1
	Rat	120	Muscle	13	16

If thus the experimental production of lung cancers in animals by the mechanism and route of exposure evidently operating in the causation of cancers of the respiratory tract by the inhalation of coal tar fumes and dust has remained a disappointing procedure, this methodologic inadequacy is shared with that of most other known human respiratory carcinogens (Hueper). However, such shortcomings in experimental test methods do not negate the convincing and conclusive evidence provided by clinical and epidemiological data obtained on human population groups exposed to the inhalation of coal tar and pitch fumes and dust and developing cancers of the respiratory system because of it.

10. Petroleum — Mineral Oil — Wax — Asphalt — Petroleum Carbon — Carbon Black — Methylated Naphthalene — Combustion Products — Shale Oil and Derivatives

a) Technological Aspects

Mineral oils and related products, such as waxes, tars, asphalts, and pitches, can be obtained by the distillation and fractionation of various natural raw products, such as petroleum, oil shale, bituminous coal, natural asphalts, and hydrogenated coal (HUEPER; GOLDBLATT and GOLDBLATT; PAGE et al.; LIJINSKY). Since these raw products vary according to their derivation among each other as well as among members of the same group in their chemical composition, and because this quality is distinctly influenced for their derivatives by the types of processing procedures used, the great majority of these products lacks any definite chemical uniformity and standardization. Nevertheless, the general rule can be applied that derivatives which have been obtained by the application of high temperatures resulting in the formation of cyclic compounds (AULD) or are the result of cracking processes (HOLT et al.) contain polycyclic aromatic hydrocarbons, some of which are recognized and potent chemical carcinogens to man and animals (HIEGER and WOODHOUSE; TWORT and FULTON; EBY, PRIESTLEY, REHNER and HALE; SHUBIK, SAFFIOTTI, LIJINSKY, PIETRA et al.; LIJINSKY, DOMSKY and RAHA; EICHHOFF and TITSCHACK; TEBBENS, THOMAS and MUKAI).

Although it has been claimed that only such products having a high boiling point are carcinogenic, human and experimental observations definitely show that also derivatives distilling over at a boiling point below 700 °C. such as methylated naphthalenes, may possess carcinogenic properties (SHUBIK and SAFFIOTTI; HUEPER and CAHNMANN; ANDERVONT; POEL; HORTON, DENMAN and TROSSET; KOTIN, FALK and THOMAS; LUSHBAUGH; LUSHBAUGH and HACKETT).

In fact, there exists an increasing amount of evidence incriminating not only aromatic components of mineral oils and related chemicals in the production of cancers, but also aliphatic chemicals such as paraffins, aliphatic epoxides (ozonized gasoline) and nitro olefins (SHUBIK, SAFFIOTTI, LIJINSKY et al.; KOTIN, FALK and McCAMMON; KOTIN, FALK and THOMAS; KOTIN and FALK; JULSRUD; DEICHMANN).

The carcinogenic properties of these materials is being attested by numerous reports relating the development of cancers of the skin, including scrotal skin, in various types of worker groups having an occupational contact with them (lubricating oil, paraffin oil, cooling oil, waxes, fuel oil, asphalt and coke of stills, plasticizers in tiles, fillers in rubber, electrode component, etc.) as well as in several species of experimental animals to which they were applied or injected (HENDRICKS, BERRY, LIONE and THORPE; LIONE; SOUTHAM and WILSON; HENRY; WADE; ECKARDT; HOLT; PAGE et al.; SMITH and SUNDERLAND; CRUICKSHANK and GOUREVITCH; CRUICKSHANK and SQUIRE; AULD; BROCKBANK; SQUIRE, CRUICKSHANK and TOPLEY; FIFE; GILMAN and VESSELINOVITCH; MASTROMATTEO; SPINK; BAYNES and TOMBLESON; HUEPER and PAYNE; SIMMERS; HUEPER and CAHNMANN; STEINBRUCK and CARL; WYNDER; SUNDERLAND, SMITH and SUGIURA; TWORT and TWORT; VOSAMAE; COOK, CARRUTHERS and WOODHOUSE; WOODHOUSE; LIJINSKY et al.; WADE; MacKENNA and HORNER). The great majority of the occupational oil cancers of the skin were reported from Great Britain. Not more than 10% of the observations originated from the United States despite their much more extensive production and use and a greatly higher production of petroleum derivatives in the U.S.A. than in Great Britain. As a partial explanation of this astounding phenomenon, reference may be made to a remark of ECKARDT who stated that, "the carcinogenicity of cutting oils is of such a low degree that good personal and industrial hygiene practices should eliminate any cancer hazard associated with these materials". The perhaps industrially unpleasant fact nevertheless exists — despite this admonition of taking rather lightly possible cancer hazards from such agents — that cancers of the skin from occupational contact with cutting oils have been observed in American metallurgical establishments. They regrettable, however, have not been made a matter of public record although such effects were demonstrated also in experimental animals (HUEPER and PAYNE). Litigations regarding such cases were rather settled out of court. The occurrence of skin cancers in man and experimental animals from exposure to cutting oils, on the other hand, has been reported by Canadian investigators (MASTROMATTEO; GILMAN and VESSELINOVITCH).

Only one American oil company has chosen to publish its more recent experiences on the occurrence of cancers of the scrotal skin in paraffin pressers (HENDRICKS, BERRY, LIONE, and THORPE; LIONE and DENHOLM) and has done this only after a delay of ten years when the paraffin pressing process for obtaining waxes had been replaced by the solvent process, although wax cancers have been known for many years (DAVIS; LONGMUIR; HUEPER). Since similar conditions of exposure to carcinogenic oils from which crude or "slack" wax is pressed have prevailed in other oil companies, according to reliable observations, it stands to reason that some such cancers must have occurred also in employees of these companies. Whether many of the victims of these occupational petroleum wax cancers received compensation for having contracted an often fatal occupational paraffin oil cancer, appears to be doubtful because of the statutory time clause which limits the making of such claims. It is also symptomatic of the general policy adopted in the management of information on such matters that the very extensive experimental data on carcinogenic properties of petroleum products obtained at a Midwestern university under the sponsorship and with the financial support fo the American Petroleum Institute during twelve years of research, have not been published in printed form but seem to be considered still as "privileged information" if ECKART's philosophy in such matters should have been adhered to. The observation on oil cancers has suffered the same fate, which was assigned to a similar study on coal tar cancer hazards, which was conducted at the same university during the same period, and which was carried out under the sponsorship of a group of coal tar producers who had been stimulated by HUEPER to engage in such research in 1950.

A disconcerting amount of human and experimental evidence attests to a carcinogenic effect of fully-refined hard, soft and liquid paraffin products not only on animal tissues but also on human tissues when applied to the skin, ingested, inhaled, implanted into the lumen of the urinary bladder, or parenterally injected (COLOMB; SCHOCK; SCHMÄHL and REITER; BOYD and DOLL; HUEPER; DRUCKREY, SCHMAHL and PREUSSMANN; NEUKOMM; SHUBIK et al.; BONSER, BOYLAND, BUSBY and CLAYSON; BONSER, CLAYSON, JULL and PYRAH; QUERY; MEIGS; BONSER, CLAYSON and JULL; POTTER and ROBERTSON; IRVING, GUTMANN and LARSON). SHUBIK et al. reported the presence of 1.2.5.6-dibenzanthracene in fully refined paraffins used for the coating of milk containers, and PROKHOROVA and ZNAMENSKY recorded the demonstration of 3,4-benzpyrene in paraffins of Russian make. While petroleum waxes meeting certain physicochemical specifications are permitted in the food industry of the U.S.A., the two Russian investigators recommended that the foodstuff industry should be subject to controls in regard to the use of such waxes. The experimental production of cancers in the subcutaneous tissue of mice receiving implants of pellets of fully refined paraffin in which such impurities of carcinogenic aromatic hydrocarbons were not demonstrable with the most sensitive available methods — indicates that a carcinogenic effect of paraffin seems to depend on both aromatic and aliphatic chemical constituents of crude, semi-refined and fully-refined waxes.

Apart from the various contacts which human population groups have with these carcinogenic agents for occupational and economic-environmental reasons, such exposures may occur also because of the pollution of some natural media with native petroleum oils. Such petroleum oils and the polycyclic aromatic hydrocarbons contained in them have been demonstrated in the sediments of the Gulf of Mexico (WHITEHEAD and BREGER; SMITH; BAKER; MULIK and ERDMANN) as well as in South African asbestos (crocidolite) (HARINGTON), and in manganese nodules of the western North Atlantic (THOMAS and BLUMER). These findings indicate a rather wide range of natural occurrence of polynuclear hydrocarbons related to natural types of mineral oils and their prolonged preservation in strongly oxidized sediments over many thousands of years. Natural crude petroleum, moreover, has seeped in and contaminated in some areas of the United States, local drinking water supplies. Petroleum and mineral oils from natural sources, as well as from dumping ship fuel oil and escape of engine exhausts into ocean, lake and river waters, especially in or near harbor areas, has been polluting to an increasing degree all bodies of water within or near industrialized countries (CAHNMANN and KURATSUNE; HUEPER).

It is noteworthy in this connection that non-processed natural bitumen or asphalt, such as that mined from the "asphalt lake" in Trinidad, has not displayed any carcinogenic properties in man (ZEGLIO) and experimental animals (HUEPER), although crude natural petroleum oils, particularly those rich in aromatic compounds, have induced cancers when applied to the skin of mice and rabbits (HIEGER and WOODHOUSE; TWORT and FULTON) and may have been involved in the causation of skin cancers in oil field workers (SCHWARTZ, TULIPAN and BIRMINGHAM).

Carcinogenic constituents of mineral oils and derivatives are emitted into the air in numerous occupational activities where they are used in the manufacture of numerous products (rubber, plastics, steel, linoleum, etc.) or as lubricants, coatings and as fuels. They are present in automobile exhausts and in the effluents of oil refineries and filling stations.

Exposure to various types of petroleum products is rather widespread for the populations of industrialized countries for both occupational and environmental reasons (dietary, cosmetic, medicinal, atmospheric, aquatic, sanitary, etc.) (HUEPER). They form constituents of polishes, paints, pesticide preparations, paper and food container coatings, printing materials, water repellents of brick walls and textiles, lubricants, fuel oils, and many other products used in plants and homes (Division of Air Pollution; HENDRICKS).

b) Epidemiology

Occupational respiratory contact with these products may be due to an inhalation of oil fogs, mists and sprays, such as those encountered under occupational condi-

tions in paraffin pressing sheds, metal lathe operations, spraying of pesticide preparations, investment casting, high pressure lubrication, diesel jet testing, paraffin oil
spraying of brick construction, textile spinning, and printing, and complication also
exposures to combustion products in automobile and diesel engine exhausts (Jones;
Tubich et al.; Humperdinck; Meyer-Brodnitz). A habitual and occupational inhalation or ingestion of mineral oil containing nasal and laryngeal sprays creates a
similar respiratory contact with paraffin oils and also may cause an oil pneumonia
(Foe and Bigham; Proudfit et al.; Jampolis et al.; Sante; Wood). While it has
often been asserted that the ingestion of such oils for laxating purposes may lead to
an aspiration of such oils into the lungs and thereby to the development of an oil
pneumonitis, it is more likely that the oil droplets retained under such conditions in
the lungs enter the body through resorption by the intestinal mucosa from where they
are transported into the blood of the vena cava inferior, the thoracic duct and the
pulmonary arterial system. Here they are retained finally within the pulmonary
capillaries (Daniel, Frazer, French and Sammons; Hueper; Meyers and Griffith; Schneider; Editorial) and thereby give rise to inflammatory and possibly
cancerous reactions.

Lung and larynx cancer hazards from occupational exposure to finely dispersed
or nebulized oil in the inhaled air have been recorded by Huguenin, Fauvet and
Bourdin for metallurgical workers, chauffeurs, garage mechanics and engineers.
Kennaway and Kennaway noted a relatively high ratio of laryngeal cancers, but
not of pulmonary cancers, in mulespinners having contact with shale oil and showing
a high attack rate of cancers of the skin, especially the scrotum and vulva. Southam
mentioned that mulespinners developed occasionally multiple primary cancers involving the lung and stomach in addition to the skin. Roesch observed a combination of
three primary cancers (skin, lung and stomach) in a paraffin presser; Touraine and
Bour also attributed the development of cancer of the lung in members of some
occupations to their inhalation of lubricating oil mists. Such exposures may account
also in part for the excessive lung cancer mortality among male metal grinders
observed by Turner and Grace. A similar observation concerning a special liability
to cancer of the lung by metal turners, mechanics, fitters and wood workers was
reported by Berndt. From an epidemiologic analysis of the relation of occupation
to cancer of the lung in Japan, Tsuchiya concluded that the only occupational group
showing a higher risk to lung cancer were workers exposed to petroleum products.

Additional suggestive evidence on such relationships involving an occupational
exposure to oil mist was advanced by Huguenin, Fauvet and Bourdin, and
Huguenin, Fauvet and Mazabraud. The epidemiologic analysis of employees of a
large Public Utility Company by Christian also provided evidence in support of
the view that an inhalation of oil mists and fumes created an excessive liability to
lung cancer since substation operators exposed to oil fumes from interruptors, had a
lung cancer rate of 433 per 100,000, chauffeurs had one of 238 and mechanics one of
215, while the average rate was 35.4.

Respiratory exposures to mineral oil fogs, mists and fumes are doubtlessly sustained by workers employed in automobile service stations and garages (Fredde), in
rolling mills using the cold reduction of steel strip (Jones), in iron casting operations
and steel plants (Larson) where mineral oil baths are employed for quenching purposes; in asbestos-cement plants where mineral oils are used as molding oils (Enge-

BRIGTSEN); in textile spinning establishments (EICKHOFF); in manufactures of roofing felt (GOLDFIELD and McANLIS), in industrial establishments in which mineral oil is used as an air filtering agent in air conditioning equipment (HECHT), and in large-scale spraying of pesticide preparations which are dispensed in methylated naphthalene. It is interesting to note that EICKHOFF could not detect any special cancer hazard from contact with mineral oils in German textile workers. Drinker even ventured the opinion that there was no scientific support for apprehension on the breathing of oil mists, either from machine shop work or from insecticide spraying where a gasoline-type vehicle is the vehicle.

While HENDRICKS et al. recently concluded from a review of the literature and from their own observations in oil refineries that "there is no evidence to suggest any relation between the inhalation of oil mist and lung cancer" and that paraffin pressers do not show an excessive liability to lung cancer, it is noteworthy that the existence of such causal associations are clearly demonstrated among the workers of one of the refineries included in the study of HENDRICKS et al. as evident from the data of Table 68 (HOLT).

Table 68. *Comparison of Lesions Among Pressmen with 10 Years or More Service with the Normal Male Population Using Adjusted Rates for Both the Pressmen and the Normal Population* (HOLT et al.)

Site of Lesion	Adjusted Rate per 100,000		% of Total Lesions Adjusted	
	Normal Population	Pressmen	Normal Population	Pressmen
Lung	30	271	7.3	13.3
Stomach	68	407	16.3	20.0
Intestines	35	135	8.7	6.6
Rectum	34	135	8.3	6.6
Scrotum	0.15	1080	—	53.0

According to HOLT, the probabilities of the observed cancer cases occurring in the normal population were as follows: Lung: One in 10,000; Stomach: Five in 10,000; Scrotum: Less than 3 in ten trillion. These findings are in general agreement with those made in another oil refinery in which a survey revealed that of 19 cases of lung cancer occurring among the total number of employees of all types, 17 cases involved workers engaged in manufacturing processes and only two (2) affected white collar workers, although their ratio was 1 : 2.

Apart from the fact that cancers have developed at times from cosmetic paraffinomas present in various human organs (BAUER; BAADER; SCHMAEHL and REITER), such developments have been reported occasionally also as sequelae of medicinal oil pneumonia (WOOD; SANTÉ). The recent observations of BONSER et al. on the development of cancers of the bladder in rats with intravesically placed paraffin pellets and of similar neoplasms in the bladder of mice equally treated (MEIGS) and the production of subcutaneous sarcomas around paraffin implants in mice (SHUBIK et al.) give convincing testimony of the carcinogenic properties possessed by even fully refined paraffin waxes and paraffin oils. They support the view that the inhalation of such products in nebulized form should create a serious respiratory cancer hazard to the millions of workers employed in many industries, and different occupations, and exposed to oil mists, fogs and sprays (HUEPER and PAYNE).

Of even more serious and general significance in this respect is the inhalation of exhaust fumes emitted from gasoline motors and diesel engines, since such effluents contain not only often unburned fuel in the form of oil droplets but also appreciable amounts of newly created carcinogenic combustion products. The atmospheric pollution with these carcinogenic constituents of the exhausts of automobiles, busses and trucks as well as of many types of industrial machines and airplane motors, is responsible for a considerable fraction of the rapidly increasing smog formation in all metropolitan areas (KOTIN and FALK; LYONS; KATZ; COMMINS; COOPER; WALLER; COMMINS and LAWTHER; WYNDER; MILLS; FITTON).

During recent years repeated attempts have been made to minimize the cancer hazards to respiratory organs which might result from the release of diesel engine exhaust into the air of workshops as well as of the general environment, by claiming that such effluents while being toxic, do not contain any carcinogenic polycyclic aromatic hydrocarbons if the operation of a diesel engine is well adjusted (COMMINS, WALLER and LAWTHER; COMMITTEE ON MEDICAL SCIENCE, EDUCATION, and RESEARCH). Support for this general allegation has been provided by the failure of several experimental investigations in obtaining skin and lung cancers in mice or rabbits, respectively, which were either painted with diesel engine exhaust soot or inhaled it (MITTLER and NICHOLSON; SCHMIDTMANN).

Such assertions should not be accepted as valid for the following reasons. Since the type of exhaust released from diesel engines depends upon the type of engine and the fuel supplied to it as well as on the conditions under which an engine is operated (availability of oxygen, workload), there probably does not exist any typical diesel pollution (BATTIGELLI). The ideal operating conditions used for demonstrating the carcinogenic innocuousness of diesel engine exhaust do not exist under many "normal" conditions of operation of diesel engines and many of these engines are not kept in proper working condition. This is visibly apparent from the frequent release of dark black soot from the exhaust pipes of diesel trucks. Such soot does not contain only carbon but also carcinogenic polycyclic aromatic hydrocarbons (KÜHN; SULLIVAN and CLEARY; BATTIGELLI; KOTIN, FALK and THOMAS; CLEMO). The carcinogenic chemicals present in the diesel engine exhaust therefore, can be expected to be present whenever a diesel engine is subjected to excessive strain usually caused by an overload or when it is operated in an environment with limited oxygen supply (mines, tunnels) (WALLER, COMMINS and LAWTHER; HOLTZ; CROOK; SULLIVAN and CLEARY). Such pollutions are likely to exist also in inadequately ventilated diesel engine test rooms and repair shops (CALBIANI).

While the available human evidence does as yet not definitely establish whether an occupational inhalation of diesel engine fumes has solely been responsible for the production of lung cancers in man, the carcinogenic constituents in their exhaust certainly would tend to aggravate the total load of inhaled carcinogenic chemicals in all individuals exposed to such atmospheric pollutants. Diesel engine exhausts thus may significantly contribute to the development of lung cancers among members of such population groups. The epidemiologic studies by KAPLAN and by RAFFLE on the lung cancer liability of operating railroad workers in the United States and in England have led these investigators to the conclusion that the lung cancers observed among these railroad workers did not have any apparent causative relationship to diesel fume inhalation. The statistical methods used by KAPLAN and the control groups chosen by him to prove this claim, however, are of a type which destroys any scientific value of the conclusions reached by KAPLAN from his data. The negative evidence by KAPLAN, moreover, is refuted by observations published by HUEPER on this subject, who found that 75% of all lung cancers among railroad empoyees of two large American companies were found among operating railroad workers who constituted only 25% of the total number of employees. KAPLAN's findings also disagree with the data obtained by Ross from an analysis of the rapid growth of the lung cancer rate among members of the Brotherhood of Railroad Trainmen between 1935 and 1952 (Table 69) (10 fold).

Table 69. *Incident of Cancer other than of the Lungs from Insurance Records of the Brotherhood of Locomotive Engineers, Brotherhood of Locomotive Firemen and Enginemen, and Brotherhood of Railroad Trainmen*

Year	Deaths from Cancer other than that of the Lungs			
	Firemen (per 50,000)	Trainmen (per 100,000)	Engineers (per 50,000)	Total
1942	77	164	75	316
1943	79	161	83	323
1944	88	190	93	371
1945	74	176	88	338
1946	92	215	91	398
1947	91	229	76	396
1948	70	200	82	352
1949	85	240	86	411
1950	77	206	74	357
1951	87	230	109	426
1952	81	238	80	399
Totals	901	2,249	937	4,087
Increase Cancer (less lung) comparing 1942—1953	5.19%	45.12%	6.67%	26.27%
Increase Cancer (less lung) comparing 1942—1951	12.99%	40.24%	45.33%	34.81%
Average Increase of Cancer (less lungs) for 10 years, 1942—1951, incl.	6.49%	22.56%	14.67%	16.77%

January 25, 1954, E. S. Ross, M. D., Chief Medical Director, Brotherhood of Railroad Trainmen.

Chemically similar exposures are sustained by petroleum asphalt workers, road construction and repair workers, tile makers, carbon electrode manufacturers and users, and many others who inhale petroleum asphalt dust and fumes with demonstrated carcinogenic properties (LOCKHART; MALY and MADER; HUEPER and PAYNE; SIMMONS).

Such pollutions with carcinogenic hydrocarbons generated by the incomplete combustion of gasoline and motor oil may recently have been intensified by the introduction of possibly carcinogenic additives, such as lead naphthenate, carbon tetrachloride, 1:1:1-trichlorethane, etc. to gasoline (BALDWIN, CUNNINGHAM and

PRATT; DOOLEY). A similar observation was made also in regard to additives used in cutting oils which, when applied to the skin of mice, induced cancer formation (GILMAN and VESSELINOVITCH).

Finally, attention may be called to types of exposure to petroleum products which may create respiratory cancer hazards for workers employed in tobacco sheds in which tobacco leaves are cured by exposing them to the heat and soot generated by the burning of carcinogenic residual fuel oils, or for workers in and residents of quarters which are heated with stoves and burners using kerosene or petroleum oil as fuel (DIKUN), or for agricultural laborers employed in or living near orchards and vege-table fields protected against cold spells by the burning of old rubber tires and fuel oil in smudge pots, by the production of large amounts of soot. The failure to produce skin cancers in mice (MIESCHER and SCHWARZ) treated with a concentrated benzol extract of oil soot from a domestic oil burner in an ointment base cannot be con-sidered as a competent type of experimental study since the maximal duration of the experiment was only 272 days and was, therefore, insufficient for covering even half of the minimal latent period of a bona fide carcinogenic bioassay on test materials of the type used (HUEPER and CONWAY; HUEPER and PAYNE; KURATSUNE and HUEPER).

The numerous observations on the causative role of polycyclic aromatic hydro-carbons present in various carbonaceous materials widely used for the production of heat and energy in the human economy and discharged often into the air of work rooms and communities without any consideration of the possible and even actual respiratory cancer hazards created thereby, deserve serious attention by all public health agencies if any rational prevention of respiratory cancers is to be attempted (SULA).

11. Ionizing Radiations

a) Technological Aspects

Exposure of man to ionizing radiations (alpha-, beta-, and gamma rays) occurs from natural as well as man-made sources. Natural radiations act either from exter-nal sources, such as cosmic radiation and radiations arising from radioactive elements present in the crust of the earth and as potassium 40 and carbon 14 in organic matter, including foodstuffs. Radioactive matter present in the atmosphere in the form of gas (radon) or dust may be inhaled or ingested and may consist of natural elements or, if the product of atomic nuclear operations, may be of man-made origin. X-radiation or Roentgen-radiation generated by many devices such as cathode tubes, x-ray tubes, electron guns, x-ray diffraction apparatus, radioactive static eliminators, television tubes and radar apparatus, is essentially a product of man-made activities.

While all living matter, including man, has been exposed since time immemorial to usually minor doses of natural ionizing radiations from external sources and has withstood such influences without any apparent major biologic injury, this situation has undergone, since the turn of the century with the discovery of radioactive chemi-cals and x-radiation, and particularly since the more recent development of atomic energy during the last 20 years, fundamental changes. During this period, health hazards and especially cancer hazards to man from contact with radioactive chemicals from various sources have grown from rather modest importance of often local proportions to problems of major and worldwide significance involving mankind at large.

Several large worker groups and population groups have become affected by this development to an exceptional degree because of their employment in occupations entailing the production of radioactive materials or on account of their exposure to radioactive matter and ionizing radiations released by the detonation of nuclear devices. As the result of the last mentioned events occurring in different parts of the world, the human environment — including food, water and air — have become contaminated with radioactive matter of different types and with different biologic affinities and effects. The increasing use of ionizing radiations in medicine for diagnostic and therapeutic purposes has added to and intensified these exposures for many individuals. Because all types of radiation exert eminent carcinogenic effects on man and experimental animals, this development has been associated with the appearance of a rapidly rising number of cancers in man affecting a variety of organs and tissues which depend on the specific type of radioactive materials active and upon their external or internal route of exposure. Such radiation cancers have been induced as the result of occupational, cosmetic, dietary, medical, military and environmental exposures (HUEPER; AUB; EVANS; HEMPELMANN and MARTLAND; MEDICAL RESEARCH COUNCIL; GLUCKSMANN, LAMERTON and MAYNEORD; ZUPPINGER; TULLIS; WARREN). Organs of the respiratory system have become involved whenever gases or dust emitting ionizing radiations were inhaled or radioactive matter was directly introduced into the ducts and cavities of the respiratory tract or when penetrating ionizing radiations acted from the outside upon respiratory organs.

b) Epidemiology

Up to some 20 years ago, occupational exposures of the respiratory organs to radioactive agents were limited to relatively small groups of industrial and professional workers (miners and refiners of radioactive ores, especially pitchblende, industrial and medical consumers of radioactive substances, such as gas mantle manufacturers, luminous dial painters, radio tube makers, physicists and radiologists). Non-occupational, medicinal exposures of these tissues to ionizing radiations (x-rays), on the other hand, involved a considerably larger group of individuals, particularly those receiving large doses of x-rays for therapeutic purposes delivered over the chest or neck because of malignant tumors or tuberculous lymph nodes in these regions. Since the advent of nuclear energy production, the manufacture of radioactive isotopes and the explosion of nuclear devices, the number and variety of persons inhaling radioactive gases and dusts have not only grown in the occupational fields but also have become practically universal as the result of radioactive fallout as far as the general population is concerned. Occupational exposures are not infrequently unsuspected by investigators not familiar with industrial practices. They may affect sometimes a much larger number of workers than the ones directly concerned with the operation of diverse devices emitting radioactive energy and particles (undertakers, employees of pathologic institutes, printers, textile and paper makers, cleaning personnel of research laboratories and industrial facilities where radioactive isotopes are employed, sewage disposal workers, etc.).

a) Respiratory Cancers in Radioactive Ore Miners and Millers

aa) Radioactive, Non-Uranium Miners
aβ) Lung Cancer in Schneeberg Miners

The oldest known occupational respiratory cancer hazard has been associated for several centuries with the mining of radioactive ores although its exact causal mechanism, i.e., inhalation of radioactive gases and dust, has been recognized only rather recently. The original observations on the frequent occurrence of a chronic pulmonary disease fatal during the prime of life among the miners of the Erzgebirge, on both the Saxon and Bohemian sides, had been noted since the Middle Ages (AGRICOLA in 1500; MATTHESIUS 1559; PANSA in 1607; SCHEFFLER in 1770, etc.) (PIRCHAN and SIKL; LÖWY). The Schneeberg mines located on the northern or Saxon slope of the Erz Mountains were worked since 1410 first for copper and iron, since 1740 for silver, zinc, tin, lead, manganese and magnesium, and at present for bismuth, arsenic, nickel and cobalt, i.e., they were not mined for radioactive ores, such as pitchblende (uranium ore), although such operations may have been introduced since the end of World War II.

The pulmonary ailment affecting the miners at Schneeberg was known for many years before its actual neoplastic character was recognized, as "Bergsucht" (miners' phthisis, or mountain disease). The anatomic nature of this disorder was not discovered until 1879, when HÄRTING and HESSE proved it to be of neoplastic nature. It was diagnosed at that time as a "lymphosarcoma fibromatodes". Since 1926 the studies of ROSTOSKI, SAUPE and SCHMORL established definitely these pulmonary tumors as carcinomas of the lung, after ARNSTEIN in 1913 had first diagnosed some of these cancers as squamous cell carcinomas. During the interval these occupational pulmonary radiation cancers had become the subject of investigation by various German scientists (COHNHEIM, 1882; ANCKE, 1884; ARNSTEIN, 1913; UHLIG, 1920; RISEL, 1921).

The Schneeberg mines employed at an average 650 miners during the years 1869 to 1877. There was some labor turnover. Death from miners' disease, which, was estimated as cancerous in about 75%, according to HÄRTING and HESSE, removed between 1869—1871, 63 miners, between 1872—1874, 47 miners and between 1875—1877, 40 miners. KOELSCH noted that between 1875 and 1912, out of 469 deaths of miners, 276 were due to cancer of the lung (10 to tuberculosis and 183 to other causes). An enquiry among 143 working and retired miners conducted in 1913 by ARNSTEIN revealed that cancer of the lung still existed among the miners. This disease, on the other hand, was absent among 176 workers employed in the ultramarine cobalt factory at the nearby Oberschlema. SAUPE found radiographic evidence of lung cancer in eight (8) out of 143 working miners examined.

By 1922 the erroneous opinion prevailed in authoritative circles, that this occupational cancer hazard had ceased to exist (ROSTOSKI). What actually had occurred during these years was a progressive reduction in the number of miners (ARNSTEIN) which had dropped by 1928 from formerly some 800 men to only 116 actually at work, and 38 former miners (total 154), thereby decreasing the size of the effectively exposed worker group. During the preceding three (3) years, 21 of the 154 miners had died. Autopsies performed on 13 of them revealed the presence of a lung cancer in all of them, while clinical evidence indicated the existence of additional lung cancers in two (2) of the eight (8) cases in which a post mortem examination was not made. Thus lung cancer was found in 15 of 21 miners (71 per cent). By 1939, there were only approximately 70 miners employed in the Schneeberg mines. In about 75 to 80 per cent, lung cancer was the cause of death in members of this relatively old worker group (HUECK). The rather frequent multifocal origin of the Schneeberg lung cancers noted by SCHMORL and by BEYREUTHER (25% of the cases) was not evident at that time among the seven cases examined by HUECK. Epidemiologie studies performed at that time on control worker groups, including miners working in non-radioactive or weakly radioactive mines and in plants as well as in the general population in the vicinity of Schneeberg, did not reveal any excessive lung cancer incidence (ROSTOSKI, SAUPE and SCHMORL; HUECK; ROSTOSKI). Schneeberg lung cancers were still observed in 1957 according to a report of SEPKE.

The statistical data on lung cancer rates among Schneeberg miners together with comparative figures for lung cancer rates in the population of Vienna presented by PELLER in 1939 demonstrate adequately the scope of the cancer hazard existing at Schneeberg (Table 70).

Table 70. *Crude Cancer Mortality per 1,000 in Schneeberg Miners*

	Miners in Schneeberg		Vienna Males 15—79 years of age 1932—1936
	1875—1894	1895—1912	
Lung Cancer	12.7 ± 1.0	16.5 ± 1.5	0.34
Cancer of Other Organs	2.4 ± 0.4	2.1 ± 0.6	2.1

The exposure time ranged from 10 to 45 years and averaged 25 years. The lag period varied in several former miners between 10 and 17 years (ROSTOSKI; SCHMORL). The average age was during the early period (before 1904) 38 years (UHLIG) and rose to 55 years by 1926 (range 37—69 years (ROSTOSKI, SAUPE and SCHMORL). It was noted by HÄRTING and HESSE that drillers and hewers developed lung cancer at an earlier age and with a higher frequency than other underground workers, such as carpenters and masons. Drillers and hewers, therefore, sustained apparently the most severe exposure to the causal agents (radioactive dust and gas in addition to silica dust, arsenic, etc.) (NEITZEL).

Among 41 cases which were analyzed for their specific histologic type, 26 were squamous cell carcinomas, 14 were small cell carcinomas, some with giant cells (Fig. 44), and one (1) was a multifocal carcinoma which exhibited both small cell and adenocarcinomatous structures. Radiation cancers of the lung as observed among Schneeberg miners thus adhered to the general pattern of histologically diverse responses to the same etiologic agent.

Etiology: During the early period after the discovery of these lung cancers when radioactivity of chemicals was still unknown, it was supposed that the development of these neoplasms was related to the heavy exposure to silica dust, i.e., to silicotic pneumoconiosis sustained by these miners. However, silicosis was, as a rule, not very extensive in miners with lung cancer (ROSTOSKI; SEPKE) and HUECK noted that silicosis had no causal relation to these cancers. Also speculations as to a contributory role of an occupational contact with water in the mines causing a tendency to the frequent occurrence of colds were advanced (HÄRTING and HESSE). SCHMORL pointed out that such cancers seemed to originate from pulmonary scars. After the chemical composition of the ore had been ascertained, various metals contained in the ore, such as cobalt, bismuth, nickel, chromium and arsenic, were considered as being causally involved in the production of these tumors (HÄRTING and HESSE; ROSTOSKI and SAUPE). Arsenic attracted special consideration in this respect since the ore contained 0.5 per cent of this mineral (RISEL; ROSTOSKI). It was assumed that fungal growth might tend to volatilize the arsenic present in the ore and thus cause it to be inhaled. However, the miners had no signs of arsenic poisoning and the molds proved to be inactive. This etiologic concept was later more or less

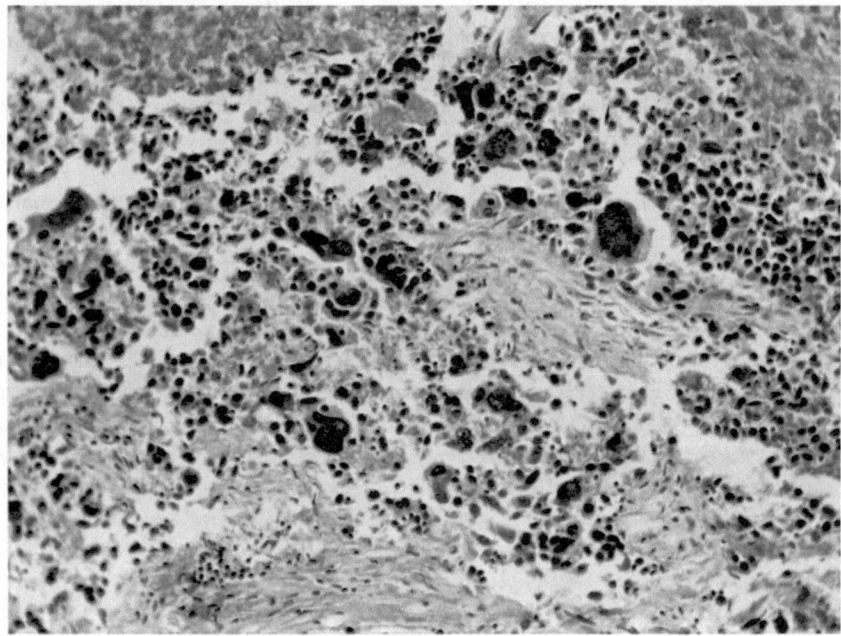

Fig. 44. Anaplastic carcinoma of the lung in a Schneeberg miner

abandoned (SCHMORL; LOUTIT), and arsenic remained merely for some time as a possible contributory factor in the speculations entertained by several investigators on the etiology of these cancers (LORENZ).

VESIN, as well as LORENZ, proposed the hypothesis that also genetic, hereditary factors associated with an assumed inbreeding of the population at Schneeberg might represent a contributory factor. Considering the fact that Schneeberg, around the turn of the century, was a town of 10,000 inhabitants and was supplied with railroad connections with the rest of the world, "inbreeding" as a cause of endemic predisposition in such a community can scarcely be taken seriously.

Following the discovery of radioactivity in the air and dust of the Schneeberg mines after the turn of the century, the causal importance of this factor has received increasing attention. The prolonged inhalation of radioactive matter present in the mine air seems to be at present generally accepted as the real cause of the lung cancers observed for so many years and at such a high incidence among the miners at

Schneeberg (LUDEWIG and LOSENSER; SCHMORL; ROSTOSKI; BRANDT; ROSTOSKI; TELEKY; PELLER; ROSTOSKI and SAUPE; NEITZEL; WEBER; FISCHER-WASELS; RAJEWSKI; LISCO; SCHMORL; GLUCKSMANN et al.). It is remarkable, therefore, that in 1944 LORENZ still claimed that radon was not the sole factor operating in the induction of the lung cancer among Schneeberg miners and that other influences, such as chronic irritation, arsenic, and hereditary susceptibility also played a primary role. He tried to support this opinion by pointing out that studies on other groups exposed to radon or radium, including radium plant workers, presented no clear-cut evidence that radium or radon had ever induced lung cancer in man outside the mining district of Schneeberg and Joachimsthal. Since a similarly negativistic assessment as to the predominant significance of inhaled radon and its radioactive solid daughters attached to the mine dust was adhered to and practically applied in regard to the control of these occupational lung cancer hazards (HUEPER) in the Rocky Mountain region of the Colorado Plateau, it should be pointed out that in more recent years the evidence on hand at the time and to an even greater and more convincing and conclusive degree hence contradicted definitely the scientific and rational validity of such peculiar conclusions.

Determinations of the radioactivity of the air in various mines in the Schneeberg region were made first by LUDWIG and LORENSER; and RAJEWSKY. There were distinct fluctuations in the radioactive content of the air in different mines, in different parts of the same mine and in the same location in the same mine at different times. The water in the mines also contained radioactive material. The radioactivity in the mine air ranged, according to LUDWIG and LORENSER, from 3.6×10^{-10} to 1.8×10^{-8} curies per liter. The highest values were obtained in places where the air was stagnant and, especially, at the head of the mine ducts where drilling was carried out and when thereby new pockets of radioactive gases were opened. The radioactivity at such places varied from 3.6×10^{-9} to 9×10^{-9} curies per liter. RAJEWSKY obtained in general, similar measurements (7×10^{-12} to 7×10^{-9} curies per liter) with the exception of values recorded for one mine (Siebenschlehen) known as the "Death Mine" because of the high incidence of lung cancer among the miners employed in this particular mine (HUEPER). RAJEWSKY found here values up to 5.4×10^{-8} curies per liter. The springs in the mines exhibited a radioactivity similar to that found in the air. The air which the miners exhaled also was radioactive (RAJEWSKY; LORENZ). Lung tissue of fifteen miners who had died with cancer of the lung exhibited a degree of radioactivity which increased with age, ranging from 0.06×10^{-12} gm. radium equivalent per gram of fresh lung tissue to 2×10^{-12} radium equivalent. LORENZ pointed out that the data of RAJEWSKY indicated that the amounts of radon inhaled by miners during 18 years of work and 8 hours daily in the mine, and in part retained in the lungs, approached the lower limit of the toxic dose of inhaled radon (9.5×10^{-8} curies per liter of air). RAJEWSKY concluded from these findings — and LORENZ seemed to have accepted such a conclusion — that it cannot be denied that the damage produced by the inhalation of the air of the mines containing radon was one of the causes of the disease of Schneeberg. The evidence in fact is, however, much more significant because it is well established from experiences on man and experimental animals that the carcinogenic dose of a chemical agent is as a rule well below its minimal toxic dose. Neither RAJEWSKY nor LORENZ apparently were aware of this biologic principle which supports the view that the radon content of the mine air is actually the predominant cause of the lung cancer in Schneeberg miners — unless it is postulated that lung tissue is exceptionally resistant to the carcinogenic action of ionizing radiation.

The dose calculations mentioned suffer from an additional fallacy. The inhalation of radioactive aerosols results in an eminently non-homogenous retention and deposition of solid particles on the bronchial mucosa. Such contacts, therefore, tend to create through a localized preferential precipitation of radioactive particles on the bronchial mucosa, multiple circumscribed foci of high intensity radiation. Under these conditions of exposure, a reliable and proper quantitative assessment of the focal radiation dose received by the mucosa in relation to that required for the focal induction of a bronchiogenic carcinoma cannot be made (HUG). Calculations of a minimal effective carcinogenic dose of inhaled radon and its solid daughters based on the concept of a homogeneous distribution and action of the inhaled carcinogenic matter on the bronchial mucosa thus are bound to yield distorted values.

αγ) Radioactive Lung Cancer Hazard in a Fluorspar Mining Community in Newfoundland

Epidemiology. Confirmatory epidemiologic evidence concerning a causal role of ionizing radiation inhaled by miners employed in radioactive non-uranium mines, was recently reported from Canada (DE VILLIERS and WINDISH; PARSONS, DE VILLIERS, BARTLETT and BECKLAKE). These mines were operated since 1933. The

Table 71. *Expected and Observed Deaths Due to Malignant Neoplasm of the Trachea, Bronchus, and Lung. Among Male Underground and Surface Mine Workers at St. Lawrence, Newfoundland, 1952—1960 Inclusive* [1]

Number of Deaths	All Ages	15−24	25−34	35−44	45−54	55−65	65−74	75+
a) Death from all causes, Newfoundland, less death among St. Lawrence miners (1952—1960)	15,264	385	432	602	984	1,545	2,814	3,570
b) Death due to malignant neoplasm of trachea, bronchus, and lung, Newfoundland, less death due to this cause among St. Lawrence miners (1952—1960)	157	1	4	18	29	61	31	13
c) Death from all causes, St. Lawrence miners (1952—1960)	71	—	5	19	17	16	9	5
Expected death, St. Lawrence (b/a) × c	0.7303	—	0.0463	0.5681	0.5010	0.6317	0.0991	0.9182
Observed death, St. Lawrence (1952—1960)	21	—	2	6	8	5	—	—
Ratio of observed death to expected death	28.76	—	43.20	10.56	15.97	7.92	—	—

[1] Cases in categories 1 to 3 only.

evidence recorded was related to the observation that since 1952 two to three deaths from primary cancer of the lung have occurred regularly each year among the male inhabitants of a small fluorspar mining community of St. Lawrence, Newfoundland. These deaths constituted 23 of the 51 deaths that occurred during the 10-year period

Table 72. Comparison of St. Lawrence, Jachymov and Schneeberg, Colorado Plateau, and South Africa Data

	Fluorspar Mines — St. Lawrence		Uranium Mines			
	Dead-end Areas	Ventilated Areas	Jachymov & Schneeberg — Abandoned Mine	Working Mine	Colorado Plateau Working Mines	South Africa Working Mines
Radon (pc per litre) Average Range	270—25,000*	<5—1,510	?—54,000[1]	2,900[2] / 360—18,000[3] / 7—7,000[1]	70—59,000[7]	25—500[9]
Radon daughters (multiples of 1.3 × 10^5 Mev per litre) Average Range	0.4—193	2.5—10** / 0—12				
Gamma radiation (mr./hr)	0.03—0.50					
Incidence of lung cancer as % of miner deaths	33 (1933 61) / 45 (1952—61)		43 (1875—1939)[4] / 52 (1921—39)[4]		11.4[8]	3.5[9]
Duration of underground exposure (years) Average and range	12.5 (5.5—21.3)		17 (13—23)[5]		7, 8, 9, 10, 12	17.3 (3—30)[10]
Induction period (years) Average and range	19.1 (11.5—25.0)		25 (15—43)[5] / 50 (40—67)[5] / 55 (37—69)[6]			
Age at death (years) Average and range	46.8 (33—56)					58 2 (45—73)[9]

* Estimated, on basis of highest radon daughter concentration found.
** Estimated.
[1] RAJEWSKY (1939), quoted by LORENZ (1944); measurements made between 1936 and 1939.
[2] EVANS and GOODMAN (1940).
[3] LUDEWIG and LORENSER (1924) qroted by LORENZ (1944).
[4] After LORENZ (1944).
[5] Nine cases — PIRCHAN and ŠIKL (1932).
[6] Thirteen cases — ROSTOSKI and others (1926) quoted by LORENZ (194
[7] HOLADAY et al. (1957); data collected in 1952.
[8] Miners with three or more years underground experience—five cases — ARCHER et al. (1962).
[9] OOSTHUIZEN et al. (1958).
[10] Based on 14 of 23 cases reported by OOSTHUIZEN et al. (1958).

(1952—1961) among employees with one or more years of underground mining experience. A shift to a younger average age at death from lung cancer and an association between age at entry into risk and age at death were observed. The observed death rate from lung cancer of this population group was about 29 times the expected one as determined by comparison with a control community of similar size in the same geographical region, and with the population of the rest of New-foundland. These epidemiologic findings were characteristic of an occupational exposure to a carcinogenic agent.

Table 73. *Relation Between Age at Entry in Occupation and Age at Death*

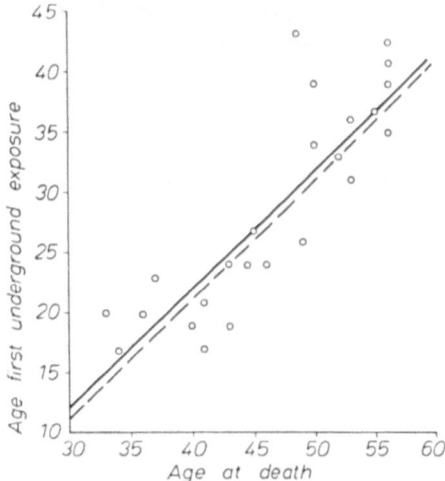

The following tables present the essential data on the lung cancer deaths among this miner population (Table 71 and 72) (DE VILLIERS and WINDISH).

Etiology. The ore mined was fluorspar (calcium fluoride, CaF_2) which contained very small amounts of other minerals (0.002—0.4% of manganese; 0.002—0.01% of nickel; less than 0.01% of chromium; 0.27% of yttrium). Arsenic and cerium were absent. Minute amounts of radioactive samarium-147 were present. In addition to air-borne dust containing quartz and calcium fluoride, radon daugthers were found in the mine air, as well as in the air of the processing plants (Table 73). These values were within the general range of those reported from the Schneeberg and Joachimsthal mines, considering the rather variable character in the amounts of radioactive matter a different times.

While the evidence recorded points definitely to the radioactivity of the mine air as the main factor causing the high incidence of carcinoma of the lung among these fluorspar miners (PARSONS et al.), it was deemed advisable to assess in this respect also the smoking habits of the miners because of the claims made by various investigators (DOLL and HILL) concerning the major role of cigarette smoking as a cause of lung cancer. After citing the observation of DOLL and HILL that lung cancer is 20 times as frequent among heavy smokers as among nonsmokers, the Canadian investigators noted that, "the 20 times greater incidence of carcinoma of the lung in St. Lawrence compared with the rest of Newfoundland might be considered attributable to smoking only if all the population of St. Lawrence smoked heavily (25 g. or more of tobacco daily), while the population of the rest of Newfoundland were non-smokers. Since this is not the case, factors besides heavy smoking habits of the St. Lawrence population must be operating to produce a high incidence of lung carcinoma."

αδ) *Miscellaneous Non-Uranium Mines*

Metal Ore Miners of the Colorado Plateau. The recently published results of epidemiologic studies on the lung cancer frequency among uranium ore miners and metal ore miners of the Colorado Plateau which were initiated by HUEPER in 1948, and after 1952, continued by the Division of Occupational Health, U.S. Public Health Service, and the Epidemiology Branch, National Cancer Institute, suggest that similar exposure conditions may account in toto or in part for the excessive frequency of pulmonary cancer among non-uranium metal miners of this region. The original epidemiologic investigations conducted on this subject by HUEPER in cooperation with the Division of Industrial Medicine, University of Colorado (PRINCI and WARING; CHURCH) and the Colorado State Health Department (CLEERE; JACOE) between 1948 and 1952, demonstrated that the highest lung death cancer rates for males were present in the central section of the State where industrial and mining activities were prevalent (Fig. 45) and that lower rates were found in the eastern and western sections of this State.

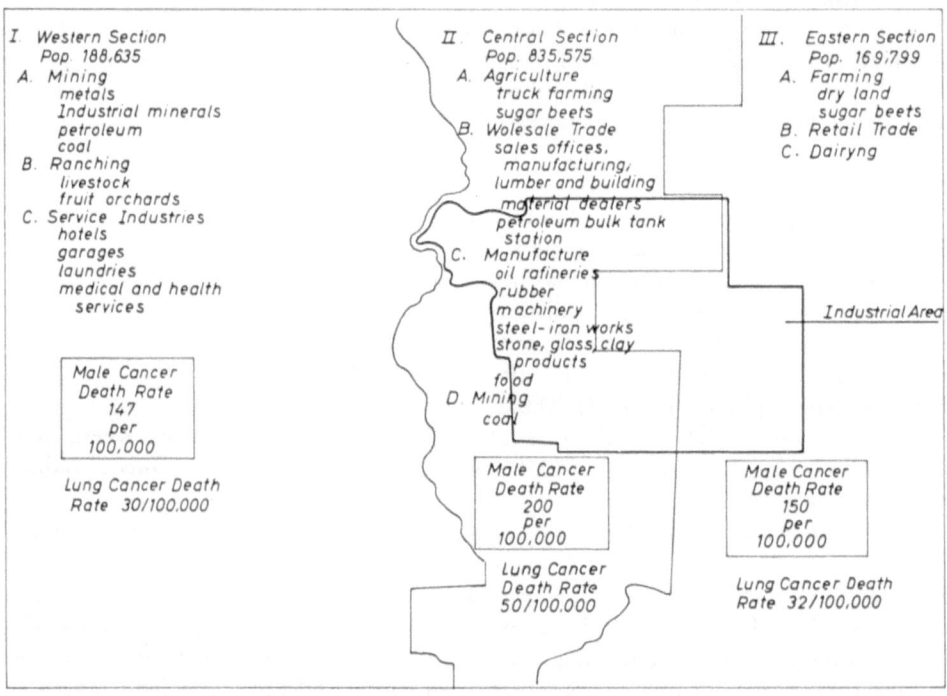

Fig. 45. Cancer death rates for males, 1943 to 1948, in three sections of Colorado

It is an established fact that many of the non-uranium mines in the Rocky Mountains are radioactive although usually only to a minor degree (JACOE). The metal mines studied by JACOE contained mainly gold, silver, lead, zinc and tungsten bearing ores. The highest concentration of radioactivity found was 2100 uuc/l and in only one location in a single lead mine no radon was found, however 30—60 uuc/l was found elsewhere in the same mine. A study of lead and zinc mines in a specific area gave such a variety of results that no relationship could be established. A group of these mines showed radon concentrations as follows: 119, 201, 151, 26, 126, 259, 1440 and 258 uuc/l, and a similar group in the same district — 160, 180, 340, 320, and 120 uuc/l. The next group in this area however showed only 0—60, 30, 50 uuc/l.

This particular district has never produced uranium ores and is situated about 80 miles from the nearest uranium producing mine. In addition to a pollution of the underground mine air with radioactive matter, such mines usually are also contaminated with arsenic containing dust, since arsenic is present in most of the non-ferrous metal ores. It is probable that the inhalation of this atmospheric pollutant may also significantly be involved in the causation of occupational lung cancers (WAGONER, MILLER, LUNDIN, FRAUMENI and HAIJ) among non-uranium ore miners. The excessive incidence of these tumors in this occupational group is evident from the data of Table 74 (WAGONER et al.). This table, moreover, shows that in contrast to observations on

Table 74. *Comparison of Foreign-Born with Native-Born Metal Miners (Standardized Cancer Mortality Ratios, with Numbers of Expected and Observed Deaths According to Organ System, January 1, 1937, through December 31, 1959).*

Cause of Death	Foreign Born			Native Born		
	Ex-pected Deaths	Ob-served Deaths	Standard-ized Mortality Ratios	Ex-pected Deaths	Ob-served Deaths	Standard-ized Mortality Ratios
All malignant neoplasms .	41.9	78	186 *	32.0	57	178 *
Digestive system	19.8	39	197 *	14.4	12	83
Respiratory system	8.6	21	244 *	7.5	26	347 *
Other systems	13.5	18	133	10.1	19	188 **

* Significant at 1% level.   ** Significant at 5% level.

higher lung cancer rates in members of foreign born groups than in native ones, native miners have a higher lung cancer rate than foreign born miners. The other factor which may account for this excessive liability to lung cancer among metal miners in the Rocky Mountains region is arsenic.

In critically analyzing these observations, WAGONER et al. noted that histories of cigarette smoking were not obtained in their study; however, it seemed to them unlikely that they would differ substantially from those of uranium miners (WAGONER, ARCHER, CARROLL, HOLADAY and LAWRENCE). These differed from the general population only enough to raise the lung-cancer mortality by an estimated 10 percent. They stated, moreover, that it is unlikely that socioeconomic distribution could account for the excess respiratory cancer rate in their study group, and that any genetic factors might not be suspected of having been operative.

The evidence on an excessive lung cancer frequency among radioactive non-uranium mines deserves global attention despite these uncertainties as to the actual role which an atmospheric pollution of the mine air with radioactive matter may play in this phenomenon, because the existence of similar radioactive air pollution has been recorded for mines of several other countries and states (South Africa; Egypt; Germany; New York) (DE VILLIERS and WINDISH; HUBACHER; HARRIS AWAAD, EL-SHERBINI, HAMMOND, HAZAA, KHARADLY and VALIC; CHEMICAL and ENGINEERING NEWS). Such occupational exposures, however, have as yet not been associated with any demonstrated excessive liability to pulmonary cancer by the miners employed in such mines. Some studies have dealt with the influence which radioactive mine air might have on the development of silicosis in the lungs of miners (ROSTOSKI; ULMER, NICOLAS, MUTH, OBERHAUSEN and ONSTEAD).

β) Uranium Ore Miners
βα) Lung Cancer in Joachimsthal Miners

Epidemiology. Uranium ore mining was carried out until World War II mainly for extracting the radium contained in such ores, and less for obtaining the uranium to be used in the production of pigments, glazes, etc. During and after World War II, uranium ore mining was greatly expanded for the manufacture of military explosive devices and subsequently also for exploring the usefulness of nuclear energy for non-destructive, particularly commercial and medical — purposes. Uranium or carnotite or pitchblende mining is carried out in Bohemia, the Congo, Canada, the U.S.S.R., the United States of America, and various other countries. While the German investi-gators of the Schneeberg situation suspected for many years that the miners' disease known as "radium disease" and frequently observed among the pitchblende miners of Joachimsthal (JACHYMOV) — which lies 30 km. south of Schneeberg on the southern slope of the Erzgebirge — (SCHMORL), was identical with the disorders affecting the Schneeberg miners, it was only in 1929 that LÖWY substantiated this old supposition when he reported the first cases of lung cancer found in three (3) former uranium ore miners of Joachimsthal, in a radium plant with 60 employees. This first observation was followed by others in rapid succession (SIKL, 1930; ZIEL, 1930; BEUTEL, 1931; PIRCHAN and SIKL, 1932; PELLER, 1939; SAUPE, 1939; TELEKY, 1937; BEHOUNEK and FORT, 1941; MAHLER and ZIEL, 1930; BEHOUNEK, 1927; WAELSCH, 1946). The mines at Joachimsthal employed in 1929 about 400 workers, of whom approximately 100 were miners (LÖWY); 320 miners in addition to 80 pensioners were employed in 1931 (SIKL) in these mines.

SIKL reported in 1930 the presence of carcinomas of the lung in eight (8) out of 15 miners and pensioners who came to autopsy and estimated their incidence at 50% in all deaths in members of this occupational group. An additional case was published by BEUTEL in 1931. In a comprehensive report of PIRCHAN and SIKL appearing in 1932, nine (9) new cases of lung cancer in Joachimsthal miners were placed on record. They occurred among 323 miners during the years 1929—1930, and were seen among 19 deaths and in 13 necropsies. SAUPE found in 1939 among 398 active or former miners subjected to a physical examination, three (3) cases of lung cancer. When in 1939, PELLER reviewed the accumulated evidence, he established the fol-lowing statistical correlations with lung cancer in Joachimsthal miners which are given in Table 75.

Table 75. *Cancer Mortality in Joachimsthal Miners per 1,000*

Cancer of	Joachimsthal Miners		Vienna, Males 15--79 years 1932—1936
	1929—1938	1929—1938 Autopsies only	
Lung	9.8 ± 1.5	8.3 ± 1.6	0.34 ± 0.01
Larynx . . .	0.2	0.3	0.07
Skin	0.2	0.3	0.05
Bone	0.2	0.3	0.12
All other organs	0.45 ± 0.3	0.0	1.86 ± 0.02
All organs . .	10.9 ± 1.6	9.2 ± 1.6	2.44 ± 0.03

PELLER concluded from his epidemiologic studies that the miners of Joachims-thal have, 1. a high percentage of malignancies (53%) among their deaths; 2. a several-times-increased cancer mortality rate due to an enormous frequency of pulmonary cancers in the age period 35—54; 3. an exceptionally high proportion of primary lung cancers; 4. a reduced incidence of cancer in non-respiratory organs; and 5. an increased mortality from causes other than cancer in younger age groups. He noted, like SCHMORL for lung cancers in Schneeberg miners, an increased incidence of multiple primary tumors of the lungs among Joachimsthal miners.

In 1950, SIKL recorded a total of 20 cases of lung cancer in Joachimsthal miners which had been observed between 1933 and 1938, and finally WAELSCH noted in 1946 that cancer of the lung accounted for the death of such miners in 45.4% of a total of 63 cases.

The distinct shift in the age at death from lung cancer among these miners is evident from the data collected by GLUCKSMANN et al. on this subject: 2 cases were in the age 20—39 class; 11 cases in the 40—49 class; and 7 cases were in the 50-and-over class. The average age at death was given as 47.6 years, which agrees approximately with that noted by SIKL, which was 49 years. The exposure time varied from 9 to 23 years and was given as 17 as an average. The lag period after cessation of employment in the mines was up to 23 years. Among 26 cancers histologically examined, there were 10 squamous cell carcinomas and 15 round cell carcinomas. In one case, the primary site was apparently not the lung, but the pleura and its type was given by PIRCHAN and SIKL as undifferentiated atypical carcinoma. While some degree of silicosis was seen in all lungs with cancer, silicosis on the whole was not a prominent feature in cases of cancer. In fact, lungs most heavily affected with silicosis were generally free from malignant growth (SIKL; PIRCHAN and SIKL). These observations were in general agreement with those made in Schneeberg miners.

Pertinent to this problem of the role of silicosis and cancer of the lung in radioactive ore miners are the experimental observations of WATANABE and of ENGELBRECHT, THIART and CLAASSENS. WATANABE exposing rodents to radioactive feldspar dust, obtained a fibrosing pneumoconiosis, while this condition did not appear when a non-radioactive feldspar was administered. WATANABE concluded from this observation that the natural radioactivity of inhaled rock dust alone may cause the development of fibrotic nodules in the lung. In the experiment of ENGELBRECHT et al., rats inhaled a radioactive silica-containing dust of gold mines for testing the premise whether the radioactivity adds to the fibrosing effect of silica on the lung. The investigators concluded that the radioactivity in the dust enhanced the fibrogenic action of silica on the lungs of rats. Radiation cancers in other organs, especially the hematopoietic organs and bones, were absent in Joachimsthal miners.

Etiology. The degree of atmospheric pollution with radioactive matter in the Joachimsthal mines was stated to be 30 times the tolerance dose (EDITORIAL; PELLER). It was noted that under such conditions of exposure it is scarcely surprising that in the past, more than half of the miners died of lung cancer (EDITORIAL, 1952). This statement contrasts sharply with the allegation of TSCHELNITZ (1935) who studied the physical conditions present in the mines in relation to the etiology of the lung cancer. TSCHELNITZ claimed that it is grossly erroneous that radium introduced into the body by drinking water or air, as found in Joachimsthal, can produce any body injury. He pointed out in support of this astounding contention, that radon inhaled is completely exhaled within 7 hours and that the work-free-interval of 17 hours between shifts is completely sufficient to remove any permanent exposure. TSCHELNITZ incriminated as the principal causal factor the injury to the structure of the lung induced by the inhaled silica. BEHOUNEK and FORT, on the other hand, after a critical analysis of the exposure conditions present in the Joachimsthal mines came to the conclusion that the excessive incidence of lung cancer is attributable to the prolonged inhalation of radium emanation present in the mine air. The radio-activity of the air near drill holes was found to be up to 8×10^{-8} curies per liter. The activity of the springs in the mines ranged from 1×10^{-9} to 2×10^{-6}. The lung tissue of some miners contained 1×10^{-12} gm. of radium per gm. of tissue (LORENZ; EVANS and GOODMAN).

The lung cancers in radioactive uranium miners of Joachimsthal, Czechoslovakia and in the radioactive ore miners of Schneeberg, Germany, have been accepted for many years past as occupational diseases to which compensation laws are applicable (HUECK; LÖWY; ZIEL; OFFICIAL REPORT).

ββ) Lung Cancers in Uranium Ore Miners of the Colorado Plateau

Epidemiology. The initial attempt to obtain information on the probable exist-ance of lung cancer hazards in uranium ore miners of the Colorado Plateau was organized by HUEPER in 1948 with the cooperation of the Colorado State Health Department and the Division of Industrial Medicine, University of Colorado, School of Medicine, Denver, Colorado. It was planned at that time to ascertain the causes of death not only for uranium ore (carnotite) miners and millers, but also for workers engaged in the mining and milling of various arsenic containing non-ferrous metal (silver, copper, zinc, etc.) ores — an activity carried on for many years in the same region. Because of administrative difficulties encountered in the continuation of this epidemiologic survey, it was appropriated in 1951 by the Division of Occupational Health, USPHS, which operated this exploration from then on in conjunction with the Colorado State Health Department and the Atomic Energy Committee.

These shifts in management of the epidemiologic survey in Colorado were brought about by the fact that at that time some Government scientists still believed that the lung was refractory to the carcinogenic action of inhaled radioactive matter and that for this reason, such exploratory studies were not indicated. These officials indeed went so far as claiming that scientists recommending such fact finding epidemiologic procedures in Colorado were displaying "bad scientific judgment" and deserved to be dismissed from the Government service (HUEPER). They insisted, moreover, that any mentioning of the extensive experiences made since 1879 on occupational lung cancer hazards in Saxon and Bohemian radioactive mines at Schneeberg and Joa-chimsthal at medical conferences be suppressed as not being in the "public interest".

The mining of uranium ore on the Colorado Plateau had been a relatively small-scale operation until the latter part of World War II, when uranium ore became in great demand for the production of military explosive devices. The production of this ore rose rapidly after the war, and amounted for the year 1956 to approximately 3 million dry tons yielding one-fourth of one (1) per cent uranium concentrate or about 8000 tons by the end of 1956. In 1957, there were a total of 12 uranium mills operating in the United States. All except one were privately owned. The completion of construction of eight additional mills was scheduled for the end of 1957 or early 1958.

The uranium ore mining industry soon expanded from the Colorado Plateau into adjacent regions (Utah, Arizona, New Mexico, Montana, South Dakota and Wyoming) and employed a rapidly rising number of miners and millers. The study of the health hazards of this occupational group which was started in 1951 comprised about 5,400 miners and millers.

In addition to periodic medical examinations performed on the miners and millers, determinations of the quantity and quality of the ionizing radiations present in the various mines (in 1959 samples were examined of 302 out of a total of 371 mines which employed 3,619 miners) were made (GOVERNORS' Conference). When in 1961 a preliminary report on the results of these studies was rendered, it appeared that among 907 white miners with more than 3 years of underground experience, death from respiratory cancer (6 deaths) accounted for nearly five times the normal rate (ARCHER, MAGNUSON, HOLADAY and LAWRENCE). A cytological examination of the sputum of uranium miners started in 1957, provided additional evidence suggesting the existence of a radiation specific lung cancer hazard. In 1960, the sputums of 1,788 miners were examined. In the first 272 reports, the sputum of 230 miners was negative, that from 33 was doubtful, and that of nine (9), or 3.3 per cent, was positive for cancer cells.

The subsequent analysis of such correlations published by WAGONER, ARCHER, CARROLL, HOLADAY and LAWRENCE in 1964 which covered an observation period extending from 1950 to 1962, yielded confirmatory evidence concerning an excessive liability of lung cancers in American uranium ore miners (Table 76).

Table 76. *Number of Expected and Observed Deaths from Respiratory Cancer in Relation to Duration of Underground Uranium and Underground Nonuranium Mining Experience (White Miners) 1950 Through 1962*

Duration of underground nonuranium mining experience (years)	Duration of Underground Uranium Mining Experience					
	Less than 5 years		5 years or more		Total	
	Expected	Observed	Expected	Observed	Expected	Observed
0	0.7	0	0.6	5 [2]	1.3	5 [1]
1—4	0.3	0	0.1	0	0.4	0
5 and more . .	0.7	1	0.4	6 [2]	1.1	7 [2]
Total	1.7	1	1.1	11 [2]	2.8	12 [2]

[1] Significant at 5 percent level (8).   [2] Significant at 1 percent level (8).

For testing the validity of their conclusion that the cumulative dose of airborne radiation contained within the uranium ore mines was responsible for the excess of respiratory cancers among the miners, WAGONER et al. calculated 3 measures of radon-daughter exposure for a number of miners (Table 77).

They found that the mean number of months of underground experience and the mean dose rate of miners with respiratory cancer were greater, though not significantly so, than those of other groups used for comparison. The value of these observations is accentuated by the fact that there was a significant excess of respiratory cancers even among uranium miners with no prior hard-rock mining experience.

Considering the fact that the uranium mines in the Rocky Mountain region are in operation for only a relatively short time, that the peak values of radioactivity in some of these mines were several-fold those noted in the "death mine" of Schneeberg, and that protective technologic measures, i.e., mainly ventilation, were introduced into the operation of most of these mines only after 1950 and did not invariably produce a satisfactory improvement of the exposure conditions, it is safe to predict that many additional cases of lung cancer and a considerably higher incidence rate of these tumors will become apparent for this worker group during the decades to come.

Table 77. *Disease Classification of Uranium Miners According to Radon-Daughter Exposure*

Disease classification	Number of miners	Mean age	Mean respiratory exposure		
			Under-ground duration in months	Dose rate [1]	Cumulative dose [2]
1. Malignant neoplasms of the respiratory system	25	53.9	88.9	30.9	2,878.4 ($\overline{X}_1$)
2. Respiratory diseases other than respiratory neoplasm (includes pneumoconiosis and conditions contributing to cor pulmonale)	24	53.5	74.9	22.6	1,826.2 ($\overline{X}_2$)
3. Diseases other than those of the respiratory system (arteriosclerotic heart disease and "other neoplasms")	51	55.0	63.3	16.6	1,107.7 ($\overline{X}_3$)
4. Living miners matched with respiratory neoplasms on basis of year of birth, year of initial examination, and race	50	55.1	63.9	22.3	1,136.6 ($\overline{X}_4$)

t value for $\overline{X}_1 - \overline{X}_2 = 1.19$ t value for $\overline{X}_1 - \overline{X}_4 = 2.04$ [3]

t value for $\overline{X}_1 - \overline{X}_3 = 2.15$*** t value for $\overline{X}_2 - \overline{X}_3 = 1.80$

[1] Average working level $= \dfrac{\sum\limits_{i=1}^{m} \dfrac{Xi}{K}}{n}$

[2] Average working level months $= \dfrac{\sum\limits_{i=1}^{m} \dfrac{Xi}{K} \times Yi}{n}$

[3] Significant at 5 percent level-because of the multiple comparison, i. e. 4 groups taken 2 at a time, the exact level of significance is unknown.

where
X = radon-daughter level.
Y = months of exposure at radon-daughter level.
K = $1.3 \cdot 10^5$ MeV of potential alpha energy from radon-daughter per liter of air.
i = $1.2 \ldots m$ = number of radon-daughter level measurements.
n = number of miners.

Etiology. In etiologic respects it is important that WAGONER *et al.* stated that in contrast to the European uranium mines and to the U.S. metal mines, only minimal amounts of constituents of the ore suspected of carcinogenic activity in man (arsenic, chromium, nickel, iron) are present in the U.S. uranium ores. Their data showed, moreover, no relationship between the number of cigarettes smoked by these miners and the type and duration of uranium mining experience. They considered it, therefore, unlikely that smoking alone accounted for the excess of respiratory cancer among the long-term uranium miners.

There is general agreement among several groups of investigators who determined the quality and quantity of ionizing radiation in 371 uranium ore mines of the Colorado Plateau and adjacent regions that in many of these mines the working level of radiation was excessive in many mines and in some highly excessive (HOLADAY et al.; ARCHER and SIMPSON; GOVERNORS' CONFERENCE; TORREY and JACOE; MORRILL; TSIVOGLOU and AYER; MILLER, HOLADAY and DOYLE). In 1959, thirty-three per cent of the samples taken of the mine atmosphere had concentrations of less than one time the accepted working level of tolerance; 22 per cent had between 1 and 3 times the working level; 23 per cent had between 3 and 9 times the working level, and 22 per cent had concentrations of more than 10 times the working level. The primary hazard involved in mining uranium arises from the alpha emitters, RaA, and RaC[1].

While NEUMANN and ALERCIO, WELFORD and MORSE proposed to use the amount of urinary uranium excreted in the Friday urine as a measure of exposure hazard, SULTZER and HURSH recommended that urinary polonium might serve as a rough measure to estimate the cumulative lung exposure to radon and its daughters. They mentioned in this connection that the radon daugthers decay to lead[210], a lead isotope with a long effective half-life in the body and a decay scheme producing polonium[210]. HOLADAY et al.; AURAND et al.; SHAPIRO; and JECH devised methods for determining roughly the radioactive dose, i.e., radon decay products retained in the lung, from tests on exhaled air.

Because of the role which a radioactive type of lead assumes in determining these carcinogenic exposures of uranium ore miners, it may be mentioned that BLACK in 1943, raised the question of a possible lung cancer hazard for lead miners, smelter workers, lead solderers, plumbers, and members of many other occupations having contact with lead dust and fumes, because he observed lung cancers in two lead workers which developed many years after cessation of exposure to lead. BLACK pointed out in support of his claim that commercial lead contains radium D and is the most radioactive of all common metals. Its radioactivity was said to vary with the ore from which lead is obtained and with the age of the lead (BLACK). It is uncertain, however, whether this claim is valid since DINGWALL-FORDYCE and LANE reported in 1963 that lead workers seem to have a slightly substandard mortality rate from cancer of all sites. This renewed interest in a potential carcinogenic effect of lead on man was generated in part by the observation that lead fed to rats will cause carcinoma of the kidney (ZOLLINGER; BOYLAND, DUKES, GRIVER and MITCHLEY; VAN ESCH, VAN GENDEREN and VINK; KILHAM et al.). It is not likely that the excessive incidence of lung cancer among English boiler scalers is attributable to the 5 per cent of lead contained in the ash of the creosote-pitch fuel often used (SHERWOOD and BEDFORD).

Information is lacking whether more than one of the American uranium ore miners who developed lung cancers have received compensation (McADAMS), although the existence of causal relations to their job specific exposure to ionizing radiations is recognized (INGRAM; LISCO).

No official data are available as to the occurrence of lung cancers among the uranium ore miners of Katanga, Canada, and the U.S.S.R. (JACOBS; WARSCHOWSKI; EDITORIAL).

γ) Lung Cancer Hazards for Employees of Uranium Ore Refiners,
Radium Laboratories, Nuclear Installations and Power Plants and
Similar Establishments

Epidemiology. Individuals employed in uranium ore mills become exposed to fumes and dust of uranium, which is an alpha emitter. The radioactivity (alpha particles) of uranium presents its greatest hazard when the material is present as an insoluble compound, and lodges in the lungs for a long time (HARRIS and KINGSLEY). Uranium is the basic fuel of the nuclear reactors. It occurs naturally or artificially in various isotopes (U 233, U 234, U 235, U 238 and U 239). U 239 decays to plutonium 239. It has been claimed that so far no significant ill effects which could be attributed either to the chemical or radioactive toxicity of uranium have been seen in humans in personnel employed in nuclear energy installations (HARRIS and KINGSLEY). Whether the same holds true for workers employed in uranium refining plants, however, remains to be determined. Without any doubt such workers had at least ten years ago, definite and considerable exposure to uranium dust and fumes because of lack of any significant protective measures (HUEPER). The actuality of these conditions is well illustrated by pictures contained in an article by DOYLE. That metallic uranium when parenterally introduced into rats is capable of inducing cancers was shown by HUEPER, ZUEFLE, LINK and JOHNSON.

A similar absence of incriminating evidence concerning the presence of an occupational respiratory cancer hazard in nuclear reactor facilities is implied by reports published on this aspect although poor ventilation design in some such plants has been admitted (HELD). Emission of radioactive matter from the reactor stack causing atmospheric radioactive contamination resulting therefrom has been observed (LOWRY; GELLER, WORDEN, CASSIDY and BARTHOLOMEW). It is remarkable that LOVE in 1951 noted from a survey of an atomic pile site that a much higher than expected incidence of primary lung carcinoma prevailed at the Brookhaven National Laboratory. He claimed, however, that this phenomenon was not attributable to any occupational radiation exposure. MOSHMAN and HOLLAND made in 1949, a similar observation for the employees of the Oak Ridge installation and proposed that this finding merely reflected the normal trend in lung cancer rates.

Since at the time of the two reports all atomic energy installations had been operating for only a few years, it is unlikely that lung cancers among the employees of such establishments could justly be attributed to occupational factors at that time.

The respiratory radiation hazards related to such industrial activities resemble in many respects those associated with the burning of radioactive wastes in incinerators of institutions, laboratories, hospitals and related establishments and the operation of batteries of radioactive static eliminators (MACHIS and GEYER; COREY, PERRY and SCHWARTZ; BERMAN and ERNEST). Whether such atmospheric environmental pollution with radioactive wastes constitutes a respiratory cancer hazard to the neighborhood is likewise at present problematical.

Observations made in workers employed in radium factories and laboratories, on the other hand, strongly indicate that radioactive atmospheric pollutants (SAUPE; SCHLUNDT, McGAVOCK and BROWN; MORRIS) inhaled by such employees represent the primary causal factor in the development of lung cancers as well as of leukemia in some of them. The occurrence of lung cancer in members of this occupational group was reported by LÖWY (2 cases — one of them having also leukemia);

TELEKY (1 case); NEITZEL (1 case and 3 cases of pulmonary fibrosis (RAJEWSKY); STEIN (3 cases); BAADER, moreover, received information on four cases of occupational lung cancer in workers employed in Belgian radium ore refineries. It is obvious from this evidence that radioactive respiratory cancer hazards extend from the miners to the millers of uranium ores.

No information is available at this time whether the bathing in radioactive water practiced for the alleged protection and restoration of health in Germany, Bohemia and the U.S.A. and associated with an inhalation of radioactive mist and gas, consti-

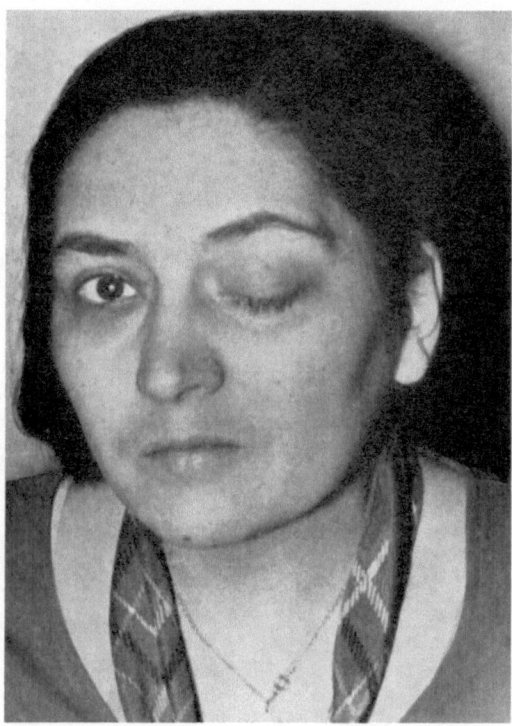

Fig. 46. Carcinoma of the maxillary paranasal sinus in a luminous dial painter (courtesy of Dr. AUB)

tutes an effective lung cancer hazard (LANGE; NEITZEL; SIKL; BEHOUNEK; HUECK) although the drinking of such water has caused in some individuals radiation sarcomas of the bone (HUEPER).

While the pulmonary cancer hazard related to the introduction of radioactive material into the lung is well known, considerably less attention has been given to the fact that occupationally inhaled radioactive chemicals or their direct injection for therapeutic or diagnostic purposes (thorium dioxide) into the paranasal sinuses also has been followed by the development of carcinomas of the paranasal sinuses. Such cancerous reactions have been observed in five former luminous dial painters (MARTLAND; AUB, EVANS, HEMPELMANN and MARTLAND; HASTERLIK, MILLER and FINKEL) (Figs. 46 and 47) as well as 5 patients receiving thorotrast injections into the maxillary sinus (HOFER; TULLIS; GROSS; FRUHLING and KEILING; BUDA, CONSLEY and RANKOW). The latent period of these radiation cancers which were squamous cell carcinomas, was from 15 to 20 years.

A successful production of maxillary sinus carcinomas (squamous cell carcinomas) in rhesus monkeys which received intrasinusoidal implants of Ag^{110} and Co^{60} was reported by MELNIKOV. These observations demonstrate that various parts of the respiratory tract are capable of reacting with the development of cancers when adequately exposed to ionizing radiations.

The validity of this statement is further attested to by several observations on the occurrence of lung cancer in patients following a diagnostic parenteral injection of

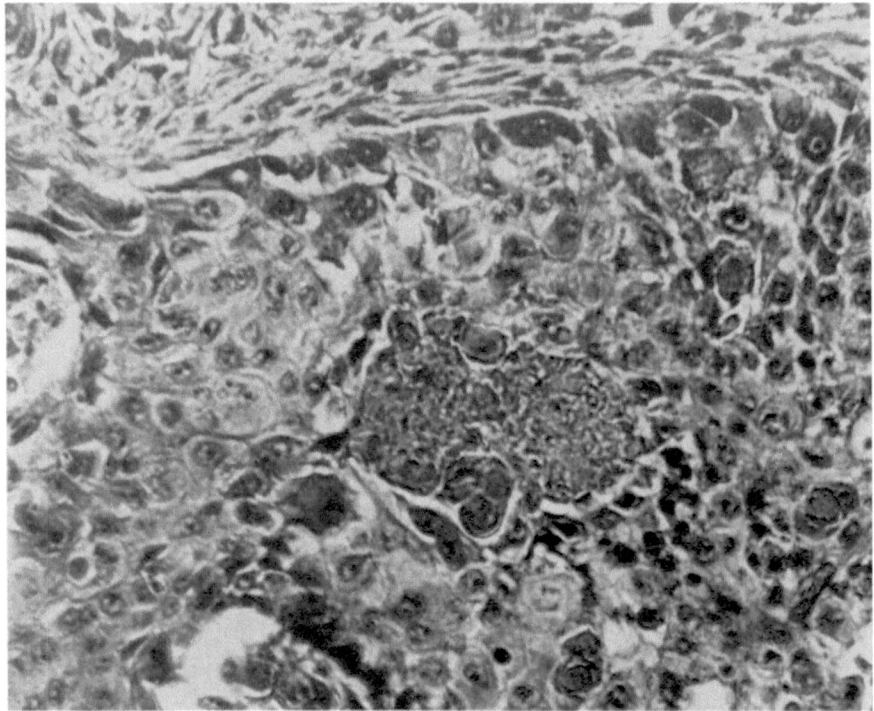

Fig. 47. Squamous cell carcinoma of the maxillary sinus (above)

thorotrast (FRUHLING, GROSS, BATZENSCHLAGER and DORNER). Bronchial carcinomas have been seen many years after a bronchographic examination entailing an intra-bronchial introduction of thorotrast by ROTH and by VÖGTLIN et al., while five additional such cases were reported after an angiographic use of thorotrast by HACKENTHAL; ABRAHAMSON et al., HOLTHUSEN; BATZENSCHLAGER; and NIELSEN and KRACHT. Although there exists scarcely any doubt concerning the existence of causal interrelations for the two carcinomas developing after an intrabronchial introduction of thorium dioxide, such associations are less sure for the carcinomas of the lung following an intravascular injection of this agent. It must be pointed out, however, that reliable experimental evidence demonstrates that various colloidally dispersed particulate or macromolecular materials intravenously injected are retained in the capillaries of the lung. A part of such matter is subsequently excreted into the alveolar lumens enclosed in histiocytes (HUEPER). This process has been observed also following an intravenous injection of thorotrast. Since the decay of thorium dioxide is associated with the production of alpha-, beta-, and gamma-radiations the basic conditions exist in such cases for an ultimate development of pulmonary cancers.

Reports in the medical literature indicate that such cancerous responses to radiations have lately been observed also in other parts of the respiratory system, especially the larynx, in an appreciable number of patients who received some 20 to 40 years previously, x-ray treatments to the neck for malignant and non-malignant diseases, particularly those affecting the thyroid (HOLINGER and RABBETT; KING et al.; GOOLDEN; MAJOROS, DEVINE and PARKHILL; VAN NIEUWENHUYSE; JACQUES; VON EICKEN; GARRETT).

A similar potential connotation is attached to the development of fibrosis of the lung following an occupational and, especially, a therapeutic exposure of the chest to large doses of x-radiation, emitted by radioactive chemicals as well as from x-ray tubes (DOENECKE; IRMSCHER; TÖNGES and KALBFLEISCH; BELT; WARREN and GATES; WARREN; HAMPERL; BAUDISCHE; CHU, PHILLIPS, NICKSON and McPHEE; FLEMING, FILBEE and WIERNIK; BAUER and SCHRAER; FREID and GOLDBERG; BERGMANN and GRAHAM; LOUGHEED and MAGUIRE). In only one of these cases of chronic radiation pneumonia with fibrosis present in a worker inhaling radioactive industrial dust of a FISCHER-TROPSCH process did the histologic examination reveal an initial carcinoma after an exposure-free interval of 18 years (IRMSCHER). In none of the many hundreds of persons who developed this radiation pneumonitis after the administration of x-radiation for malignant conditions of the chest, especially carcinoma of the breast, on the other hand, has so far been seen a secondary cancerous development. It is not unlikely, however, that the great majority of these persons of usually adult age succumbed to their primary disease long before the latent period for radiation cancers of the lungs had elapsed.

Corresponding time relations may account likewise in part for the present absence of reliable observations on a causal relation between an inhalation of atmospheric radioactive pollutants and a delayed development of pulmonary cancers in members of populations most severely exposed to such carcinogens, since these usually act in a greatly reduced concentration, and, therefore, presumably require a much longer latent period for cancerous reactions to appear than that observed in uranium ore miners for cancer of the lung (mean value about 19 years) (DUNHAM; MEDICAL RESEARCH COUNCIL, 1956; 1960; EISENBUD and HARLEY; LOCKHART; TAJIMA and DOKE; CARMICHAEL and TUNNICLIFFE; SIENKO and COCCONI; SETTER; ZIMMER, LICKING and TABOR; DAWSON; HUBER; WEGST; PELLETIER and WHIPPLE; HOLLISTER). In assessing the potential carcinogenic significance of such exposures to the human lung, it must be emphasized that the absolute amounts entering the respiratory tract from such sources is very small when compared with the quantity of radioactive matter introduced into the lung from the various occupational activities cited. If such environmental radioactive atmospheric exposures should be effective in man, it must be supposed that because of the prospective very long latent period, only those individuals may develop some 40 to 50 years hence lung cancers who were in their early youth when being exposed. At the present, any incriminating claims represent for these reasons, mere speculations based on factually unfounded suppositions and dealing with possibilities. These, nevertheless, because of the general evidence available on such matters, deserve serious consideration.

Experimental Carcinogenesis. The large amount of human evidence concerning a carcinogenic action of ionizing radiations on the tissues of the respiratory system has received lately ample support from experimental observations.

The production of cancers of the lung in experimental animals (mice, rats, dogs, rabbits) by radioactive chemicals, intratracheally, intrabronchially, intravenously or intrapulmonarily introduced has successfully been accomplished with a variety of such agents by an appreciable number of investigators (WARREN and GATES;

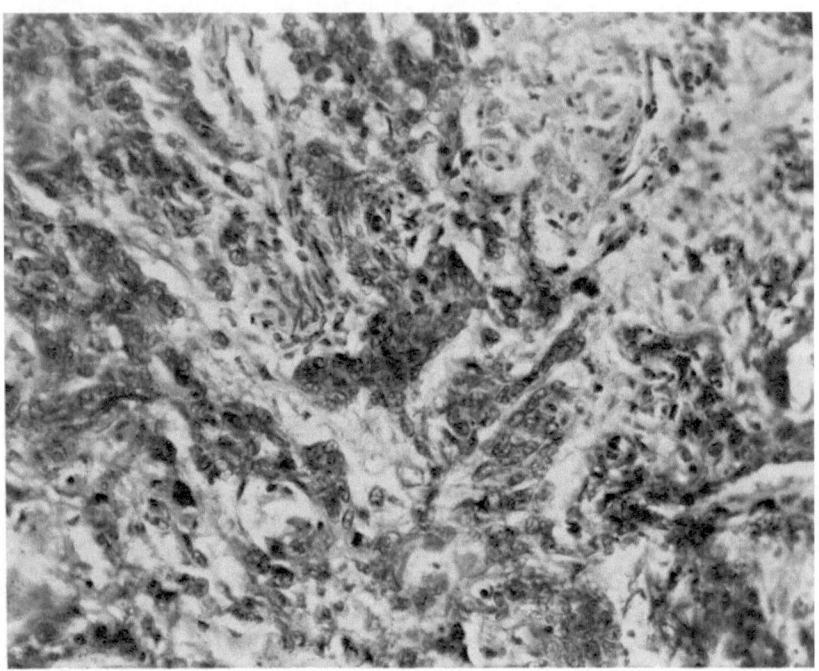

Fig. 48. Immature cell carcinoma in the lung of a rat intratracheally insufflated with radioactive cerium (courtesy by Dr. CEMBER)

WILLARD, MARKS and BAIR; ALTMANN, HUNSTEIN and STUTZ; CEMBER, WATSON and NOVAK; CEMBER; PARK, BAIR and CLARKE; GUIMARAES, LAMERTON and CHRISTENSEN; CEMBER and STEMMER; KOCHETKOVA, AVRUNINA and SAGAIDAK; LASKIN, KUSCHNER, NELSON, ALTSHULER, HARLEY and DANIELS; KOTSCHETKOWA and AWRUNINA; KUSCHNER; KURSHAKOVA and IVANOV). The following radioactive chemicals were used in these experiments: Cobalt[60]; Strontium[90]; Plutonium[239]; Ruthenium[106]; Yttrium[90]; Cerium[144]; Sulfur[35]; Phosphorus[32]; Gold[198]; Iron[59]; and Rhodium[106]. The bronchial carcinomas produced were usually squamous cell carcinomas and undifferentiated carcinomas (Fig. 48). While these experiments provided ample proof of the fact that pulmonary tissue when exposed to various types of ionizing radiation, reacts with the development of bronchogenic carcinomas, they did not duplicate the type of exposure to radioactive matter present in man.

The results obtained when such chemicals were inhaled as a gas or dust must be considered of possessing more conclusive value.

In the first experiments of this type reported, SCHMIDTMANN failed to elicit any epithelial bronchial proliferations in experimental animals exposed to the inhalation of dust of 6 drill holes from Schneeberg mines. Attempts of ROSTOSKI and SAUPE to induce lung cancers in mice inhaling radium emanation (radon) were unsuccessful because of an early death of the mice. DÖHNERT, who exposed white mice to the mine gases and dust by keeping them within the Schneeberg mines noted that after one year in the mines, seven (7) of the 26 mice histologically examined had pulmonary tumors (25%), of which two (2) were diagnosed as papillary adenocarcinomas. Since some strains of white mice develop spontaneously lung adenomas in a much higher percentage of older animals, the significance of these findings is doubtful. However, some support for suggesting causal relations between exposure and lung tumor formation may be deduced from the results obtained by CAMPBELL who exposed mice to the inhalation of dust from Joachimsthal mines and noted that tumors of the lung were present in 20.3% of the test series, while they were found in only 2.1% of the untreated controls. Similarly positive observations were subsequently reported by RAJEWSKY, SCHRAUB and KAHLAU and by KAHLAU, who exposed mice to the inhalation of radium emanation and noted the presence of many pulmonary adenomas and adenocarcinomas in these mice. However, the experimental conditions used, particularly the employment of a non-inbred strain of mice and a relatively small number of mice, impair the value of their observations. It must be mentioned, however, that experimental studies of UNNEWEHR on mice inhaling radon yielded similar neoplastic responses in the lung, i.e., the development of bronchial carcinomas. LISCO and FINKEL, moreover, reported similar results when animals inhaled an aerosol of radioactive cerium (Ce^{144}).

Finally, it may briefly be mentioned that mice given either gamma radiation emitted from radium or x-radiation over prolonged periods of time exhibited an increased number of pulmonary tumors (LORENZ, ESCHENBRENNER, HESTON and DERINGER; LORENZ, HESTON, ESCHENBRENNER and DERINGER; ESCHENBRENNER and MILLER; LORENZ; HESTON, LORENZ and DERINGER). The results obtained in guinea pigs and rabbits simultaneously and identically exposed to two types of radiations, however, were equivocal.

12. Miscellaneous Respiratory Carcinogens

In addition to the different recognized or strongly suspected human respiratory carcinogens of occupational and/or environmental significance, there exists a group of chemicals which either have shown such properties when introduced into experimental animals only and for which so far any corresponding experience in man is lacking — although man becomes, for various reasons, exposed to these agents — or have exhibited carcinogenic qualities for other organs in experimental animals, while a few isolated observations in man suggest that they may elicit cancers of the respiratory tract in this species. The evidence on these chemicals is presented so as to alert all interested parties in such potential relationships, to stimulate intensified study of these chemicals, and to provide whatever basic information is available on the carcinogenic action of these chemicals which may be valuable for any medicolegal purposes. The observations cited, though representing mere clues of possible respiratory cancer hazards, are nevertheless important since the discovery of the majority of the presently known occupational cancers has resulted from further studies of such filamentous evidence.

a) Isonicotinic Acid Hydrazide (Isoniacid)

During the first decades of this century, tuberculous scars of the lung were regarded by many investigators as a cause of pulmonary cancer developing on the basis of a derailment of regenerative processes in the adjacent lung tissue (HUEPER). This concept became distintly less popular after 1930 following the discovery of specific chemical carcinogens and with improvements in the epidemiologic-statistical methods of analysis. During the past decade, however, a definite revival in the scientific interest of causal connections between pulmonary tuberculosis and lung cancer has occurred. In fact, the concept of a scar cancer of the lung has again found wider acceptance (ROESSLE; CARROLL). ROESSLE proposed that cancer formation at such sites was attributable to the carcinogenic action of the accumulated cholesterol.

BALO has reported, moreover, on the development of atypical epithelial proliferations and of lung cancers in the marginal areas of old infarcts, while PANSA and MOLLO have observed similar abnormal epithelial growth in the lungs of rabbits following the experimental production of hemorrhagic infarcts. These lesions were suggestive in their morphologic characteristics of early carcinomatous changes.

Recent experimental findings of STANTON and BLACKWELL have thrown additional light on the possible causal mechanism operating in the development of the so-called "scar" cancers of the human lung. These investigators injected intravenously into rats a mixture of a halogenated hydrocarbon (hexachlorotetrafluorobutane), which causes the development of multiple infarcts in the lung, together with a carcinogenic hydrocarbon (methyl-cholanthrene) and observed invasive epidermoid carcinomas derived from regenerating epithelium in the periphery of such infarcts. If methyl-cholanthrene was given in tricaprylin which does not produce infarcts, the development of massive keratinized cysts in the lungs only were obtained which, however, did not become cancerous. While STANTON et al. assumed that the regenerative epithelial proliferation elicited by the process of infarction played an important role in determining the cancerous sequelae induced, it is more likely that the infarcts with their interrupted vascular supply served as localizing and concentrating mechanisms for the carcinogenic chemical and that thus the carcinogenic effects associated with infarction reflect actually a quantitative dose phenomenon affecting circumscribed parts of the lung. The histologic observation made by HUEPER on the preferential accumulation of oil droplets around scars, tubercles, bronchopneumonic foci, and similar areas with interrupted blood supply and blocked vascular lumens of the pulmonary system of man following an intravenous injection of camphorated oil strongly suggests this action mechanism. The lack of cancerous transformation of the frequently occurring squamous-cell metaplasias with cyst formation in the lung of old rats with chronic pneumonic conditions, on the other hand, attest to the fact that squamous-cell metaplasia of the bronchial epithelium as such is not necessarily a precancerous condition.

Associated with this recent change in the reaction toward the existence of causal relations between pulmonary subpleural scarring and the subsequent development of lung cancer has been the appearance of numerous reports on the frequency of coexistence of pulmonary tuberculosis and cancer and on the suspected causal relations between the two conditions (CRINQUETTE and HAMEL; GEBEL, EPSTEIN, FULKERSON and SPARGER; BODENSTAB and QUARZ; WOLFORD, WEBB and STAUSS; SOCHOCKY; KHEIFETS, HERMANN and HEIM). TONELLI, however, has recently challenged the validity of such claims by pointing out that the so-called scars are pleural depressions, not preexisting to the tumor but caused by it. They, moreover, do not correspond to previous infarcts, are not tubercular and occur mostly in persons 40 to 50 years old.

Despite these criticisms of TONELLI it may nevertheless be possible that the increased interest in the association between pulmonary tuberculosis and cancer reflects at least in part, a real and recent change in the therapeutic management of pulmonary tuberculosis which is related to the introduction of chemical tuberculostatic agents, especially isonicotinic acid hydrazide (isoniacid).

Experimental observations made by several investigators during the past decade have shown that isoniacid is a chemical carcinogen to mice in which it is capable of producing benign and malignant tumors of the lung as well as cancers in other organs (JUHASZ, BALO and KENDREY VIALLIER and CASANOVA; SCHWAN, MORI, YASUNO and MATSUMOTO; BIANCIFIORI and RIBACCHI). FUKUI, NEGATA, IMAMURA and TAGASHIRA have drawn attention to the fact that, according to MORI et al., compounds capable of inducing pulmonary tumors in mice (isonicotinic acid hydrazine, ethyl carbamate, semicarbazid, pyrazinamide) have a remarkable similarity of their molecular structure in containing a carbamyl group (NH_2—C—).

$$\underset{O}{\overset{\|}{}}$$

While it is possible that the two developments cited are merely chronologically related, the fact that the tuberculostatic chemical, isoniacid, is a pulmonary carcinogen nevertheless suggests that there might exist a causal relation between the two events, and that the therapeutic use of isoniacid in patients with tuberculosis of the lung may have played an active and essential part in the subsequent development of pulmonary cancer in some of them. The evidence on hand in support of such a hypothesis deserves to be tested for its validity through conducting a critical analysis of all cases of lung cancer in tuberculous individuals whether or not they had been treated with isoniacid or any other tuberculostatic chemical and whether the quality and quantity of the chemical used as well as the latent period and any other circumstantial evidence point to the existence of a relation between the treatment given and the following pulmonary carcinogenesis.

The potential occupation significance of these experimental observations is suggested by the fact that hydrazines are employed as rocket propellants and oxidizers in the production of which the carcinogenically highly potent nitrosamines are used (BOYSEN).

b) Nitrosamines

Nitrosamines are compounds frequently used in or generated during chemical processes of industrial importance since nitrosamines are formed when dialkylamines are acted upon by nitrous oxide or nitric acid (DRUCKREY, PREUSSMANN and SCHMAEHL). The rocket propellant, dimethylhydrazine, thus is a reduced derivative of dimethylnitrosamine (BOYSEN; ARGUS, LEUTZE and KANE; ARGUS and HOCH-LIGETI). While so far no human observations are on record indicating that any one of the various nitrosamines found to be carcinogenic for mice, rats, guinea pigs and hamsters exerts a similar action on man, DRUCKREY has suggested that such chemicals might be contained in cigarette smoke and thus account for some of the carcinogenic properties exhibited in animals by cigarette tar.

The following experimental observations demonstrate the high carcinogenic potency of nitrosamines and specifically their carcinogenic action on the trachea, bronchi and alveolar structures of the lungs and nasal sinuses of animals (DRUCKREY, PREUSSMANN and SCHMAEHL; SCHOENTAL; DONTENWILL and MOHR; ARGUS and HOCH-LIGETI; DRUCKREY, PREUSSMANN, SCHMAEHL and MUELLER; SCHOENTAL and MAGEE; DRUCKREY and PREUSSMANN; ZAK, HOLZNER, SINGER and POPPER; DONTEN-WILL, MOHR and ZAGEL; HERROLD and DUNHAM).

Although the various nitrosamines differ among each other in their organotropic carcinogenic action (liver, stomach, esophagus, trachea, lung, kidney, bladder, brain) depending upon their chemical constitution and the particular species used, many of them induce the development of squamous cell carcinomas and adenocarcinomas of the trachea and bronchi and alveolar carcinomas of the lung (dimethylnitrosamine, diethylnitrosamine, N-N-diamylnitrosamine, N-nitrosopiperidin, N-nitrosomorpho-lin, N-nitroso-N-methyl-urethane). The relatively high cancer attack rates, the re-markable organ specificity of some of these chemicals and the organic and species pluripotentiality of some members of this group of chemical compounds indicate their potential importance as possible human carcinogens. The experimental observations on hand are sufficiently serious and adequate for justifying thorough investigations of occupational and general population groups specifically exposed to these chemicals or their reduction and oxidation products. While the reduction product, dimethyl hydrazine, has proved to be noncarcinogenic, the oxidation product, dimethylnitra-min, when fed to rats has produced kidney cancers.

c) Nitroquinolines and Related Nitro- and Amino-Compounds

Another potential human respiratory carcinogen is 4-nitroquinoline-1-oxide, which was developed as a fungicide (URI, BOGNAR and BEKESI; NAKAHARA). This chemical and some of its nitro- and aminoderivatives induce when applied to the skin, squam-ous cell carcinomas, and sarcomas when injected subcutaneously into mice and rats (TAKAYAMA; SHIRASU and OHTA; SHIRASU; NAKAHARA and FUKUOKA; NAKAHARA, FUKUOKA and SAKAI; ENDO and KUME; CHINO; LACASSAGNE, BUU-HOI and ZAJDELA). Subsequent studies yielded the fact that mice subcutaneously injected with this chemi-cal developed also benign and malignant epithelial tumors (adenocarcinomas) of the lung (MORI; MORI and YASUNO). It is noteworthy that similar neoplastic responses in the lungs were evoked in mice when they were painted, with, or inhaled para-benzoquinone (HAYASHI, KANIZAWA and IDE; TAKIZAWA; TAKIZAWA and KANIZAWA; KISHIZAWA).

The administration of acetylaminofluorene to rats, but not to hamsters, has also resulted in the development of bronchial carcinomas (BIELSCHOWSKY; DONTENWILL, MOHR and ZAGEL), and N,N'-2,7-fluorenylenebisacetamide has been shown to induce cancers of the lung in rats in addition to cancers of the liver, mammary glands, glandular stomach, jejunum, ear duct, uterus, skin, salivary glands, kidney, cranial nerves, adrenal cortex pancreas and hematopoietic tissues (MORRIS; WAGNER; RAY, STEWART and SNELL). A comprehensive experimental and epidemiologic in-vestigation of aromatic and aliphatic amino- and nitro-compounds for carcinogenic properties exerted on tissues of the respiratory system of man and animals is urgently needed as a part of the general study on the etiologic factors responsible for the causation and rise in frequency of cancers of the lung in man. Such investigations are especially indicated for the large group of aromatic amino- and nitro-chemical workers, because UEBELIN and PLETSCHER noted not only an excessive incidence of bladder cancer but also of lung cancer among Swiss benzidine workers.

d) Carbamates

The tumorigenic action on various tissues, especially the lungs of mice and rats by ethyl carbamate (urethane) and the demonstration of this effect in the offspring of mice which received urethane during the last stage of pregnancy (NETTLESHIP and HENSHAW; LARSEN and HESTON; LARSEN; HADDOW and SEXTON; SCHOENTAL; FIORE-DONATI; RITCHIE; MOSTOFI and LARSEN; BERENBLUM and HARAN-GHERA; KLEIN; JAFFÉ; GUYER and CLAUS; ROSIN; etc.), has given rise to speculations whether or not the use of urethane and other carbamates in medicine and in the various chemicals widely employed as pesticides, insect repellents, and herbicides (BALL and COWEN; BARTALINI; SHABAD and NAUMOVA; ESKOLA; KYLE, SCHWARTZ, OLINER and DAMESHEK; CRAMER) might have played a role in the rise of lung cancers during recent decades (BALO). This suspicion received lately some support by the fact that ethyl carbamate and isopropyl-n-phenyl carbamate (VAN ESCH, VAN GENDEREN and VINK) were shown to be carcinogenic initiators and capable of producing cancers of the skin, liver and other internal organs of mice (TANNENBAUM). A weaker neoplastic effect upon the mouse lung was demonstrated for several closely related carbamates (propyl carbamate; N-methylethylcarbamate; N-hydroxy-ethylcarbamate) (FUKUI, NAGATA, IMAMURA and TAGASHIRA). The production and use of polyurethane plastics in the human economy have recently created another source of widespread contact of occupational and general population groups to polymerized carbamate derivatives which have been found to be carcinogenic when implanted into rats (HUEPER and PAYNE). The incriminating experimental evidence on hand is sufficiently serious for justifying the following investigations:

1. Surveys on the occurrence and incidence of cancers of the respiratory system, especially the lung, should be conducted among producers and users of carbamate pharmaceuticals, pesticides, herbicides and insect repellents for establishing factual evidence on the neoplastic action of such compounds in man.

2. Similar epidemiologic surveys should be made on worker groups engaged in the production and processing of polyurethane plastics especially where fumes and dusts from such products are inhaled.

e) Chlorinated Hydrocarbons

Chlorinated hydrocarbons are mainly known for their toxic effect upon the liver in man and animals and for their hepatocarcinogenic action in mice, rats and hamsters (chloroform, carbon tetrachloride, DDT, Aldrin, Dieldrin, Aramite) (EDWARDS and DALTON; DELLA PORTA, TERRACINI and SHUBIK; RUDALI and MARIANI; ESCHENBRENNER and MILLER; STOWELL, LEE, TSUBOI and VAILASANA; FITZHUGH and NELSON; DAVIS and FITZHUGH). AN DER LAN, moreover, has recently demonstrated that DDT, methoxychlor, Rothane (dichloro-diphenyl-dichlorethane) and Kelthane (Di-p-diphenyl-trichlor-ethanol) like the carbamate insecticide, Sevin (l-naphthyl-N-methyl-carbamate), when applied to the invertebrate, Turbellaria or Tricladida, elicit abnormal cell growth of the epidermis and tumor formation.

The observation of a cancer of the lung in a laboratory technician, 23 years old, who had worked with DDT for nine years previously (RANDIG) and in a chemist-entomologist who had been engaged for a number of years in the development of DDT preparations (HUEPER) suggest the possibility that these hepatocarcinogenic agents when inhaled in sufficient quantities over an adequate length of time might exert also a carcinogenic effect upon the respiratory organs. For this reason, it seems to be advisable to undertake epidemiologic studies on producers and the industrial and agricultural users of chlorinated hydrocarbons inhaling these chemicals in the form of dust, mists, suspensions and gases sustaining identical types of exposure for their relative liability to cancer of the respiratory organs.

f) Formaldehyde

Since formaldehyde is a mutagen (AUERBACH) and because GARSCHIN and SCHABAD (1935) produced atypical proliferations of the bronchial epithelium in mice following the introduction of formalin, the suspicion has prevailed that the inhalation of formaldehyde vapors might lead to the development of lung cancer in man (bakelite makers, undertakers, histologic technicians, wrinkle proofers of clothing, etc.) (FISHER, KANOF and BIONDI; GLASS; HENSON; LUTZ; BOURNE and SEFERMAN). Some experimental support of such a suspicion may be deduced from observations of WATANABE and SUGIMOTO, who obtained subcutaneous sarcomas in rats following the subcutaneous injection of urotropin, a formaldehyde releasing urinary antiseptic. Experiments of HORTON, TYE and STEMMER who subjected mice to the inhalation of gaseous formaldehyde, did not result in the production of pulmonary tumors although the tracheal and bronchial mucosa of such animals showed hyperplastic and atypical metaplastic changes which, however, did not progress to an invasive cancer. In contrast, some of the mice subjected to repeated inhalation of an aerosol of coal tar developed squamous cell cancers of the bronchi. Formaldehyde vapors applied simultaneously with the inhalation of aerosol of coal tar did not hasten or potentiate tumor formation in the lung.

There is not sufficient experimental and human epidemiologic evidence indicating that exposures to formaldehyde vapors constitute a significant and actual lung cancer hazard.

g) Natural and Man-Made Polymers

Several isolated observations suggest that an occupational and habitual inhalation of various natural and man-made carbon polymers might causally be related to the development of cancer of the lungs. The coexistence of bagassosis and lung cancer was reported by ONUIGBO. KOTIN and FALK recorded two cases of lung cancer in workers exposed to fiberglass and plexiglass dust or fumes generated during the synthesis and manufacture of these products. Fragments of the polymers were present in the tumor tissue. BRESLOW, studying the role of different occupational factors in pulmonary carcinogenesis, found that deep-fat frying cooks had a statistically excessive liability to lung cancer. It may be of significance that fatty acids undergo polymerization when subjected to high temperature and oxidation and that such fats contained material which when injected into rats displayed carcinogenic properties. The demonstration of carcinogenic qualities in various aliphatic diepoxides when applied to the skin of mice furnishes additional evidence that polymerization products might be involved in the cancerization process elicited by some chemicals since diepoxides exhibit a tendency to polymerize and to influence the degree of polymerization of chemicals with which they come in contact (HENDRY, HOMER, ROSE and WALPOLE; WEIL, CONDRA, HAUN and STRIEGEL; ORRIS, VAN DUUREN and NELSON; HINE, GUZMAN, COURSEY, WELLINGTON and ANDERSON; KOTIN and FALK). Since HINE et al. found in tests on animals that two epoxy-resins possessed carcinogenic properties, it may be pertinent to point to the excessive attack rate of lung cancer in painters (PIPER; WYNDER). Mention also may be made in this connection of the local and systemic carcinogenic effects elicited in rats by parenterally introduced carboxymethyl cellulose, polyvinyl pyrrolidone and several dextrans (NELSON; HUEPER), since these and similar water-soluble polymers are widely used as active ingredients in hair lacquers and have induced in some individuals (beauticians especially) multifocal granulomatous reactions in the lungs (EDELSTON; BERGMANN, FLANCE, CRUZ, KLAM, ARONSON, JOSHI, and BLUMENTHAL; BRUNNER, GIOVACCHINI, WYATT, DUNLAP and CALANDRA; BERGMANN; BRUNNER; DRAIZE, NELSON, NEWBURGER and KELLY; DEAN; DOYLE; CARES).

1. The spreading practice of deep-fat frying for commercial and home purposes and the thereby conditioned exposure of cooks, kitchen personnel and housewives to fumes and mists of repeatedly heated and oxidized fats which have undergone polymerization, provides an urgent indication to survey employees of commercial deep-fat frying operations for their relative liability to cancers of the respiratory organs.

This type of respiratory exposure may also be present as a part of the carcinogenic hazards connected with charcoal broiling of meats and fish, although the major part of carcinogenic exposures is probably connected here with the inhalation of carcinogenic combustion products of coal or wood and of burned meat and fish.

2. Employees in beauty parlors and women and men applying frequently to their hair and without precautions, nebulized hair lacquers furnish another group of people in need of comprehensive and critical epidemiologic analysis for occupational and habitual lung cancer hazards.

3. A third class of individuals who should be analyzed in this direction are the large and diverse groups of industrial producers, processers, and users of water-soluble and insoluble, solid and liquid plastics inhaling dusts, fumes, and mists of various natural and man-made polymers and developing in part as the result of such exposures, irritations of the lung (chemical pneumonia) or pneumoconioses.

D. Prevention and Control of Occupational Respiratory Cancer Hazards

The evidence presented establishes definitely the fact that numerous man-made and man-used respiratory carcinogens have been introduced into the human environment during the past 150 years and that they are responsible not only for a rapidly growing number of occupational cancers of the lung, pleura, larynx, nasal cavity and paranasal sinuses, but evidently also play a significant role in the causation of such cancers in the general population through their direct or indirect, local and general spread into the atmosphere, especially of urban and industrialized regions. Since cancers of the respiratory system are still among the least therapeutically controlled malignant tumors and have alarmingly increased in frequency during the last 60 years, they represent an important problem for applied cancer prevention.

A practical approach to occupational respiratory cancer control by preventive and prophylactic measures has to include two aspects representing different problems of technology, public health, and law. The primary, but not always principal hazard affects the various types of workers engaged in the production, processing, handling, transportation, shipping, consuming and using of such carcinogenic materials. It is obvious that this group of workers includes often a considerable number of individuals who are not ordinarily and readily suspected of having such contacts. Many of them, moreover, are being exposed to such agents while working either on other jobs within the plant area or while handling such products, usually intermittently, in transit (stevedores, truckers, shipping clerks, laundresses, salesmen, delivery men, etc.). There can be little doubt that under ordinary circumstances, occupational exposures to respiratory carcinogens go often unnoticed for the last group of individuals listed. They are usually also not subjected to any control measures. Cancers resulting from such contacts for these reasons do, as a rule, not become causes of compensation procedures even if existing occupational compensation laws would apply to occupational diseases contracted under such circumstances.

The second and often much larger group of individuals exposed to occupational or industrial respiratory carcinogens, comprises the persons who have contact with these agents following their dissemination in the immediate environment of industrial establishments (fume zone), i.e., persons who work, live, play or attend school near such plants and later in life and often after a lag period of many years, develop the so-called "neighborhood cancers". A variety of these cancers are represented by those which occur in individuals living or working near the roads of transportation of carcinogenic materials and inhale, therefore, the dust from roads accidentally contaminated with such materials or reside along roads paved with slags containing carcinogenic residues (asbestos, radioactive chemicals, nickel, etc.). An additional group of persons having environmental exposures to respiratory carcinogens consists of members of the household of workers who have occupational contact to carcinogens and who bring home their dusty and dirty work clothes for cleaning, and thereby spread contact with such carcinogens to other members of the household ("household cancers"). The definite demonstration of such respiratory "neighborhood" and "household cancers" is of rather recent date and has remained limited essentially to only two types of carcinogens (beryllium, asbestos). Their recognition was facilitated by the fact that these carcinogens produce pulmonary changes of etiologically characteristic nature. While the environmental dissemination of respiratory carcinogens has been made the subject of some control legislation, it is doubtful whether any number of these cancers appearing in members of the general population from such events has ever been made the subject of litigation or of criminal prosecution.

A preventive control of occupational respiratory cancer hazards can be achieved by either eliminating the carcinogenic agent from the work environment, i.e., by discontinuing its further production and use, or by employing production and handling procedures which preclude any contact of workers with the hazardous material. The practical application of the first mentioned method of control which obviously is the most effective one, encounters often distinct difficulties because of the unavoidable need for many of the carcinogenic products mentioned, such as chromium, nickel, carbonaceous fuel, etc. It is, moreover, obvious that such procedures would always result also in the closure of the plant and thereby in the loss of employment of the workers involved. Safety, therefore, is bought under such circumstances with unemployment through elimination of the hazardous jobs.

A similar result is likely to occur in many instances if hazardous occupational exposures to respiratory carcinogens are controlled by the introduction of safer and more effective technologic production measures. Such procedures usually are associated with the introduction of extensive automation which again results in a reduction in labor force. The use of and insistence on technologic preventive measures against respiratory cancer hazards, as against any other industrial cancer hazards thus create serious social and economic repercussions for the workers employed in such operations. The safety obtained under such circumstances for the workers retained in their jobs is, moreover, rarely absolute. There usually remains some unavoidable degree of hazard for such workers. Unless special precautions are taken, it is also possible that the use of effective preventive measures within a plant may result in a more marked pollution of the periplant environment, i.e., air, soil and water, through a more massive release of plant wastes with exhaust air and waste water. It is obvious from these considerations that also a control of respiratory cancer hazards by technologic means is available only for a price. It is up to human society to decide whether or not it is willing and able to pay the entire price or whether it prefers to make a compromise at some level of partial safety which does not endanger its present economic existence, but which at the same time provides only incomplete and probably not maximally possible safety.

It is apparent, moreover, from the preceding discussion that in any attempt to secure relative protection against occupational and industry-related respiratory cancer hazards, human society is faced with the practical and moral problem that such efforts might result in the substitution of one social inequity by another one and that the enforcement of justice thereby might become a two-faced measure. Any attempt at improving radically this complex situation and to unravel the complicated relationships will confront mankind with the perplexing dilemma of finding new means for promoting progress and prosperity without human sacrifice and for restraining those of its members who continue to adhere to the old principle of dubious morality that the ultimate purpose of organized mankind is the accumulation of physical, monetary assets and not the acquisition of moral values and the protection of the well-being of its individual members as well as of mankind as whole.

References

Nonspecific Respiratory Irritants
Exclusive of Silicosis

ADELHEIM, R.: Beiträge zur pathologischen Anatomie und Pathogenese der Kampfgasvergiftungen. Virchows Arch. path. Anat. 236, 309—360 (1922).
Advisory Committee to the Surgeon General of the Public Health Service: Report on smoking and health. Public Health Service Publ. No. 1103, Washington, D. C., 1963, p. 387.
ALLEN, M. L.: Bronchiogenic carcinoma associated with pneumoconiosis. Report of 2 cases. J. Indust. Hyg. Toxicol. 16, 346—347 (1934).

BALO, J., E. JUHASZ, and J. TEMES: Pulmonary infarcts and pulmonary carcinoma. Cancer 9, 918—922 (1956).

BRINKMANN: Über Lungenkarzinom. Inaug. Diss. Leipzig 1924.

BROCKBANK, W.: Occupational incidence of primary lung cancer. Quart. J. Med. 1, 31—40 (1932).

BURGESS, S. G., and C. SHADDICK: Bronchitis and air pollution. Roy. Soc. Prom. Hlth J. 79, 10—24 (1959).

CAMPBELL, A. H., and E. J. LEE: The relationship between lung cancer and chronic bronchitis. Brit. J. Dis. Chest 57, 113—119 (1963).

CASE, R. A. M., and A. J. LEA: Mustard gas poisoning, chronic bronchitis and lung cancer. Brit. J. prev. soc. Med. 9, 62—72 (1955).

CUNNINGHAM, G. J., E. NASSAU, and J. B. WALTER: The frequency of tumor-like formations in bronchiectatic lungs. Thorax 13, 64—68 (1958).

DRUCKREY, H., R. PREUSSMANN, and D. SCHMÄHL: Carcinogenicity and chemical structure of nitrosamines. Acta Un. int. Cancr. 19, 510—511 (1963).

DUBLIN, L. P., and R. J. VANE: Metropolitan Life Insurance Company Survey, 1937—1939.

DUGUID, J. B.: The incidence of intrathoracic tumors in Manchester. Lancet 2, 111—113 (1927).

DUNNER, L., and M. S. HICKS: Bronchial carcinoma in dusty occupations in boiler scales and grain dockers. Brit. J. Tuberc. 47, 145—151 (1953).

DYER, N. H.: Cancer as related to the mining industry in West Virginia. W. Va med J. 48, 187—189 (1952).

ENGER, Inaug. Diss. Leipzig 1923.

FALK, H. L., H. M. TREMER, and P. KOTIN: Effect of cigarette smoke and its constituents on ciliated, mucus-secreting epithelium. J. Nat. Cancer Inst. 23, 999—1012 (1959).

FEIL, A.: Pneumoconiose et cancer. Presse méd. 43, 212 (1935).

FINKE, W.: Chronic pulmonary disease as a possible factor in lung cancer. Internat. Rec. Med. 169, 61—72 (1956).

FRIEDRICH, G.: Periphere Lungenkrebse auf dem Boden pleuranaher Narben. Virchows Arch. path. Anat. 304, 230—247 (1939).

FULTON, J. S: Carcinoma of the lung. Proc. roy. Soc. Med. 42, 775—782 (1949).

GERBE, H.: Über das Bronchuscarcinom auf Grund statistischer Erhebungen im Heinrich Braun Krankenhaus, Zwickau, i. Sa. Z. Krebsforsch. 49, 667—676 (1939/40).

HAMPELN, P.: Häufigkeit und Ursache des primären Lungenkarzinoms. Grenzgeb. Med. 36, 145—150 (1923).

HIRSCH, E. F., and H. B. RUSSELL: Chronic exudative and indurative pneumonia to inhalation of shellac. Arch. Path. 39, 281—286 (1945).

HUEPER, W. C.: Über die intravenöse Kampferölinjektion auf Grund pathologisch-anatomischer Untersuchungen. Med. Klin. 18, 373—376 (1922).

— Occupational tumors and allied diseases. Springfield, Ill.: C. C. Thomas 1942.

—, Occupational and environmental pulmonary cancer with special reference to pneumoconiosis. Proc. Seventh Saranac Symposium on Pneumoconiosis. 1952, pp. 154.

—, Trauma and cancer. Trauma 1, 47—110 (1959).

—, Methodologic explorations in experimental respiratory carcinogenesis. Arzneimittelforsch. 14, 814—822 (1964).

JAMES, W. R. L.: Primary lung cancer in South Wales coal-workers with pneumoconiosis. Brit. J. industr. Med. 12, 87—91 (1955).

KENNAWAY, E. L., and N. M. KENNAWAY: The incidence of cancer of the lung in coal miners in England and Wales. Brit. J. Cancer 7, 10—18 (1953).

KIKUTH, W.: Über das Lungencarcinom. Virchows Arch. path. Anat. 255, 107—128 (1925).

KOUWENAAR, W.: On cancer incidence in Indonesia. J. Nat. Cancer Inst 11, 642—643 (1950).

KREYBERG, L.: Occupational infiuences in a Norwegian material of 235 cases of primary epithelial lung tumours. Brit. J. Cancer 8, 605—612 (1954).

KUSCHNER, M.: The response of the lung to carcinogens. Arch. environm. Hlth 6, 118—121 (1963).

LICKINT, F.: Ätiologie und Prophylaxe des Lungenkrebses. Dresden: T. Steinkopff (1953).

Löhr, B., and A. Wagner: Relations of type of tumor and localization of bronchial carcinoma to pulmonary ventilation and changes in their relationship to exogenous influences (chronic bronchitis, pneumonia, smoking). Arch. klin. Chir. 280, 592—708 (1955).

Lüders, C. J., and K. G. Themel: Die Narbenkrebse der Lunge als Beitrag zur Pathogenese des peripheren Lungencarcinoms. Virchows Arch. path. Anat. 325, 499—551 (1954).

Morgan, J. G.: Some observations on the incidence of respiratory cancer in nickel workers. Brit. J. industr. Med. 15, 224—234 (1958).

Müller, F. H.: Tabakmißbrauch und Lungencarcinom. Z. Krebsforsch. 49, 57—85 (1939).

National Survey: Chronic bronchitis in Great Britain. Brit. med. J. 2, 973—979 (1961).

Onuigbo, W. I. B.: Metastasizing lung cancer associated with past bagassosis. Am. Rev. resp. Dis. 86, 723—725 (1962).

Passey, R. D.: Some problems in lung cancer. Lancet 2, 107—112 (1962).

Pemberton, J.: Air pollution as a possible cause of bronchitis and lung cancer. J. Hyg. Epidem. (Praha) 5, 189—194 (1961).

Rössle, R.: Die Narbenkrebse der Lungen. Schweiz. med. Wschr. 73, 1200—1203 (1943).

Schmorl, G.: Über die Beziehungen anthrakotischer bronchialer Lymphknoten zu Bronchialerkrankungen und zur Bronchitis deformans. Münch. med. Wschr. 72, 757—758 (1925).

Schulte, G.: Pneumokoniosen der Ruhrbergleute und Lungenkarzinom. Fortschr. Röntgenstr. 41, 444 (1930).

Schulz, O.: Die Beurteilung der schweren Staublungenerkrankungen nach der Verordnung von 11. 2. 1929 unter besonderer Berücksichtigung der Frage einer Entschädigungspflicht von Begleiterkrankungen. Arch. Gewerbepath. Gewerbehyg. 6, 117—143 (1935).

Seyfahrt, C.: Lungenkarzinom in Leipzig. Deut. med. Wschr. 50, 1497—1499 (1924).

Staemmler, M.: Beruf und Krebs. Münch. med. Wschr. 85, 121—125 (1938).

Stofer, A. B.: Lungenschädigungen durch feste und flüssige organische Substanzen. Path. et Microbiol. (Basel) 24, 107—139 (1961).

Teleky, L.: Occupational cancer of the lung. J. industr. Hyg. 19, 73—85 (1937).

Versluys, J. J.: Cancer and occupation in the Netherlands. Brit. J. Cancer 3, 161—185 (1949).

Woodruff, C. E., and H. C. Nahas: Pulmonary tuberculosis, bronchiectasis and calcification as related to bronchogenic carcinoma. Am. Rev. Tuberc. 64, 620—629 (1951).

Wynder, E. L., and E. A. Graham: Etiologic factors in bronchogenic carcinoma with special reference to industrial exposures. Arch. industr. Hyg. 4, 221—235 (1951).

Silicosis

Adamo, M.: Silicosi e cancro polmonare. Medicina legale e delle assicurazioni, Vol. II, Geneva, 1954.

Ahlendorf, W.: Silikose und Bronchialkarzinom. Z. Krebsforsch. 41, 125—129 (1959).

Allen, M. L.: Bronchiogenic carcinoma associated with pneumoconiosis. J. industr. Hyg. 16, 346—347 (1934).

Anderson, C. S., and J. H. Dible: Silicosis and carcinoma of the lung. J. Hyg. 38, 185—204 (1938).

Astorri, P.: Cancro del polmone in soggetto silicotico. Contributo casistico e considerazione clinica. 14 (1953).

Balo, J.: Lungenkarzinom und Lungenadenom. Akademiai Kiado Budapest, 1957, pp. 363.

Bauer, A.: Kieselsäure und Krebs. Zbl. allg. Path. path. Anat. 86, 67—68 (1950).

Berblinger, W.: Zunahme des Lungenkrebses und Staublungenkrankheiten. Med. Klin. 27, 1337—1342 (1931).

Becker, B. J. P.: University of Witwatersrand, Rep. South Africa. Personal communication, 1958.

Bonser, G. M., J. S. Faulds, and N. J. Stewart: Occupational cancer of the urinary bladder in dyestuffs operatives and of the lung in asbestos textile workers and in iron-ore-miners. Amer. J. clin. Path. 25, 126—134 (1955).

Bossi, E.: Silicosi e cancro polmonare. Sicurezza Sociale. 12, (1957).

Bradshaw, H. H., and R. J. Chodoff: Anthracosilicosis simulating pulmonary carcinoma. Amer. Rev. Tuberc. 39, 817—824 (1939).

Braun, H.: Silikose und Bronchialcarcinom. Med. Klin. 51, 1863—1865 (1956).

158 References

CAMPBELL, J. A.: Cancer of the human lung and animal experiment. J. industr. Hyg. 19, 449—462 (1937).

CHARR, R.: Carcinoma of the bronchus in association with anthracosilicosis. A study of four cases. Amer. J. med. Sci. 194, 535—541 (1937).

CHATGIDAKIS, C. B.: A study of the bronchial mucous glands in white South African miners. Arch. environm. Hlth 1, 335—342 (1960).

CHIURCO, G. A.: Silicosi-morbo sociale e professionale rapporto con il ca. polmonare. Sicurezza Sociale. 16, 129—224 (1961).

DI BIASI, W.: Die Staublungenerkrankungen. In Jötten und Gärtner. Dresden: Steinkopff 1950.

DIKSHTEIN, E. A.: Changes of the bronchial tree in pneumoconiosis combined with bronchial carcinoma. Vopr. Onkol. 7, 20—26 (1961).

DIBLE, J. H.: Silicosis and malignant disease. Lancet. 2, 982—983 (1934).

DOGLIONI, L.: Su tre casi di silicosi associata a carcinoma polmonare. Riv. anat. pat. 1137—1163, 1954.

DRUCKREY, H., u. D. SCHMAEHL: Cancerogene Wirkung von Quarz bei Implantation an Ratten. Naturwissenschaften 41, 534 (1954).

FAULDS, J. S.: Haematite pneumoconiosis in Cumberland miners. J. clin. Path. 10, 187—199 (1957).

—, and M. J. STEWART: Carcinoma of the lung in haematite miners. J. Path. Bact. 72, 353—366 (1956).

FINE, M. J., and J. V. JASO: Silicosis and primary carcinoma of the lung. J. Amer. med. Ass. 104, 40—43 (1935).

FISCHER, W.: Der Lungenkrebs. Zbl. Path. 85, 193—212 (1949).

FISCHER-WASELS, B.: Die Ursachen des primären Lungencarcinoms. Frankfurt. Z. Path. 49, 145—154 (1936).

FRUEHLING, L., et A. OPPERMANN: Cancer pulmonaire et silicose pulmonaire. Strasbourg, med. 3, 389—394 (1952).

GHISLANDI, E., e M. FINULLI: Su due casi di silicosi massiva associata a neoplasia polmonare. Med. d. Lavoro, 50, 426—431 (1959).

GOLDING, C. G.: Pneumoconiosis in South Wales anthracite miners. Lancet 2, 891—896 (1946).

GROSSE, H.: Silikose und Lungenkrebs. Arch. Gewerbepath. Gewerbehyg. 9, 357—372, 1956.

HOLSTEIN, E.: Lungenkrebs bei chronischen gewerblichen Lungenschädigungen. Zbl. inn. Med. 62, 569—580, 1941.

HUEPER, W. C.: Über die intravenöse Kampferölinjektion auf Grund pathologisch-anatomischer Untersuchungen. Med. Klin. 18, 373—376 (1922).

— Occupational tumors and allied diseases. Springfield, Ill.: C. C. Thomas 1942.

— Silicosis, asbestosis and cancer of the lung. Amer. J. clin. Path. 25, 1388—1389, 1955.

—, and W. W. PAYNE: Carcinogenic studies on petroleum asphalt, cooling oil and coal Tar. Arch. Path. 70, 372—384 (1960).

JAMES, W. R. L.: Primary lung cancer in South Wales coal workers with pneumoconiosis. Brit. J. industr. Med. 12, 87—91 (1955).

JOHNSTONE, R. T.: Silicosis and cancer. J. Amer. med. Ass. 176, 81 (1961).

KAHLAU, G.: Der Lungenkrebs. Ergebn. allg. Path. path. Anat. 37, 258—419 (1954).

KENNAWAY, E. L., and N. M. KENNAWAY: The Incidence of cancer of the lung in coal miners in England and Wales. Brit. J. Cancer. 7, 10—18 (1953).

KERGIN, Fr. G.: Silicotic and tuberculosilicotic lesions simulating bronchiogenic carcinoma. J. thorac. Surg. 24, 545—567 (1952).

KIKUCHI, K., and T. KODAMA: Silicosis and lung cancer in Hokkaido. III. Jap. J. Chest Dis. 23, 620—628 (1964).

KLOTZ, M. O.: Association of silicosis and carcinoma of the lung. Amer. J. Cancer 35, 38—49 (1939).

—, and W. SIMPSON: Silicosis and carcinoma of the lung. Emmanuel Libman Anniversary Vol. 2, 685—696 (1932).

LAVENNE: cited by Puccini.

LEICHER, F.: Über die Silikosis der mediastinalen Lymphknoten und ihre Komplikationen. Virchows Arch. 315, 341—374 (1948).

MEIKLEJOHN, A.: Silicosis in sandstone workers. Brit. J. industr. Med. 6, 241—244 (1949).
MEREWETHER, E. R. A.: Annual report of the chief inspector of factories for the year 1947. Medical section. London: H. K. Stationery Office 1948.
MITTMANN, O.: Über die Unabhängigkeit von Lungenkrebs und Silikose. Forschungs-Arbeiten aus dem wissenschaftlich-statistischen Sektor der Krebsforschung NW. Bonn 1959.
MOREL, L., SENDRAIL-PESQUÉ, H. BOUISSOU, J. COLL, M. GIRARD, et J. DIRAT: Association de silicose et de cancer bronchique. Arch. Mal. prof. 21, 225 (1960).
MULLER, M., A. MARCHAND-ALPHAND, P. CUALLACCI, P. NADIRAS, et P. H. MULLER: A propos de 6 observations de silicose avec cancer pulmonaire. Lille méd. 5, 36—40 (1960).
PARKES, G. D.: Mellor's Modern Inorganic Chemistry. New York: Langmans, Green and Co. 1939.
PAUL, R.: Silicosis in Northern Rhodesia copper miners. Arch. environm. Hlth 2, 96—109 (1961).
PIAZZA, G.: Occlusione bronchiale da cancro in silicosi. Rad. Med. 41, 307 (1955).
PUCCINI, C.: Il problema della cancro-silicosi. Med. d. Lavoro. 51, 18—36 (1960).
RACUGNO, V., e G. CARTA: Contributo allo studio dell'associazione silicosi e carcinoma del polmone. Med. d. Lavoro. 48, 478—484 (1957).
ROESSLE, R.: Die Narbenkrebse der Lungen. Schweiz. med. Wschr. 73, 1200 (1943).
ROSTOSKI, O., u. E. SAUPE: Gewerbehygienische und klinisch-röntgenologische Untersuchungen an den Erzbergleuten des Johanngeorgenstädter Grubenbezirkes. Arch. Gewerbepath. 1, 731—734 (1931).
RUETTNER, J. R.: Kann der Silikose eine ätiologische Bedeutung für die Geschwulstbildung zugesprochen werden? Oncologica 2, 115—122 (1949).
— Die Silikose in der Schweiz, 1945—1960. Suppl. Pathologia et Microbiol. 23, 150 (1960).
SCHAUTZ, R., und W. KLEIN: Bronchial-Carcinom und Silikose. Chirurg 31, 135—141 (1960).
SCHOCH, H.: Silikose und Lungenkrebs. Z. Unfallmed. Berufskr. 47, 138—184 (1954).
SCHULTE, G.: Pneumokoniosen der Ruhrbergleute und Lungenkarzinom. Fortschr. Röntgenstr. 41, 444 (1930).
SCHULZ, O.: Die Beurteilung der schweren Staublungenerkrankungen nach der Verordnung vom 11. 2. 1929 unter besonderer Berücksichtigung der Frage einer Entschädigungspflicht von Begleiterkrankungen. Arch. Gewerbepath. 6, 117—143 (1935).
SLADDEN, A. F.: Silica content of the lung. Lancet 2, 123—125 (1933).
SPOERLEIN, S.: Schützt die Silikose vor Lungenkrebs. Zbl. allg. Path. path. Anat. 89, 197—200 (1952).
STAEMMLER, M.: Beruf und Krebs. Münch. med. Wschr. 85, 121—125 (1938).
SWEANY, H. C., J. D. PORSCHE, and J. R. DOUGLAS: Chemical and pathologic study of pneumoconiosis. Arch. Path. 22, 593—633 (1936).
TAKEDA, K., K. KIKUCHI, H. KOBAYASHI, M. ALZAWA, T. KODAMA, and Y. TOYOFUKU: Silicosis and cancer of the lung in Hokkaido. I. Report of 50 cases of silicosis. Jap. J. Cancer Clin. 10, 627—636 (1964).
VORWALD, A. J., and J. W. KARR: Pneumoconiosis and pulmonary carcinoma. Amer. J. Path. 14, 49—58 (1938).
WAETJEN, J.: Zur Kenntnis der Quarzitstaublunge. Arch. Gewerbepath. 11, 551—574 (1942).
WEDLER, H. W.: Asbestose und Lungenkrebs. Münch. med. Wschr. 19, 296 (1943).
WEISSMANN, H.: Silicosis and bronchogenic carcinoma. Amer. Rev. Tuberc. 76, 1088—1093 (1957).
WILLIS, H. S., and P. BRUTSAERT: Tumor-like structures in the lungs of Guinea pigs artificially exposed to silica dust. Amer. Rev. Tuberc. 17, 268—278 (1928).

Specific Occupational Respiratory Carcinogens

ALWENS, W.: Lungenkrebs durch Arbeit in Chromat-herstellenden Betrieben. Proc. 9. Kongress f. Unfallmed. u. Berufskr. 973—982, 1938.
BERNDT, M.: Cancer and occupation. Statistical investigation. Krebsarzt 18, 289—296 (1963).
BIDSTRUP, P. L., and R. A. M. CASE: Carcinoma of the lung in workmen in the bichromate-producing industrie in Great Britain. Brit. J. industr. Med. 13, 260—264 (1956).
BOURNE, H., and W. R. RUSHIN: Atmospheric pollution in the vicinity of a chromate plant. Industr. Med. 19, 568—569 (1950).

BUECHLEY, R., J. E. DUNN, G. LINDEN, and L. BRESLOW: Excess lung cancer mortality rates among Mexican women in California. Cancer 10, 63—66 (1957).

BUELL, P., J. E. DUNN, and L. BRESLOW: The occupational-social class risks of cancer mortality in man. J. chron. Dis. 12, 600—621 (1960).

CLEMMESEN, J., and A. NIELSEN: The social distribution of cancer in Copenhagen, 1943 to 1947. Brit. J. Cancer 5, 159—171 (1951).

COHART, E. M.: Socioeconomic distribution of cancer of the lung in New Haven. Cancer 8, 1126—1129 (1955).

COMMINGS, B. T.: Polycyclic hydrocarbons in rural and urban air. Int. J. Air Pollut. 1, 14—17 (1958).

CURWEN, M. P., E. L. KENNAWAY, and N. M. KENNAWAY: Cancer of the lung and larynx in town and country. Acta Un. int. Cancr. 10, 104—109 (1954).

DEAN, G.: Lung cancer among white South Africans. Brit. med. J. 2, 952—857 (1959).

— Lung cancer among white Sout Africans. Report on a further study. Brit. med. J. 2, 1599—1605 (1961).

— The complex aetiology of lung cancer. Acta Un. int. Cancr. 19, 721—723 (1963).

DORN, H. F., and S. J. CUTLER: Morbidity from cancer in U. S. Part I. Variation in incidence by age, sex, race, marital status and geographic region. Publ. Hlth Monograph No. 29. 1955, p. 121. Washington, D. C.

EASTCOTT, D. F.: The Epidemiology of lung cancer in New Zealand. Lancet 1, 37—39 (1956).

ECKARDT, R. E.: Air pollution, lung cancer and chronic lung disease. J. occup. Med. 6, 184—188 (1964).

EISENBUD, M., R. C. WANTA, C. DUSTAN, L. T. STEADMAN, W. B. HARRIS, and N. WOLF: Nonoccupational berylliosis. J. industr. Hyg. 31, 282—294 (1949).

FERSHTUDT, V. L.: Cancer of the lung: Incidence in a major industrial center. Acta Un. int. 19, 745—748 (1963).

FIRKET, J.: The problem of cancer of the lung in the industrial area of Liège during recent years. Proc. roy. Soc. Med. 51, 347—352 (1959).

FISHER, R. G., and P. W. RICKERT: Lung cancer in chromate workers. Amer. J. Path. 35, 699 (1959).

GAFAFER, W. M.: Health of workers in chromate producing industry. Publ. Health Service Publ. No. 192. Government Printing Office, 1952, Washington, D. C., p. 131.

GRAHAM, S., M. LEVIN, and A. M. LILIENFELD: The socioeconomic distribution of cancer of various sites in Buffalo, N. Y., 1948—1952. Cancer 13, 180—191 (1960).

GRISWOLD, M. H.: Lung cancer in Connecticut on increase. Conn. Hlth Bull. 70, 4—12 (1956).

GROSS, E., and F. KOELSCH: Über den Lungenkrebs in der Chromatfarbenindustrie. Arch. Gewerbepath. 12, 164—176 (1943).

GOLDBLATT, M. W., and J. GOLDBLATT: Industrial carcinogenesis and toxicology. In E. R. A. MEREWETHER: Industrial medicine and hygiene. Vol. 3. London: Butterworth & Co. (1956).

HAMMOND, E. C.: Lung cancer death rates in England and Wales compared with those in the U. S. A. Brit. J. Med. 2, 649—654 (1958).

HAMPELN, P.: Häufigkeit und Ursache des primären Lungenkarzinoms. Grenzgeb. Med. 36, 145—150 (1923).

HERDAN, G.: The increase in the mortality due to cancer of the lung in the light of the distribution of the disease among the different social classes and occupations. Brit. J. Cancer 12, 492—506 (1958).

HUEPER, W. C.: Über die intravenöse Kampferölinjektion auf Grund von pathologisch-anatomischen Untersuchungen. Med. Klin. 18, 373—376 (1922).

— Occupational tumors and allied diseases. Springfield, Ill.: C. C. Thomas 1942.

— Environmental carcinogenesis in man and animals. Ann. N. Y. Acad. Sci. 108, 963—1038 (1963).

— Berufskrebse. Gerichtsmedizinische Betrachtungen. Leipzig: Steinkopff 1963.

— A quest into the enviromental causes of cancer of the lung. Publ. Hlth Monograph No. 36. 1955, p. 54.

— The role of occupational and enviromental air pollutants in the production of respiratory cancers. Arch. Path. 53, 427—450 (1957).

HUEPER, W. C.: Methodologic explorations in experimental respiratory carcinogensis. Arznei-mittelforsch. 14, 814—822 (1964).
— Epidemiologic, experimental and histologic studies in metal cancers of the lung. Acta Un. int. Cancr. 15, 424—436 (1959).
—, and W. D. CONWAY: Chemical carcinogenesis and cancers. Springfield, Ill.: C. C. Thomas 1965.
—, P. KOTIN, E. C. TABOR, W. W. PAYNE, H. FALK, and E. SAWICKI: Carcinogenic bioassays on air pollutants. Arch. Path. 74, 89—116 (1962).
HURWITZ, C.: Primary carcinoma of the lung in the Bantu. Acta Un. int. Cancr. 20, 648—651 (1964).
KENNAWAY, E. L.: The data relating to cancer in the publications of the general register office. Brit. J. Cancer 4, 158—172 (1950).
—, and N. M. KENNAWAY: Studies of the incidence of cancer of the lung and larynx. Brit. J. Cancer 5, 153—158 (1951).
KIMINA, S. N.: Cancerogenic substances in the atmosphere and the incidence and mortality of lung cancer. Abstr. 8. int. Cancer Congr. Moscow, 1962, p. 183.
KIVILUOTO, R.: Pleural calcification as roentgenologic sign of non-occupational endemic anthophyllitic-asbestosis. Acta radiol. Suppl. 194, 1—67 (1960).
KREYBERG, L.: Histologic lung cancer types. A morphological and biological correlation. Acta path. microbiol. scand. 157, 7—92 (1962).
— 3:4-Benzpyrene in industrial air pollution. Some reflexions. Brit. J. Cancer 13, 618—622 (1959).
— Occupational influences in a Norwegian material of 235 cases of primary epithelial lung tumours. Brit. J. Cancer 8, 605—612 (1954).
LEW, E. A.: Cancer of the respiratory tract. Recent trends in mortality and morbidity. J. int. Coll. Surg. 24, 12—27 (1955).
MANCUSO, TH. F., and E. J. COULTER: Methodology in industrial health studies. Arch. environm. Hlth 6: 210—226 (1963).
— — Methodology in industrial health studies. The demographic approach. Arch. environm. Hlth 6, 515—524 (1963).
— — Cancer mortality among native white, foreign white and non-white male residents of Ohio: Cancer of the lung, larynx, bladder and central nervous system. J. Nat. Cancer Inst. 20, 79—105 (1958).
MORRISON, S. L., Occupational mortality in Scotland. Brit. J. industr. Med. 14, 130—132 (1957).
NEWHOUSE, M. L., and H. THOMPSON: Epidemiological studies of patients with mesothelial tumors in the London. Area. Proc. conference on biological effects of asbestos. 1964. Ann. N. Y. Acad. Sci. 132, 519—588 (1965).
NIEBERLE: Über endemischen Krebs im Siebbein von Schafen. Z. Krebsforsch. 49, 137—141, (1939—1940).
OETTEL, H.: Rauchen und Gesundheit. Ärztebl. Rheinland-Pfalz. 217—241 (1965).
PARSONS, W. D., A. J. DE VILLIERS, L. S. BARTLETT, and N. R. BECKLAKE: Lung cancer in a fluorspar mining community. II. Prevalence of respiratory symptoms and disability. Brit. J. industr. Med. 21, 110—116 (1964).
PHILLIPS, A. J.: Cancer mortality trends in Canada: 1941-to 1958. Brit. J. Cancer 15, 1—9 (1961).
— The increase in lung cancer mortality in Canada. Brit. J. Cancer 13, 589—594 (1959).
POCHE, R., O. MITTMANN, and O. KNELLER: Statistische Untersuchungen über das Bronchial-carcinom in Nordrhein-Westfalen. Z. Krebsforsch. 66, 87—108 (1964).
PYBUS, F. C.: Cancer and atmospheric pollution. Newc. med. J. 28, 31—66 (1963).
SARUTA, N., S. YAMAGUCHI, N. ISHINISHI, T. TSUTSUMI, and Y. KODAMA: Effects of air pollution on the health of people in Northern Kyushu, Japan. Jap. J. med. Sci. 12, 167—176 (1961).
SAWICKI, E., FR. T. FOX, W. ELBERT, T. R. HAUSER, and J. MEEKER: Polynuclear aromatic hydrocarbons composition of air polluted by coal-tar pitch fumes. Amer. industr. Hyg. J. 23, 482—486 (1962).

SAWICKI, E., T. R. HAUSER, W. C. ELBERT, F. T. FOX, and J. MEEKER: Polynuclear aromatic hydrocarbon compounds of the atmosphere of some large American cities. Amer. industr. Hyg. J. 23, 137—141 (1962).

SEGI, M., and M. KURIHARA: Cancer mortality for selected sites in 24 countries. No. 2 (1958—1959). Tohoku University Medical School, 1962, p. 127.

SELIKOFF, I. J., J. CHURG, and E. C. HAMMOND: Asbestos exposure and neoplasia. J. Amer. med. Ass. 188, 22—26 (1964).

STEINER, P.: Cancer: Race and geography. Baltimore: Williams & Wilkins 1954.

STOCKS, P.: On the relations between atmospheric pollution in urban and rural localities and mortality from cancer, bronchitis and pneumonia with particular reference to 3:4-Benzpyrene, beryllium, molybdenum, vanadium, and arsenic. Brit. J. Cancer 14, 397—418 (1960).

— Endemiology of cancer of the lung in England and Wales. Brit. J. Cancer 6, 99—111 (1952).

— The association between social class and susceptibility to cancer. In R. W. RAVEN: Cancer progress volume. London: Butterworth 1963.

—, and J. M. CAMBELL: Lung cancer death rates among non-smokers and pipe and cigarette smokers. Brit. J. 2, 923—926 (1955).

THOMSON, J. G., R. O. C. KASCHULA, and R. R. McDONALD: Asbestos as a modern urban hazard S. Afr. med. J. 37, 77—81 (1963).

TURNER, H. M., and M. G. GRACE: An Investigation of cancer mortality among males in certain Sheffield trades. J. Hyg. 38, 90—95 (1938).

WAGNER, J. C., S. A. SLEGGS, and P. MARCHAND: Diffuse pleural mesothelioma and asbestos exposure in the North-Western Cape Province. Brit. J. industr. Med. 17, 260—271 (1960).

WAGONER, J. K., V. E. ARCHER, B. E. CARROLL, D. A. HOLIDAY, and P. A. LAWRENCE: Cancer mortality patterns among U. S. uranium miners and millers, 1950 through 1962. J. nat. Cancer Inst. 32, 787—801 (1964).

—, R. W. MILLER, FR. E. LUNDIN, J. F. FRAUMENI, and M. E. HAIJ: Unusual cancer mortality among a group of underground metal miners. New Engl. J. Med. 269, 284—289 (1963).

WALTERS, L. G.: Industrial cancer in South Africa. Med. Proc. 9, 24—30 (1963).

WEBSTER, J.: Asbestosis in non-experimental animals in South Africa. Nature 197, 5—6 (1963).

WYNDER, E. L., and E. A. GRAHAM: Etiologic factors in bronchogenic carcinoma with special reference to industrial exposures. Arch. industr. Hyg. 4, 221—235 (1951).

WAGLER, F., H. MÜLLER, and M. ANSPACH: Gibt es eine endemische Asbestose. Z. Hyg. 8, 246—255 (1962).

Arsenic

ABELIUK, S., H. OYANGUREN, and V. MATURANA: Occupational arsenical dermatosis in a copper mine. Rev. Med. (Santiago) 85, 631—635 (1957).

AKAZAKI, K.: Silicosis and lung cancer at Ikuno mine. p. 2. Personal communication (1960).

ARGUELLO, R. A.. E. E. TELLO, B. A. MACOLA, and L. MANZALO: Cutaneous cancers in chronic regional endemic arsenicalism in the Province of Cordoba. Rev. Fac. Cience méd. Univ. Córdoba 8, 409—432 (1950).

ARHELGER, S. W., and A. J. KREMEN: Arsenical epithelioma of medicinal origin. Surgery 30, 977—986 (1951).

BAILEY, E. J.: The arsenic content of human lungs and tracheo-bronchial lymph glands. Brit. J. Cancer 11, 54—59 (1957).

—, E. L. KENNAWAY, and M. E. URQUHART: Arsenic content of cigarettes. Brit. J. Cancer 11, 49—53 (1957).

BAUER, K. H.: Das Krebsproblem. Berlin, Springer (1949).

BEHOUNEK and FORT: cited by Roth, F.

BELLESSINI, C.: New syndrome from industrial poisoning. Pensiero med. 25, 269—280 (1936).

BOHNENKAMP, H.: Über chronische Arsenvergiftung. Ber. 8. Internat. Kongr. f. Unfallmed. u. Berufskrankh. 2, 1069—1072 (1938).

BOUTWELL, R. K.: A carcinogenic evaluation of potassium arsenite and arsanilic acid. Agricult. & Food Chem. 11, 381—385 (1963).

BARONI, C., G. J. van ESCH, and U. SAFFIOTTI: Carcinogenic tests of two inorganic arsenicals. Arch. environm. Hlth. 7, 668—674 (1963).

BOWEN, A. L., T. L. T. LEWIS, and W. C. EDWARDS: Acute arsenical poisoning due to acetarsol pessaries, Brit. med. J. 1, 1282—1284 (1961).

BRIDGE, J. C.: Arsenic. Annual rep. chief inspector of factories and workshops, 1926, H. M. Stationary Office, London, p. 85.

BRAUN, W.: Krebs an Haut und inneren Organen, hervorgerufen durch Arsen. Dtsch. med. Wschr. 83, 870—872, 881, 903—904 (1958); Germ. med. Mth. 8, 321—324 (1958).

BUTZENGEIGER, K. H.: Die chronische Arsenvergiftung. Ärztl. Wschr. 4, 365—369 (1949).

CALNAN, C. D.: Arsenical keratoses and epithelioma with bronchial carcinoma. Proc. roy. Soc. Med. 47, 405—406 (1954).

CURRIE, A. N.: The role of arsenic in carcinogenesis. Brit. med. Bull. 4, 402—405 (1947).

DAFF, M. E., and E. L. KENNAWAY: The arsenic content of tobacco and tobacco smoke. Brit. J. Cancer 4, 173—182 (1950).

DANBOLT, N., and M. H. FOSS: Arsenical treatment as a cause of cancer of the skin and internal organs. T. norske Laegeforen. 78, 275—276 (1958).

DEROBERT, L., and A. HADENGUE: Un cas de cancer du larynx chez un ouvrier exposé aux poussières arsénicales. Arch. Mal. prof. 11, 397—398 (1950).

DOIG, A. T.: Dust diseases, excluding the fibrotic pneumoconioses. In E. R. A. MEREWETHER: Industrial medicine and hygiene, vol. 3, chapter 2, p. 123, London: Butterworth 1956.

DÖRKEN, H.: Einige Daten bei Frauen mit Lungenkrebs. Oncologia 16, 325—338 (1963).

ECKARDT, R. E.: Industrial carcinogens. New York: Grune & Stratton 1959.

Editorial: Arsenic in food. Lancet. 2, 540 (1951).

— Arsenic as a cause of cancer. Brit. med. J. 1, 912 (1948).

Food standards committee, ministry of food: Arsenic content of food. J. Amer. med. Ass. 157, 1632 (1955).

FORSSMAN, S.: cited by Wm. E. SMITH: An evaluation of claims for occupational factors in cancer of the lung. Acta Un. int. Cancr. 9, 50—58 (1953).

FROMMEL, E.: Les états pulmonaires prédisposant du cancer; considerations sur l'étiologie du cancer du poumon. Rev. Méd. (Paris) 44, 31—40 (1927).

FROST, D. V.: Arsenic and selenium in relation to the food additive law of 1958. Nutr. Rev. 18, 129—131 (1960).

—, L. R. OVERBY, and H. C. SPRUTH: Arsenical in feed. Studies with Arsanilic and Related Compounds. Agricult. and Food Chem. 3, 235—243 (1955).

GEVER, L.: Über die chronischen Hautveränderungen beim Arsenicismus und Betrachtungen über die Massenerkrankungen in Reichenstein in Schlesien. Arch. Derm. Syph. (Berl.) 43, 221—280 (1898).

GOULDEN, E., E. L. KEKNAWAY, and M. E. URQUHART: Arsenic in the suspended matter of town air. Brit. J. Cancer 6, 1—7 (1952).

HARKIM, W. D., and R. E. SWANI: The chronic arsenical poisoning of herbivorous animals. J. Amer. chem. Soc. 30, 928—935 (1908).

HALVER, J. E., and L. M. ASHLEY: Further induction of rainbow trout hepatoma with chemical carcinogens. Quart. Progr. Rep. Bureau of Sport Fisheries and Wildlife. October, 1962, p. 19—23.

HENRY, S. A.: Cancer of the scrotum in relation to occupation. London: Oxford Univ. Press 1946.

HOW, S. W., and S. YEH: Studies on endemic chronic arsenical poisoning. Rep. Institute of Pathology, National Taiwan Univ. 14, 75—105 (1963).

HESS, H.: Arseninhalation und Bronchialcarcinom bei Winzern. Dtsch. Z. Chir. 283, 274—279 (1956).

HILL, A. B., and E. L. FANING: Studies in the incidence of cancer in a factory handling inorganic compounds of arsenic. Brit. J. industr. Med. 5, 1—15 (1948).

HOFMANN, P.: Die Gefährdung der Tierwelt durch Industriegase. Arch. Gewerbepath. Gewerbehyg. 7, 670—672 (1936—1937).

HOLLAND, R. H., A. R. ACEVEDO, and D. A. CLARK: The arsenic content of bronchial mucosa and submucosa in man. Brit. J. Cancer. 14, 169—172 (1960).
—, R. H. WILSON, A. R. ACEVEDO, M. S. McCALL, D. A. CLARK, and H. C. LANZ: A study of arsenic in regular-sized unfiltered and filtered cigarettes. Cancer 2, 1115—1118 (1958).
HOLMQUIST, I.: Occupational arsenical dermatitis. A study among employees at a copper ore smelting work including investigations of skin reactions to contact with arsenic compounds. Acta derm.-venereol. (Stockh.) 31, 26 (1951).
HOPKINS, R., and M. T. SUDDIFORD: Multiple epitheliomas and pigmentary dermatosis in a Negro boy. Arch. Derm. Syph. 29, 408—421 (1934).
HUEPER, W. C.: Occupational tumors and allied diseases. Springfield, Ill.: C. C. Thomas 1942.
— Morphological aspects of experimental actinic and arsenic cancer in the skin of rats. Cancer Res. 2, 551—559 (1942).
— A quest into the environmental causes of cancer of the lung. Publ. Health Monograph No. 36, 1955.
— Epidemiologic, experimental and histological studies on metal cancers of the lung. Acta Un. int. Cancr. 15, 424—436 (1959).
— Cancer hazards from natural and artificial water pollutants. Proc. conference on physiological aspects of water quality. Division of Water Supply and Pollution Control, Public Health Service, Washington, D. C., p. 181—193, 1960.
— Berufskrebse. In E. BAADER: Handbuch der gesamten Arbeitsmedizin. Bd. 2, S. 301—385. München: Urban & Schwarzenberg 1961.
— Carcinogens in the human environment. Arch. Path. 71, 237—267, 355—380 (1961).
—, and W. D. CONWAY: Chemical carcinogenesis and cancers. C. C. Thomas, 1965.
—, and S. ITAMI: Effects of neoarsphenamine of spontaneous breast tumors in mice. Amer. J. Cancer 17, 106—115 (1933).
—, P. KOTIN, E. C. TABOR, W. W. PAYNE, H. FALK, and E. SAWICKI: Carcinogenic bioassays on air pollutants. Arch. Path. 74, 89—116 (1962).
—, and W. W. PAYNE: Experimental studies of chromium compounds. Proc. 13th Internat. Congr. Occup. Health, 1960, p. 473—486.
— — Experimental studies in metal carcinogenesis. Arch. environm. Hlth 5, 443—462 (1962).
JHAVERI, S. S.: A case of cirrhosis and primary carcinoma of the liver in chronic industrial arsenical intoxication. Brit. J. industr. Med. 16, 248—250 (1959).
JOHNSTONE, R. T., and S. E. MILLER: Occupational diseases and industrial medicine. Philadelphia, Pa.: W. B. Saunders 1960.
KAY, K.: Environmental arsenic contamination and control in smelting operations. Proc. Internat. Clean Air Conf. London, 1959, p. 86—90.
KOELSCH, F.: Die beruflichen Arsenschäden im Weinbau und in den gewerblichen Betrieben. Arch. Gewerbepath. Gewerbehyg. 16, 405—438 (1958).
— Der Arsenkrebs. Zbl. Arbeitsmed. 8, 129—134 (1958).
KRUG, H.: Ein Beitrag zum Arsen-Lungenkrebs. Z. ges. inn. Med. 14, 426—431 (1959).
LATARJET, GALY, MARET, and GALLOIS: Cancers broncho-pulmonaire et intoxication arsenicale chez les vignerons du Beaujolais. Mem. Acad. Chir. 90, 384—390 (1964).
LEITCH, A., and E. L. KENNAWAY: Experimental production of cancer by arsenic. Brit. med. J. 2, 1107 (1922).
LIEBGOTT, G.: Pathologische Anatomie der chronischen Arsenvergiftung. Dtsch. med. Wschr. 74, 855—856 (1949).
— Über die Beziehungen zwischen chronischer Arsenvergiftung und malignen Neubildungen. Zbl. Arbeitsmed. 2, 15—16 (1952).
LIPSCHUTZ, B.: Einige Beobachtungen über experimentelle Pigmenterzeugung durch Arsenzufuhr. Arch. Derm. Syph. 147, 520 (1924).
LULL, L., and A. WALLAACH: cited by Hueper, W. C.
MEESSEN, H.: Morphologische Beiträge zum Problem des Lungenkrebses. Ärztl. Forsch. 8, 481—486 (1954).
MEREWETHER, E. R. A.: Industrial health. Ann. Rep. Chief Inspector of Factories for the Year 1943, 38—56, 1944.
MONTGOMERY, H.: Arsenic as an etiologie agent in certain types of epithelioma. Arch. Derm. Syph. 32, 218—236 (1935).

MONTGOMERY, H., and M. WAISMAN: Epithelioma attributable to arsenic. J. invest. Derm. 4, 365—383 (1941).

NIEBERLE, K.: Über endemischen Krebs im Siebbein von Schafen. Ztschr. f. Krebsf. 49, 137—141 (1939—1940).

NEUBAUER, O.: Arsenical cancer: A review. Brit. J. Cancer 1, 192—244 (1947).

OSBURN, H. S.: Cancer of the lung in Gwanda. Cent. Afr. J. Med. 3, 215—223 (1957).

PEIN, H. VON: Über die Krebsentstehung bei der chronischen Arsenvergiftung. Dtsch. Arch. klin. Med. 190, 429—443 (1943).

PINTO, S. S., and C. M. McGILL: Arsenic trioxide exposures in industry. J. industr. Med. 22, 281 (1953).

PRELL, H.: Die Schädigung der Tierwelt durch die Fernwirkung von Industrieabgasen. Arch. Gewerbepath. 7, 656—670 (1937).

RAPOSO, S.: Le cancer á l'arsénic. C. R. Soc. biol. (Paris) 98, 86 (1928).

RINGERTZ, N.: Environmental factors and smoking in the causation of cancer of the lung. Proc. Fifth Internat. Congr. Geographic Pathology, Washington, D. C., 1954, Basle: S. Karger 1955.

ROCKSTROH, H.: Zur Ätiologie des Bronchialkrebses in arsenverarbeitenden Nickelhütten. Arch. Geschwulstforsch. 14, 151—162 (1959).

ROTH, F.: Über die chronische Arsenvergiftung der Moselwinzer unter besonderer Berücksichtigung des Arsenkrebses. Z. Krebsforsch. 61, 287—319 (1956).

— Arsen-Leber-Tumoren. Z. Krebsforsch. 61, 468—503 (1957).

— The sequelae of chronic arsenic poisoning in Moselle vintners. Germ. med. Mth. 11, 172—175 (1957).

— Über den Bronchialkrebs arsengeschädigter Winzer. Virchows Arch. path. Anat. 331, 119—137 (1958).

RUSSELL, B., and R. KLAGER: Two cases of multiple arsenical cutaneous carcinoma. Proc. roy. Soc. Med. 38, 128—129 (1945).

SATTERLEE, H. S.: The problem of arsenic in American cigarette tobacco. New Engl. J. Med. 254, 1149—1154 (1956).

SAUPE, E.: Carcinoma of the lung in arsenic miners; Two Cases. Arch. Gewerbepath. 1, 582 (1930).

— Discussion. Z. Krebsforsch. 32, 687 (1930).

— Über die Beziehungen zwischen Lungenkrebs und Staublungenerkrankung. Zbl. inn. Med. 54, 825—838 (1933).

SCHINZ, H. R., und E. UEHLINGER: Der Metallkrebs: Ein neues Prinzip der Krebserzeugung. Z. Krebsforsch. 52, 425—437 (1942).

SCHMORL, G.: Pathological study of Schneeberg lung cancer. Rep. Internat. Cancer Conf. London, Bristol: John Wright & Sons, Ltd. 1928.

SEMON, H. C.: A case of arsenical keratosis followed by cancer. Brit. med. J. 2, 975 (1922).

SNEGIREFF, L. S., and O. L. LOMGARD: Arsenic and cancer. Arch. industr. Hyg. Med. 4, 199—205((1951).

SOMMERS, S. C., and R. G. McMANUS: Multiple arsenical cancers of the skin and internal organs. Cancer 6, 347—359 (1953).

SOWDEN, G.: Atmospheric pollution with arsenical dust. J. State Med. 35, 668 (1927).

TELLO, E. E.: Hidroarsenicismo cronico regional endemico (hacre). Imprenta de la Universidad Cordoba, 1951, p. 162.

VALLEE, B. L., D. D. ULMER, and W. E. C. WACKER: Arsenic toxicology and biochemistry. Arch. industr. Hlth 21, 132—151 (1960).

WAGONER, J. K., R. W. MILLER, F. E. LUNDIN, J. F. FRAUMEL, and M. E. HAIJ: Unusual cancer mortality among a group of underground metal miners. New Engl. J. Med. 269, 284—289 (1963).

WERNER, K., and J. BECKER: Das Bronchus-Karzinom in strahlenklinischer Sicht. I. Teil. Strahlentherapie 101, 217—226 (1956).

WILLIAMSON, A. W. R.: Arsenical skin cancer and lung cancer. Guy's Hosp. Rep. 109, 42—45 (1960).

Asbestosis

AHLBORG, G., and C. J. HANSSON: Asbestos, en för sverige ny yrkessjukdour. Svenska Laek.-Tidn. **53**, 1376—1383 (1956).

ALVARADO, C., L. ENRIQUEZ, and D. BARRON: Asbestosis. Salud. publ. Méx. **11**, 537—566 (1960).

ALWENS, W.: Über Asbestose der Lunge. Münch. med. Wschr. **82**, 1797—1800 (1935).

ANDERSON, J., and F. A. CAMPAGNA: Asbestosis and carcinoma of the lung. Arch. environm. Hlth 1, 27—32 (1960).

BECKER, J. P.: University of the Witwatersrand, Johannesburg, R. S. A., 1958, personal communication.

BOHLIG, H.: Über das Auftreten des Lungenkrebses bei Asbestose. Kongreßber. med. wissensch. Ges. Röntg. DDR. Berlin: Akademie-Verlag 1955.

—, and G. JACOB: Neue Gesichtspunkte über den Lungenkrebs der Asbestarbeiter. Dtsch. med. Wschr. **81**, 231—233 (1956).

— — Die Häufigkeit des Lungenkrebses bei deutschen Asbestarbeitern. Dtsch. Gesundh.-Wes. **13**, 1101—1103 (1958).

— —, and B. KALLABIS: Über Morbidität und Pathologie des Asbestlungenkrebses. Ztschr. f. Unfallmed. u. Berufskr. 1, 64—78 (1959).

— —, and H. MUELLER: Die Asbestose der Lungen. Stuttgart: Georg Thieme 1960.

BOHNE, A.: Über Asbestose. Dtsch. med. Wschr. **62**, 928 (1936).

— Über Asbestose. Dtsch. med. Wschr. **66**, 1024 (1940).

— Examination of workers in an asbestos factory. Arch. Gewerbepath. **11**, 433—452 (1942).

BOEHME, A.: Asbestose und Lungencarcinom. Arch. Gewerbepath. **17**, 384—395, 457—462 (1959).

BOEMKE, Fr.: Das Lungenkarzinom in der Astbeststaublunge. Med. Mschr. **7**, 77—81 (1953).

BONSER, G. M., J. S. FAULDS, and M. J. STEWART: Occupational cancer of the urinary bladder in dyestuffs operations and of the lung in iron-ore and asbestos workers. Amer. J. clin. Path. **25**, 126—134 (1955).

BRAUN, D. C., and T. D. TRUAN: An epidemiological study of lung cancer in asbestos miners. Arch. industr. Hlth **17**, 634—653 (1958).

BUCHANAN, W. D.: The association of certain cancers with asbestosis. Excerpta Med. (Congr. Ser. Nr. 62) **2**, 617—619 (1964).

— Contribution à l'étude de l'amiantose. Arch. Malad. prof. **10**, 589—595 (1949).

CARTIER, P.: Diskussion. Arch. industr. Hyg. **5**, 78 (1952).

— Some clinical observations of asbestosis in mine and mill workers. Arch. industr. Hlth **11**, 204—207 (1955).

CAUNA, D., R. S. TOTTEN, and P. GROSS: Asbestos bodies in human lungs at autopsy. J. Amer. med. Ass. **192**, 111—113 (1965).

CHAUVET, M.: Asbestose et cancer bronchique. Presse med. **66**, 908—910 (1958).

CORDOVA, J. F., H. TESLUNK, and K. P. KNUDSOHN: Asbestosis and carcinoma of the lung. Cancer **15**, 1181—1187 (1962).

CROSSLAND, P. M.: Silicon granuloma of the skin. Arch. Derm. Syph. (Berl.) **71**, 457—461 (1955).

CURETON, R. J. R.: Squamous cell carcinoma occurring in asbestosis of the lung. Brit. J. Cancer **2**, 249—253 (1948).

DEMV, N. G.: Asbestosis. J. Amer. med. Ass. **175**, 530 (1961).

DESMEULES, R., L. ROUSSEAU, M. GIRAUX, and A. SIROIS: Amiantose et cancers pulmonaires. Sem. Hôp. Paris **23**, 1820—1823 (1947); Laval méd. **6**, 97—108 (1941).

DEWIRTZ, A. P.: Asbestwarzen. Arch. Dermat. Syph. (Berl.) **161**, 1—5 (1930).

DOLL, R.: Mortality from lung cancer in asbestos workers. Brit. J. industr. Med. **12**, 81—86 (1955).

DORN, H. F., and S. J. CUTLER: Morbidity from cancer in the United States. Publ. Health Monograph No. 56, 1959, U. S. Gov. Printing Office, Washington, D. C., pp. 207.

DREESSEN, W. C., and J. M. DALLA VALLE: A study of asbestosis in the asbestos textile industry. Publ. Health Bull. No. 241, p. 68—69, 1938. U. S. Gov. Printing Office, Washington, D. C.

Dyson, B. C., and A. E. Trentalance: Resection of primary pulmonary sarcoma. J. thorac. cardiovasc. Surg. 47, 577—589 (1964).

Editorial: Asbestos and malignancy. Brit. Med. J. 2, 202 (1964).

Egbert, D. S., and A. Geiger: Pulmonary asbestosis and carcinoma; report of o case with necropsy findings. Amer. Rev. Tuberc. 34, 143—150 (1936).

Elmes, P. C., W. T. E. McCaughey, and O. L. Wade: Diffuse mesothelioma of the pleura and asbestos. Brit. med. J. 1, 350 (1965).

Elwood, P. C., and A. L. Cochrane: A follow-up study of workers from an asbestos factory. Brit. J. industr. Med. 21, 304—307 (1964).

Enterline, Ph. E.: Mortality among asbestos products workers in the United States. Ann. N. Y. Acad. Sci. 132, 156—165 (1965).

Entickna, J. B., and W. J. Smither: Petritoneal tumours in asbestosis. Brit. J. industr. Med. 21, 20—31 (1964).

Farina, S.: Asbestosis and pulmonary neoplasias. Lavoro Um. 15, 276—281 (1963).

Fowler, P. B. S., J. C. Sloper, and E. C. Warner: Exposure to asbestos and mesothelioma of the pleura. Brit. med. J. 2, 211 (1964).

Francia, A., and G. Monarca: Asbestosi e carcinoma polmonare. Minerva med. 47, 1950—1959 (1956).

Frost, J., J. Georg, and P. F. Moller: Asbestosis with pleural calcification among insulation workers. Dan. med. Bull. 3, 202—204 (1956).

Gloyne, S. R.: The morbid anatomy and histology of asbestosis. Tubercle 14, 445, 493 and 550 (1933).

— Squamous carcinoma of lung occurring in asbestosis: two cases. Tubercle 17, 5—10 (1935).

— A case of oat-cell carcinoma of the lung occurring in asbestosis. Tubercle 18, 100—101 (1936—37).

Haddow, A. P., and E. S. Horning: On the carcinogenicity of an iron-Dextran complex. J. nat. cancer Inst. 24, 109—147 (1960).

Harington, J. S.: Occurrence of oils containing 3:4-benzpyrene and related substances in asbestos. Nature 193, 43—45 (1962).

—, and M. Smith: Studies of hydrocarbons on mineral dusts. Arch. environ. Med. 8, 453—458 (1964).

Holleb, H. B. and A. Angrist: Bronchiogenic carcinoma in association with pulmonary asbestosis. Amer. J. Path. 18, 123—135 (1941).

Homburger F.: The co-incidence of primary carcinoma of the lungs and pulmonary asbestosis. Amer. J. Path. 19, 797—807 (1943).

Hornig, F.: Klinische Betrachtungen zur Frage des Berufskrebses der Asbestarbeiter. Z. Krebsforsch. 47, 281—287 (1938).

Hueper, W. C.: Occupational tumors and allied diseases. Springfield, Ill.: C. C. Thomas 1942.

— Experimental studies in metal cancerigenesis. VI. Tissue reactions in rats and rabbits after parenteral introduction of suspensions of arsenic, beryllium, or asbestos in lanolin. J. nat. Cancer Inst. 15, 113—129 (1954).

— A quest into the environmental causes of cancer of the lung. Publ. Health Monograph No. 36, PHS Publ. No. 452, USGPO, Washington, D. C., 1955, pp. 54.

— Carcinogenic studies on water-insoluble polymers. Path. et Microbiol. (Basel) 24, 77—106 (1961).

— Environmental cancer of the lung. Acta Un. int. Cancr. 13, 97—140 (1957).

— Occupational and nonoccupational exposure to asbestos. Ann. N. Y. Acad. Sci. 132, 184—196 (1965).

Hugh-Jones, P., and B. E. Heard: Complications of asbestosis. Brit. med. J. No. 5182, 1345—1353 (1960).

Hurel, J.: Contribution à l'étude de l'asbestose. Arch. méd.-chir. Normandie 51, 98—99; 381—407; 463—493 (1960).

Isselbacher, K. J., H. Klaus, and H. L. Hardy: Asbestosis and bronchogenic carcinoma. Amer. J. Med. 15, 721—732 (1953).

Jacob, G., and H. Bohlig: Über Häufigkeit und Besonderheiten des Lungenkrebses bei Asbestose. Arch. Gewerbepath. 14, 1028 (1955).

JACOB, G., and H. BOHLIG: Die Lungenkrebserwartung der deutschen Asbestarbeiter. Krebsf. u. Krebsbek. München: Urban & Schwarzenberg 1959.
— — Das Verhalten des Bronchialbaumes bei der Asbestlungenfibrose. Arch. Gewerbepath. 18, 247—257 (1960).
JOHNSTONE, R. T., and S. E. MILLER: Occupational diseases and industrial medicine. Philadelphia, Pa.: W. B. Saunders 1960.
KEAL, E. E.: Asbestosis and abdominal neoplasms. Lancet 2, 1211—1216 (1960).
KENNAWAY, E. L., and N. M. KENNAWAY: A study of the incidence of cancer of the lung and larynx. J. Hyg. 36, 236—267 (1936).
— — Further study of incidence of cancer of lung and larynx. Brit. J. Cancer 1, 260—298 (1947).
KNOX, J. F., and J. BEATTIE: Distribution of mineral particles and fibers in the lung after exposure to asbestos dust. Arch. industr. Hyg. 10, 30—36 (1954).
KÖNIG, J.: Über die Asbestose. Arch. Gewerbepath. Gewerbehyg. 18, 159—204 (1960).
KUEHN, J.: Electron microscopy on asbestos dust and on lungs in asbestosis. Arch. Gewerbepath. 10, 473—479 (1942).
LAGUILLAUME, de B., J. CHAMPEIX, et JACQUEMENT: Arch. Anat. path. 10, 144—146 (1962).
LANZA, A. Z.: Asbestosis. J. Amer. med. Ass. 106, 368—369 (1936).
LEATHART, G. L., and J. T. SANDERSON: Some observations on asbestosis. Ann. occup. Hyg. 6, 65—74 (1963).
LEICHER, F.: Primärer Deckzellentumor des Bauchfelles bei Asbestose. Arch. Gewerbepath. 13, 382—392 (1955).
LINZBACH, A. J., and H. W. WEDLER: Beitrag zum Berufskrebs der Asbestarbeiter. Virchows Arch. path. Anat. 307, 387—409 (1941).
LUTON, P., et J. CHAMPEIX: Etude de l'asbestose. Arch. mal. prof. 7, 365—378 (1946).
— —, and FAURE: Asbestosis of the lung. Arch. Mal. prof. 7, 299—302 (1946).
LYNCH, K. M., and W. M. CANNON: Asbestosis: IV. Analysis of forty necropsied cases. Dis. Chest 14, 874—889 (1948).
—, F. A. McIVER, and J. R. CAIN: Pulmonary tumors in mice exposed to asbestos dust. Arch. industr. Hlth 15, 207—214 (1957).
—, and H. R. PRATT-THOMAS: Carcinoma of the lung in asbestosis: Report of 2 additional cases. Sth. med. J. (Bgham, Ala.) 48, 565—568 (1955).
— — Asbestosis III. Carcinoma of the lung in asbesto-silicosis. Amer. J. Cancer 34, 56—64 (1935).
—, and W. A. SMITH: Pulmonary asbestosis. I. A report of bronchial carcinoma and epithelial metaplasia. Amer. J. Cancer 36, 567—573 (1939).
MANCUSO, T. F.: Personal communication.
—, and E. J. COULTER: Methodology in industrial health studies. Arch. environm. Hlth 6, 210—226 (1963).
MEREWETHER, E. R.: Ann. Rep. Chief Inspector of Factories for the Year 1947, p. 15—17.
— Ann. Rep. Chief Inspector of Factories for the Year 1955, p. 206.
MITCHELL, Jerry: Health progress in an asbestos textile works. Arch. environm. Hlth 3, 37—41 (1961).
MURRAY, M.: Charing cross hosp. gaz. Cited by Bohlig, Jacob and Mueller, 1900.
National Cancer Institute of Canada: Annual Report, 1955—1956, p. 25.
NEWHOUSE, M. L., and H. THOMPSON: Epidemiological studies of patients with mesothelial tumors in the London area. Ann. N. Y. Acad. Sci. 132, 519—588 (1965).
NORDMANN, M.: Der Berufskrebs der Asbestarbeiter. Z. Krebsforsch. 47, 288—302 (1938).
— Lungenasbestose und Lungenkrebs. Ber. 8. Internat. Kongr. Unfallmed. u. Berufskrankh. Bd. 2. Leipzig: Georg Thieme 1939.
—, und A. SORGE: Lungenkrebs durch Asbeststaub im Tierversuch. Z. Krebsforsch. 51, 168—182 (1941).
NORDVIK, N.: La silicose et l'asbestose prédisposent-elles au cancer pulmonaire? Arch. bèlges Méd. soc. 17, 85—99 (1959).
NORO, L.: Histology of asbestosis. Acta path. microbiol. scand. 23, 53—59 (1946).
— Cited by Bohlig, Jacob and Mueller.
NOTHDURFT, H.: Experimentelle Sarkome durch reizlos einheilende Fremdkörper. Z. Krebsbekämpf. 34, 14—27 (1955).

NOTHDURFT, H.: Experimentelle Sarkomauslösung durch eingeheilte Fremdkörper. Strahlentherapie 100, 192—210 (1956).

O'DONNELL. W. M.: personal communication, 1961.

—, and R. H. MANN: Asbestose: An extrinsic factor in the pathogenesis of bronchogenic carcinoma. Amer. J. Path. 33, 610 (1957).

OLLIVIER, H., P. MORAND, and R. BRUN: Granulomas of the skin due to asbestos. Arch. Mal. prof. 10, 516—517 (1949).

OPPENHEIMER, B. S., E. T. OPPENHEIMFR, A. P. STOUT, I. DANISHEFSKY, and M. WILLHITE: Studies of the mechanism of carcinogenesis by plastic films. Acta Un. int. Cancr. 15, 659—662 (1959).

OWEN, T. K.: Carcinoma and asbestosis of the lung: Report of a case. Brit. J. Cancer 5, 382—383 (1951).

OWEN, W. G.: Diffuse mesothelioma and exposure to asbestos dust in the Merseyside area. Brit. med. J. 2, 214—218 (1964).

PARKES, G. D.: Mellor's modern inorganic chemistry. New York: Longmans, Green and Co. 1939.

PARTIGLIATTI-BARBOS, M.: Considerazioni sull'associazione asbestose e carcinoma polmonare. Gior. Acced. Med. Torino 118, 91—95 (1955).

PEACOCK, A., and P. R. PEACOCK: Asbestos as a potential carcinogen for fowls. Brit. Emp. Cancer Camp. Part. 2, 534—535 (1963). Ann. New York Acad. Sci. 132, 501—503 (1965).

PELLER, S.: Cancer in man. New York: International Universities Press, Inc. 1952.

ROMBOLA, G.: Asbestosi e carcinoma polmonare in una filatrice di amianto; sppunti sui problema oncogeno dell'asbesto. Med. d. Lavoro 46, 242—250 (1955).

ROSATO, D. V.: Asbestos: Its industrial aspects. New York: Reinhold Publ. Corp. 1959.

ROUSSEAU, L.: Quelques considerations sur l'amantiose. Sem. Hôp. (Paris) 23, 1811—1814 (1947).

SAFFIOTTI, U., F. CAFIS, L. H. KOLB, and M. I. CROTA: Intratracheal injections of particulate carcinogens into hamster lungs. Proc. Ann. Ass. Cancer Res. 4, 59 (1963). Chicago Medical School Quart. 24, 10—17 (1964).

SCHEPERS, G. W. H.: personal communication.

SCHMAEHL, D.: Cancerogene Wirkung von Asbest bei Implantation an Ratten. Z. Krebsforsch. 62, 561—567 (1958).

SELIKOFF, I. J., J. CHURG, and E. C. HAMMOND: Relation between exposure to asbestos and mesothelioma. New Engl. J. Med. 272, 560—565 (1965).

— — — Asbestos exposure and neoplasia. J. Amer. med. Ass. 188, 22—26 (1964).

SHABAD, L.: J. nat. Cancer Inst. 28, 1305—1331 (1962).

SINCLAIR, W. E.: Asbestos, its origin, production and utilization. 2nd. ed. London: Mining Publikations, Ltd. Salisbury House 1959.

SLEGGS, C. A., P. MARCHAND, and J. C. WAGNER: Diffuse pleural mesotheliomas in South Africa. S. Afr. med. J. 35, 28—34, (1961).

SMITH, Wm. E.: Survey of some current British and european studies of occupational tumor chproblems. Arch. industr. Hyg. 5, 58—79 (1952).

SMITH, W. E., L. MILLER, J. CHURG, and I. J. SELIKOFF: Mesotheliomas in hamsters following intrapleural injektion of asbestos. J. Mt Sinai Hosp. 32, 1—8 (1965).

STOLL, R., R. BASS, and A. A. ANGRIST: Asbestosis associated with bronchogenic carcinoma. Arch. industr. Med. 88, 831—834 (1951).

TELISCHI, M., and A. J. RUBENSTONE: Pulmonary asbestosis. Arch. Path. 73, 234—243 (1961).

— — Pulmonary asbestosis. Arch. Path. 72, 234—243 (1961).

TEUTSCHLAENDER, O.: Die Berufskrebse. Z. Krebsforsch. 32, 614—627 (1930).

THOMSON, J. G.: Mesothelioma of pleura or peritoneum and limited basal asbestosis. S. Afr. med. J. 36, 759—760 (1962).

VORWALD, A. J.: personal communication.

—, Th. M. DURKAN, and Ph. PRATT: Experimental studies of asbestosis. Arch. industr. Hyg. 3, 1—43 (1951).

—, and J. W. KARR: Pneumoconiosis and pulmonary carcinoma. Amer. J. Path. 14, 49—57 (1938).

WAGLER, F., H. MULLER, and M. ANSPACH: Gibt es eine endemische Asbestose? Z. Hyg. 8, 246—255 (1962).

WAGNER, J. C.: Experimental production of mesothelial tumours of the pleura by implantation of dusts in laboratory animals. Nature 196, 180—181 (1962).

— Asbestosis in experimental animals. Brit. J. industr. Med. 20, 1—12 (1963).

— Asbestos dust expsosure and malignancy. Experta med. Int. Congr. Ser. (No. 62), 3, 1066—1067 (1964).

—, C. A. SLEGGS, and P. MARCHAND: Diffuse pleural mesothelioma and asbestos exposure in the North Western Cape Province. Brit. J. industr. Med. 17, 260—271 (1960).

WALTHER, H. E.: Krebsmetastasen. Basel: Benno Schwabe & Co 1948.

WEBSTER, I.: Asbestosis in non-experimental animals in South Africa. Nature 197, 506 (1963).

— Asbestosis. S. Afr. med. J. 38, 870—872 (1964).

WEDLER, H. W.: Asbestose und Lungenkrebs. Dtsch. med. Wschr. 69, 575—576 (1943).

— Klinik der Lungenasbestose. Leipzig: 1939.

WEGELIUS, C.: Changes in the lungs in 126 cases of asbestosis observed in Finland. Acta radiol. 28, 139—152 (1947).

WEISS, A.: Pleurakrebs bei Lungenasbestose. Med. Welt (Stuttg.) 43, 93—94 (1953).

WELZ, A.: Weitere Beobachtungen über den Berufskrebs der Asbestarbeiter. Arch. Gewerbepath. 11, 536—550 (1942).

WERBER, M.: Lungen-Asbestose und Karzinom. Zbl. Arbeitsmed. 2, 179—180 (1952).

WYERS, H.: Asbestosis. Postgrad. med. J. 25, 631—638 (1949).

Chromium

Air Pollution Measurements of the National Air Sampling Network, Analyses of Suspended Particulates, 1953—1957, Public Health Service. Publication No. 637, 1958.

ANDRIEVSKAYA, Z. K., and M. M. MISLAVSKAYA: Silicosis in a chromite mine and its prophylaxis. Gig. i Sanit. 5, 28—30 (1949).

ALWENS, W.: Lungenkrebs durch Arbeit in Chromat-herstellenden Betrieben. Proc. 9, Kongreß f. Unfallmed. u. Berufskr, 973—982 (1938).

—, E. E. BAUKE, and W. JONAS: Auffallende Häufung von Bronchialkrebs bei Arbeitern der chemischen Industrie. Münch. med. Wschr. 83, 485—487 (1936).

— — — Auffallende Häufung von Bronchialkrebs bei Arbeitern der chemischen Industrie. Arch. Gewerbepath. 7, 69—84 (1936—1937).

—, and W. JONAS: Ein weiterer Beitrag zur Frage des gewerblichen Lungenkrebses. Arch. Gewerbepath. 7, 532—537 (1936—1937).

— — Der Chromat-Lungenkrebs. Acta Un. int. Cancr. 3, 103—114 (1938).

ASANG, E.: Chronische Chromatschädigung mit Entwicklung eines Lungentumors. Zbl. Arbeitsmed. 2, 181—184 (1952).

BAADER, E. W.: Der Lungenkrebs als gewerbemedizinisches Problem. Verhandl. Dtsch. Ges. inn. Med. 57, 322—332 (1951).

BAETJER, A. M.: Pulmonary carcinoma in chromate workers. Arch. industr. Hyg. 2, 487—504; 505—516 (1950).

— Relation of chromium to health. In Udy, M. J.: Chromium, vol. I., chemistry of chromium and its compounds. Am. Chem. Soc. Monograph Series. New York: Reinhold Publishing Co. 1956.

—, C. DAMRON, and V. BUDACZ: The distribution and retention of chromium in men and animals. Arch. industr. Htlh 20, 136—150 (1959).

—, J. F. LOWNEY, H. STEFFEE, and V. BUDACZ: Effect of chromium on incidence of lung tumors in mice and rats. Arch. industr. Hlth 20, 124—135 (1959).

BALL, Wm. L., et al.: Threshold limit values for 1961. Amer. industr. Hyg. Ass. J. 325—328 (1961).

BARBORIK, M., L. HANSLIAN, L. ORAL, H. SEHNALOVA, and R. HOLUSA: Carcinoma of the lungs in personnel working at electrolytic chromium plating. Pracov. Lék. 10, 413—417 (1958).

BAUKE, E., and W. ALWENS: Über röntgenologische Lungen- und insbesondere Lungenwurzel-veränderungen bei Arbeitern der chemischen Industrie. Ergebn. Dtsch. Ges. inn. Med. 48, 199—202 (1936).

BELTH, S. M., E. KAPLAN, and C. E. COUCHMAN: The collection and determination of chromium in an urban atmosphere. Arch. environ. Hlth 1, 311—315 (1960).

BIDSTRUP, P. L.: Carcinoma of the lung in chromate workers. Brit. J. industr. Med. 8, 302—305 (1951).

—, and R. A. M. CASE: Carcinoma of the lung in workmen in the bichromates-producing industry in Great Britain. Brit. J. industr. Med. 13, 260—264 (1956).

BISTER, F., G. KLAVIS, H. KOEHLER, und H. WITTGENS: Zur Gewerbetoxikologie von Anstrichstoffen auf Zinkchromatbasis. Arch. Gewerbepath. 16, 567—587 (1958).

BLUMLEIN, H.: Bösartige Tumoren nach Steckschußverletzungen. Arch. Ohr.-, Nas.-, u. Kehlk.-Heilk. 171, 239—244 (1958).

BOURNE, H., and W. R. RUSHIN: Atmospheric pollution in the vicinity of a chromate plant. Industr. Med. Surg. 19, 568—569 (1950).

—, and H. T. YEE: Occupational cancer in a chromate plant. Industr. Med. Surg. 19, 568—572 (1950).

BRINTON, I. P., E. S. FRASIER, and A. L. KOVEN: Morbidity and mortality experience among chromate workers. Publ. Hlth Rep. 67, 835—847 (1952).

BUCKELL, M., and D. G. HARVEY: An environmental study of the chromate industry. Brit. J. industr. Med. 8, 298—301 (1951).

BUESS, H.: L'enteropathie chromique, maladie professionelle peu connue, provoqueé par des chromates. Arch. Mal. prof. 12, 649—651 (1951).

— Beobachtungen und Studien über eine wenig bekannte Form von gewerblich bedingter Chromatschädigung. Helv. Med. Acta 17, 104—136 (1950).

CADOTSCH, H.: Zur Frage des Zusammenhangs zwischen Kehlkopfkrebs und Berufskrankheit. Arch. Ohr.-, Nas.-, u. Kehlk.-Heilk. 157, 68—77 (1950).

CAHNMANN, H. J., and R. BISEN: Microdetermination of chromium in blood. Analyt. Chem. 24, 1341—1345 (1952).

CAROZZI, L.: Cancer professionnel et organisation internationale du travail. Acta Un. int. Cancr. 2, 3—10 (1937).

CLARK, J. H.: The denaturation of proteins by chromium salts. Arch. industr. Hlth 20, 117—123 (1959).

DANKMAN, H. S.: Industrial exposure to chromates in New York State. Arch. industr. Hyg. 5, 228—231 (1952).

EDMUNDSON, F.: Chrome ulcers of the skin and nasal septum and their relation to patch testing. J. invest. Derm. 17, 11—19 (1951).

FISHER, R. S., and P. W. RIEKERT: Lung cancer in chromate workers. Amer. J. Path. 35, 699 (1959).

FISCHER-WASELS, B.: Cited by HUEPER. In E. BAADER (Ed.): Berufkrebse. Handbuch der gesamten Arbeitsmedizin. München: Urban & Schwarzenberg 1961.

GAFAFER, W. M., et al.: Health of workers in chromate producing industry. Publ. Health Serv. Publ. No. 192, U. S. Government Printing Office, Washington, D. C., 1953. pp. 131.

GROGAN, C. H.: Experimental studies in metal cancerigenesis. VIII. On the etiological factors in chromate cancer. Cancer 10, 625—638 (1957).

—, and H. OPPENHEIMER: Experimental studies in metal cancerigenesis III. Behaviour of chromium compounds in the physiologic pH range. J. Amer. Chem. Soc. 77, 152—157 (1955).

— — Experimental studies in metal cancerigenesis. V. Interaction of Cr^{iii} and Cr^{vi} compounds with proteins. Arch. Biochem. Biophys. 56, 204—221 (1955).

GROSS, E.: Lungenkrebs durch Arbeit in Chromat-herstellenden Betrieben. Ergebn. 8. Int. Kongr. f. Unfallmed. u. Berufskr. 966—972 (1938).

— Das Carcinom vom Standpunkt des Gewerbetoxikologen. Angew. Chem. 53, 368—372 (1940).

— Über gewerblichen Lungenkrebs. Klin. Wschr. 15, 323—325 (1936).

—, and F. KOELSCH: Über den Lungenkrebs in der Chromfarbenindustrie. Arch. Gewerbepath. 12, 164—176 (1943).

172   References

GRUSHKO, J. M.: Chromium as a cancerogenic substance. Vopr. Onkol. 7, 100—108 (1961).
— Chromium as a bioelement. Biokhim. 13, 124—126 (1948).
HATEM, S. H.: Essai sur le mecanisme de la cancerisation par les metaux. Arch. Mal. prof. 22, 40—46 (1961).
— Cancers du chrome et complexion de l'histamine par le metal. C. R. Soc. Biol. 154, 518—521 (1960).
HOSCHEK, R.: Die neue Melde- und Entschädigungspflicht bei beruflichen Chromschädigungen. Zbl. Arbeitsmed. 3, 85—88 (1953).
HUEPER, W. C.: Occupational tumors and allied diseases. Springfield, Ill.: C. C. Thomas 1942.
— Environmental lung cancer. Industr. Med. Surg. 20, 49—62 (1951).
— Environmental lung cancer. Proc. First Canadian Cancer Research Conference. Vol. I, New York: Academic Press 1955.
— Experimental studies in metal cancerigenesis. VII. Tissue reactions to parenterally introduced powdered metallic chromium and chromite ore. J. nat. Cancer Inst. 16, 447—469 (1955).
— A quest into the environmental causes of cancer of the lung. Public Health Monograph No. 36. Public Health Service. U. S. Government Printing Office, Washington, D. C. 1956, pp. 54.
— The role of occupational and environmental air pollutants in the production of respiratory cancers. Arch. Path. 63, 427—540 (1957).
— Experimental studies in metal cancerigenesis. X. Cancerigenic effects of chromite ore roast deposited in muscle tissue and pleural cavity of rats. Arch. industr., Hlth 18, 284—291 (1958).
— Epidemiologic, experimental and histological studies on metal cancers of the lung. Acta Un. int. Cancr. 15, 424—436 (1958).
— Der Chromkrebs der Menschen und Tiere. Proc. 5th Session, Commission for Occupational Cancer, Deutsche Forschungsgemeinschaft, March, 1959. Publ. 1960.
—, and W. W. PAYNE: Experimental cancers in rats produced by chromium compounds and their significance to industry and public health. Amer. Hyg. Ass. J. 20, 274—280 (1959).
— — Experimental studies in metal cancerigenesis. Chromium, Nickel, Iron, Arsenic. environm. Hlth. 5, 445—462 (1962).
— — Experimental studies of chromium compounds - - Their carcinogenicity and their importance for industrial medicine. Proc. 13th Congr. Occup. Health, 1960. U. S. Executive Committee, 1961, p. 473—486.
IMPRESCIA, S.: Bronchogenic carcinoma and chromates. Dis. Chest. 22, 347—358 (1952).
ISHIKAWA, M.: Notes on experimental anaphylaxis induced by simple chemical compounds. Jap. med. J. 1, 385—396 (1948).
KOELSCH, Fr.: Lungenkrebs und Beruf. Acta Un. int. Cancr. 3, 243—251 (1938).
KUSCHNER, M., and N. NELSON: Occupational cancer. Arch. Indust. Health 7, 29—31 (1957).
LEHMANN, K. B.: Ist Grund zu einer besonderen Beunruhigung wegen des Auftretens von Lungenkrebs bei Chromatarbeitern vorhanden? Zbl. Gewerbepath. Gewerbehyg. 9, 168—170 (1932).
LETTERER, E.: Untersuchung einer Chrom-Silikose-Lunge. Arch. Gewerbepath. 9, 496—508, (1938—1939).
—, K. NEIDHARDT, and H. KLETT: Chromatlungenkrebs und Chromatstaublunge. Arch. Gewerbepath. Gewerbehyg. 12, 323—361 (1944).
LOISELEUR, M. J.: Comparaison de l'antigenicitê molécules protéidiques, organiques et minerales. J. Méd. Bordeaux 130, 264—290 (1953).
—, et M. SAUVAGE: Characteristiques des anticorps correspondent aux antigènes minéraux. C. R. Acad. Sci. (Paris) 234, 2316—2319 (1952).
LUKANIN, W. P.: Zur Pathologie der Chromat-Pneumokoniose. Arch. Hyg. 104, 166—174 (1930).
MACHLE, W., and F. GREGORIUS: Cancer of respiratory system in United States chromate-producing industry. Publ. Hlth Rep. 63, 1114—1127 (1948).
MAGER, E.: Berufliche Erkrankungen durch Chrom und seine Verbindungen Verhandl. Dtsch. Ges. Arbeitssch. 1, 97—106 (1953).

MALOFF, Cl. C.: Use of edathamine calcium in the treatment of chrome ulcers of the skin. Arch. industr. Hlth 11, 123—125 (1955).

MANCUSO, T. E.: Occupational cancer and other health hazards in a chromate plant: A medical appraisal. II. Clinical and toxicologic approach. Indust. Med. Surg. 20, 393—407 (1951).

—, and W. C. HUEPER: Occupational cancer and other health hazards in a chromate plant: A medical appraisal. I. Lung cancers in chromate workers. Industr. Med. Surg. 20, 358—363 (1951).

MASSMANN, W., and K. PILGRIM: Das Verhalten des Lungengewebes nach intratrachealer Injektion von Mangan-IV-Oxyd und Chrom-III-Oxyd. Arch. Gewerbepath. 15, 203—212 (1956).

McDOUGALL, A.: Malignant tumor at site of bone plating. J. Bone Jt Surg. 38, 709—712 (1956).

MORRIS, G. E.: Basisches Chrom-sulfat. Ergebnisse der Epicutantestung eines Chrom-III-Salzes. Berufsdermatosen 7, 126—131 (1959).

MOSINGER, M., and H. FIORENTINI: Sur la pathologie due aux chromates. Arch. mal. prof. 15, 187—199 (1954).

— — Experiments bearing upon the idea that gastric ulcers are frequent among chrome workers. Arch. mal. prof. 16, 363—365 (1955).

NEWMAN, D. A.: Case of adeno-carcinoma of the left inferior turbinate body and perforation of the nasal septum in the person of a worker in chrome pigments. Glasgow. med. J. 33, 469 (1890).

OETTEL, H.: Discussion remarks to Hueper, Der Chromkrebs der Menschen und Tiere. Proc. 5th Session, Commission for Occupational Cancer, Deutsche Forschungsgemeinschaft, March 1959, publ. 1960.

PAYNE, W. W.: Production of cancers in mice and rats by chromium compounds. Arch. industr. Hlth 21, 530—535 (1960).

— The role of roasted chromite ore in the production of cancer. Arch. environm. Hlth 1, 20—26 (1960).

PFEIL, E.: Lungentumoren als Berufserkrankung in Chromatbetrieben. Dtsch. med. Wschr. 61, 1197—1200 (1935).

PORTIGLIATTI-BARBOS, M.: I carcinomi polmonari da cromo. Minerva med. 77, 4—5 (1957).

PRIVE, L., M. TELLEM, D. MERANZE, and R. CHODOFF: Carcinosarcoma of the lung. Arch. Path. 72, 351—357 (1961).

RIEDL, L.: Gastric ulcer developing on basis of chronic chromium poisoning. Čas. Lék. Čes. 78, 789 (1939).

RINCK, H.: Carcinoma of the lungs caused by chromates: An occupational disease. Medizinische 342—345 (1956).

SCHINZ, H. R.: Der Metallkrebs. Ein Neues Prinzip der Krebserzeugung. Schweiz. med. Wschr. 72, 1070—1074 (1942).

—, and E. UEHLINGER: Der Metallkrebs. Z. Krebsforsch. 52, 425—437 (1942).

SHIMKIN, M. H., and J. LEITER: Induced pulmonary tumors in mice. III. The role of chronic irritation in the production of pulmonary tumors in strain A mice. J. Nat. Cancer Inst. 1, 241—254 (1940).

SPANNAGEL, H.: Eine Untersuchungsmethode zur Bestimmung von Chrom in Blut und Urin. Zbl. Arbeitsmed. 1, 15—17 (1951).

— Lungenkrebs und andere Organschäden durch Chromverbindungen. Arbeitsmedizin, Heft 28. Leipzig: Johann Ambrosius Barth 1953.

STEFFEE, C. H., and A. M. BAETJER: Histopathologic effects of chromate chemicals. Arch. environ. Hlth 11, 66—75 (1965).

STRUPPLER, V.: Sarkome nach Knochennagelung. Mschr. Unfallheilk. 62, 121—127 (1959).

TABOR, E. C., and Wm. V. WARREN: Distribution of certain metals in the atmosphere of some American cities. Arch. industr. Hlth 17, 145—151 (1958).

TELEKY, L.: Krebs bei Chromatarbeitern. Dtsch. med. Wschr. 62, 1353—1354 (1936).

— Occupational cancer of the lung. J. industr. Hyg. 19, 73—85 (1937).

— Der berufliche Lungenkrebs. Acta Un. Cancr. 3, 253—273 (1938).

TEUTSCHLAENDER, O.: Die Berufskrebse mit besonderer Berücksichtigung ihrer Verhütung und der Unfallgesetzgebung. Acta Un. Cancr. 2, 67—84 (1937).

URONE, P. P., and H. K. ANDERS: Determination of small amounts of chromium in human blood, tissues and urine. Anal. Chem. 22, 1317—1321 (1950).

VIGLIANI, E. C., and N. ZURLO: Experiences of the clinica del lavoro with maximum allowable concentrations of industrial poisons. Arch. Gewerbepath. 13, 528—535 (1955).

VOLLMANN, J.: Tierexperimente mit intraossaerem Arsen-, Chrom-, und Kobaltdepot. Schweiz. Z. allg. Path. 1, 440—443 (1938—1940).

WACKMANN, J.: Pulmonary cancer in industrial workers and miners, and cancer due to chromium. Med. Lavoro 24, 189—192 (1933).

WALSH, E. N.: Chromate hazards in industry. J. Amer. med. Ass. 153, 1305—1308 (1953).

WELZ, A.: Hautkrebs durch chronische Chromschädigung. Zbl. Chir. 72, 811—817 (1947).

WORTH, G., and E. SCHILLER: Gesundheitsschädigungen durch Chrom und seine Verbindungen. Arch. Gewerbepath. 13, 673—686 (1955).

Nickel

ABMIT, H. W.: The toxicology of nickel carbonyl. J. Hyg. 7, 525—551 (1907).
— The toxicology of nickel carbonyl. J. Hyg. 8, 565—600 (1908).

ABRAHAM, H.: Asphalts and Allied Substances. 5th ed. New York: Van Nostrand Co. 1945.

AMOR, A. J.: Nickel carbonyl. Occupation and Health, Suppl., Geneva, International Labour Office. 1938, pp. 1—5.
— Growths of the respiratory Tract. VIII. Internat. Kongress Unfallmed. Berufskankh. 1938, Bd. 2, 941—962.

Ann. Report Chief Inspector of Factories for the Year 1948. London: H. M. Stationery Office 1949.

ARAKI, M., and K. MURE: Spectrographic analysis of tissues. (9). On the quantitative analysis of nickel in tumor tissues. Gann 40, 76—79 (1949).

BAADER, E. W.: Berufskrebs. Neuere Ergebnisse auf dem Gebiete der Krebskrankheiten. In Adam, C., and H. Auler: Neuere Erg. a. d. Geb. d. Krebskrankh. Leipzig: S. Hirzel 1937.

BAYER, O.: Beitrag zur Toxikologie, Klinik und pathologischen Anatomie der Nickelkarbonylvergiftung. Arch. Gewerbepath. 9, 592—606 (1938—1939).

BIDSTRUP, P. L.: Cancer of the lung in nickel, arsenic and chromate workers. Arch. belges Méd. soc. 8, 500—506 (1950).

BRIDGE, J. C.: Ann. rep. chief inspector of factories and workshops for the year 1935. London: H. M. Stationery Office 1936.

CARMICHAEL, J. L.: Nickel carbonyl poisoning. Report of a case. Arch. industr. Hyg. 8, 143—148 (1953).

CAROZZI, L.: Cancer professionnel et organisation internationale du travail. Acta Un. int. Cancr. 2, 3 (1937).

CHAUMONT, A. J., and J. J. HIMMELSBACH: Die berufliche Nickeldermatose. Kasuistische Mitteilung über Betriebsbesichtigungen in drei verschiedenen Unternehmen. Berufsdermatosen 9, 316—320 (1961).

COOPER, E. H.: An important factor in the causation of industrial cancer. Med. Press 187, 397 (1933).

DAVIS, H. W.: Nickel. In H. J. Keiser: Minerals Yearbook 1945. Washington 1947, p. 620.

DOIG, A. T.: Dust diseases, excluding the fibrotic pneumoconioses. In MEREWETHER, E. R. A.: Industrial Medicine and Hygiene. Vol. 3. London: Butterworth & Co., Ltd. 1956.

DOLL, R.: Cancer of the lung and nose in nickel workers. Brit. J. industr. Med. 15, 217—223 (1958).
— Cancer of the lung and nose in nickel workers. Med. Literature Abstr. J. Amer. med. Ass. 169, 1004 (1959).

FISCHER, M. R.: Occupation and health: nickel. Geneva, International Office, 1934, vol. 2, pp. 320—323.

FISHER, A. A., and A. SHAPIRO: Allergic eczematous contact dermatitis due to metallic nickel. J. Amer. med. Ass. 161, 717—721 (1956).

GILMAN, J. P., and P. K. BASRUR: Precancerous changes in muscle cells exposed to nickel sulphide. Proc. Amer. Ass. Cancer Res. 4, 23 (1963).

GILMAN, J. P., and H. HERCHEN: The effect of physical form of implant on nickel sulphide tumourigenesis in the rat. Acta Un. int. Cancr. 19, 615—619 (1963).
—, and G. M. RUCKERBAUER: Metal carcinogenesis. I. Observations on the carcinogenicity of a refinery dust, cobalt oxide, and colloidal thorium dioxide. Cancer Res. 22, 152—162 (1962).
GOLDBLATT, M. W., and V. A. J. WAGSTAFF: Aspects of industrial medicine and hygiene in German chemical factories. B. I. O. S. Final Report No. 1501, Item No. 24, 1948, Tech. Serv., Dept. Commerce Washington, p. 36.
GRENFELL: Le cancer professionnel. In CAROZZI, L.: La méd. du trav. 6, 1—9; 95—130 (1934).
HATEM, S.: Cancers du nickel et complexes histamine-sels de nickel. C. R. Acad. Sci. (Paris) 246, 2423—2426 (1958).
— Cancer du nickel et lésions des terminaisons nerveuses par fixation de l'histamine. C. R. Soc. Biol. 152, 1093 (1958).
— Inhibition de la cancérogénèse du nickel et libération de l'histamine engagée. C. R. Acad. Sci. (Paris) 250, 2962—2964 (1960).
— Complexion de l'histamine par le nickel, le cobalt, le chrome et le glucinium. Chimia 14, 130—133 (1960).
— Affinité de l'acide folique pour le nickel et cancers du nickel. C. R. Acad. Sci. (Paris) 254, 1177—1179 (1962).
HERCHEN, H.: Effect of duration of exposure on nickel sulphide tumorigenesis. Nature 202, 306—307 (1964).
HUEPER, W. C.: Experimental studies in metal cancerigenesis. I. Nickel cancers in rats. Tex. Rep. Biol. Med. 10, 167—186 (1952).
— A quest into the environmental cause of cancer of the lung. Publ. Hlth Monogr. No. 36, DHEW, PHS Publn. No. 452, Washington, D. C. USGPO, 1955, pp. 54.
— Experimental studies in metal cancerigenesis. IV. Cancer produced by parenterally introduced metallic nickel. J. nat. Cancer Inst. 16, 55—73 (1955).
— Experimental studies in metal cancerigenesis. IX. Pulmonary lesions in guinea pigs and rats exposed to prolonged inhalation of powdered metallic nickel. Arch. Path. 65, 600—607 (1958).
— Carcinogenic studies on water soluble and insoluble macromolecules. Arch. Path. 67, 589—617 (1959).
—, and W. W. PAYNE: Experimental studies in metal carcinogenesis. Chromium, nickel, iron, Arsenic. Arch. environ. Hlth 5, 445—462 (1962).
International Labour Office, Occupation and Health: Nickel. Geneva, 1934, vol. 2, pp. 320—323.
International Nickel Company of Canada, Ltd.: The Corporate History of the International Nickel Co. of Canada, Ltd., Canad. Mining J. 67, 311—553 (1946).
IMBUS, H. R., J. CHOLAK, L. H. MILLER, and T. STERLING: Boron, cadmium, chromium, and nickel in blood and urine. A survey of American working men. Arch. environ. Hlth 6, 286—295 (1963).
JASMIN, GAETAN: Effects of methandrostenolone on muscle carcinogenesis induced in rats by nickel sulphide. Brit. J. Cancer. 17, 681—686 (1963).
KRAFFT, K.: Nickelkarbonylpneumonien. 8. Int. Kongress Unfallmed. Berufskrankh., 1939, pp. 1054—1056.
KINCAID, J. F., J. S. STRONG, and F. W. SUNDERMANN: Nickel poisoning. I. Experimental study of the effects of acute and subacute exposure to nickel carbonyl. Arch. Industr. Hyg. 8, 48—60 (1953).
LOKEN, A. C.: Lungecarcinom hos nikkelarbeidere. T. norske Laegeforen. 70, 376—378 (1950).
MARCUSSEN, P. V.: Ecological considerations on nickel dermatitis. Brit. J. industr. Med. 17, 65—68 (1960).
MILLER, H. I., G. M. HAMA, E. C. J. URGAN, and P. DRINKER: Health hazards in metal spraying. J. industr. Hyg. 20, 380 (1938).
MITCHELL, D. F., G. B. SHANKWALKER, and S. SHAZER: Determining the tumorigenicity of dental materials. J. dent. Res. 39, 1023—1028 (1960).

MORGAN, J. G.: Some observations on the incidence of respiratory cancer in nickel workers. Brit. J. industr. Med. 15, 224—234 (1958).
— A simplified method for the estimation of nickel in urine. Brit. J. industr. Med. 17, 209—212 (1960).
NOBLE, R. L., and V. CAPSTICK: Rhabdomyosarcomas induced by nickel sulphide in the rat. Proc. Amer. Ass. Cancer Res. 4, 48 (1963).
OLSON, K. B., G. E. HEGGEN, and C. F. EDWARDS: Analysis of 5 trace elements in the liver of patients dying of cancer and noncancerous disease. Cancer. 11, 554—561 (1958).
PELLER, S.: Factor x in the carbonyl process of refining nickel. Cancer in Man. New York: International Universities Press 1952.
SAMITZ, M. H., and H. POMFRANTZ: Studies of the effects on the skin of nickel and chromium salts. Arch. industr. Hlth 18, 473—479 (1958).
SAPPINGTON, C. O.: Essentials of industrials health. Philadelphia, Pa.: J. B. Lippincott Co. 1943.
SCHÄR, M.: Epidemiologic viewpoints in the investigation of the etiology of cancer. Oncologia (Basel) 16, 179—185 (1963).
STEPHENS, G. A.: An important factor in the causation of industrial cancer. Med. Press 136, 194—200; 216—219 (1933).
STODDART, J. C.: Sensitivity to nickel a cause of infusion reactions. Lancet 2, (Oct. 1) (1960).
SUNDERMAN, F. W., Jr.: Studies of nickel carcinogenesis. Alterations of ribonucleic acid following inhalation of nickel carbonyl. Amer. J. clin. Path. 39, 549—561 (1963).
— Studies of nickel carcinogenesis. The subcellular partition of nickel in lung and liver following inhalation of nickel carbonyl. Amer. J. clin. Path. 40, 563—575 (1963).
— Studies of nickel carcinogenesis: Fractionations of nickel in ultracentrifugal supernatants of lung and liver by dextran gel chromatography. Amer. J. clin. Path. 42, 228 (1964).
SUNDERMAN, F. W, and J. F. KINCAID: Effects of exposure to nickel carbonyl. Fed. Proc. 12, 277—278 (1953).
— — Nickel poisoning. II. Studies on patients suffering from acute exposure to vapors of nickel carbonyl. J. Amer. med. Ass. 155, 889—894 (1954).
— — Nickel metabolism following multiple exposure to nickel carbonyl vapor. Fed. Proc. 14, 288—289 (1955).
— —, A. J. DONNELLY, and B. WEST: Nickel poisoning. IV. Chronic exposure of rats to nickel carbonyl. Arch. industr. Hlth 16, 480—485 (1957).
—, A. J. DONNELLY, B. WEST, and J. F. KINCAID: Nickel poisoning. IX. Carcinogenesis in rats exposed to nickel carbonyl. Arch. industr. Hlth 20, 26—41 (1959).
—, and F. W. SUNDERMAN, Jr.: Nickel poisoning. VIII. Dithiocarb: A new therapeutic agent for persons exposed to nickel carbonyl. Amer. J. med. Sci. 236, 26—31 (1958).
—, and F. W. SUNDERMAN, Jr.: Nickel poisoning. XI. Implications of nickel as a pulmonary carcinogen in tobacco smoke. Amer. J. clin. Path. 35, 203—209 (1961).
—, C. L. RANGE, F. W. SUNDERMAN, Jr., A. J. DONNELLY, and G. W. LUCYSZYN: Nickel poisoning. XII. Metabolic and pathologic changes in acute pneumonitis from nickel charbonyl. Amer. J. clin. Path. 36, 477—491 (1961).
TEDESCHI, R. E., and F. W. SUNDERMAN: Nickel poisoning. V. The metabolism of nickel under normal conditions and after exposure to nickel carbonyl. Arch. industr. Hlth 16, 486—488 (1957).
TIETZ, N. W., E. F. HIRSCH, and B. NEYMAN: Spectrographic study of trace elements in cancerous and noncancerous human tissues. J. Amer. med. Ass. 165, 2187—2192 (1957).
WASE, A. W., D. M. GOSS, and M. J. BOYD: The metabolism of nickel. I. Spatial and temporal distribution of ni[63] in the mouse. Arch. Biochem. Biophys. 51, 1—4 (1954).
WEISBURGER, J. H., P. H. GRANTHAM. and E. K. WEISBURGER. Metal ion complexing properties of carcinogen metabolites. Biochem. Pharmacol. 12, 179—191 (1963).
WEST, B., and F. W. SUNDERMAN: Nickel poisoning. VII. The therapeutic effectiveness of alkyl dithiocarbamates in experimental animals exposed to nickel Carbonyl. Amer. J. med. Sci. 236, 15—25 (1958).
— — Nickel poisoning. VI. A note concerning the ineffectiveness of edathamil calcium-disodium (calcium disodium ethylenediaminetetraacetic acid). Arch. industr. Hlth 18, 480—482 (1958).

WILLIAMS, W. J.: The pathology of the lungs in five nickel workers. Brit. J. industr. Med. 15, 235—242 (1958).

WILSON, H. T. H.: Nickel dermatitis. Practitioner 177, 303—308 (1956).

ZNAMENSKII, S. V.: Occupational bronchogenic pulmonary cancer in workers extracting, isolating and reprocessing nickel ore. Vop. Onkol. 9, 130—131 (1963) (Russian).

Iron

BARRIE, H. J., and H. E. HARDING: Argyro-siderosis of the lungs in silver finishers. Brit. J. industr. Med. 4, 225—231 (1947).

BLAHA, K.: Pachydermia of the larynx in relation to certain noxious industrial substances. Acta Univ. Carol. Med. (Praha) 10, 248—254 (1960).

BRADLOW, B. A., J. A. DUNN, and J. HIGGINSON: The effect of cirrhosis on iron storage. Amer. J. Path. 39, 221—237 (1961).

BRADSHAW, F., A. CRITCHLOW, and G. NAGELSCHMIDT: A study of the airborne dust in haematite mines in Cumberland. Ann. occup. Hyg. 4, 265—273 (1962).

BRAUN, P., J. GUILLERM, B. PIERSON et P. SADOUL: A propos du cancer brochique chez les mineurs de fer. Rev. Méd. (Nancy) 85, 702—708 (1960).

BROWER, J. W.: Personal communication (1955).

CAMPBELL, J. A.: Effects of precipitated silica and of iron oxid on the incidence of primary lung tumours in mice. Brit. med. J. 2, 275—280 (1940).

DOIG, A. T.: Dust diseases, excluding the fibrotic pneumoconioses. In MEREWETHER, E. R. A.: Industrial Medicine and Hygiene, Vol. 3. London: Butterworth & Co., Ltd. 1956.

DOLL, R.: Occupational lung cancer: A review. Brit. J. industr. Med. 16, 181—190 (1959).

DRASCHE, H.: Zur Frage der Staubgefährdung in den Sinteranlagen saarländischer Eisenhütten. Arch. Gewerbepath. 16, 666—696 (1959).

DREESSEN, W. C., H. P. BRINTON, R. G. KEENAN, Th. R. THOMAS, E. H. PLACE, and J. E. FULLER: Health of arc welders in steel ship construction. Publ. Hlth Bull. 298, 200 (1947).

DREYFUSS, T. R.: Lungencarcinom bei Geschwistern nach Inhalation von eisenoxydhaltigem Staub in der Jugend. Z. klin. Med. 130, 256—258 (1936).

DUNNER, L.: Occupational disease of the lungs in boiler scalers. Brit. J. Radiol. 16, 287—290 (1943).

—, and R. HERMON: Further observations on lung disease in boiler scalers. Brit. J. Radiol. 17, 355—358 (1944).

—, and M. S. HICKS: Bronchial carcinoma in dusty occupations: Observations in boiler scalers and grain dockers. Brit. J. Tuberc. 47, 145—151 (1953).

EHRHARDT, W., and W. HEIDEMANN: Zur Klinik und Pathologie der Ockerstaublunge. Arch. Gewerbepath. 17, 504—518 (1959).

ELLIS, J. T., I. SHULMANN, and C. H. SMITH: Generalized siderosis with fibrosis of liver and pancreas in Cooley's (Mediterranean) Anemia. Amer. Path. 30, 287—309 (1954).

FAULDS, J. S.: Pulmonary disease in iron ore miners. J. clin. Path. 25, 126—134 (1955).

— Haematite pneumoconiosis in Cumberland miners. J. clin. Path. 10, 187—199 (1957).

— Carcinoma of the lung in haematite miners. J. Path. Bact. 72, 353—366 (1956).

—, and G. S. NAGELSCHMIDT: The dust in the lungs of haematite miners from Cumberland. Ann. Occup. Hyg. 4, 255—263 (1962).

FIELDING, J.: Sarcoma induction by iron-carbohydrate complexes. Brit. med. J. 1, 1800—3 (1962).

GILMANN, Th., M. HATHORN, and P. A. S. CANHAM: Experimental dietary siderosis. Amer. J. Path. 35, 349—367 (1959).

GLIBERT: Iron, pig iron, and steel industries. Occupational Health. Vol. 2, Geneva: International Labour Office 1934.

GOLDBERG, L.: Die Wirkung von Eiseninjektionen im Tierversuch. Arzneimittel 13, 939—945 (1963).

HADDOW, A., and E. S. HORNING: On the carcinogenicity of an iron-dextran complex. J. nat. cancer Inst. 24, 109—147 (1960).

HAMLIN, L. E.: Siderosis. J. occup. Med. 1, 79—83 (1959).

HARDING, H. E., and A. P. MASSIE: Pneumoconiosis in boiler scalers. Brit. J. industr. Med. **8**, 256—263 (1951).
—, A. I. G. McLAUGHLIN, and A. T. DOIG: Clinical radiographic, and pathological studies of the lungs of electric-are and oxyacetylene welders. Lancet: 394—399 (1958).
—, D. L. TOD, and A. I. G. McLAUGHLIN: Diseases of lungs in boiler scalers with a case report and review of the literature. Brit. J. industr. Med. **1**, 247—254 (1944).
HEIMANN, H.: The health of ferrous foundry workers. Publ. Hlth Rep. **66**, 223—239 (1951).
HIGGINSON, J.: Siderosis in Southern Africa. Cent. Afr. J. Med. 1—8 (1955).
—, TH. GERRITSEN, and A. R. P. WALKER: Siderosis in the Bantu of Southern Africa. Amer. J. Path. **29**, 779—815 (1953).
HUEPER, W. C.: Occupational tumors and allied diseases. Springfield, Ill.:C. C. Thomas 1942.
—, A quest into the environmental causes of cancer of the lung. Publ. Health Monograph No. 36, U. S. Publ. Health Serv., 1955.
— Methodologic Explorations in experimental respiratory carcinogenesis. Arzneimittel-Forsch. **14**, 814—822 (1964).
—, and W. W. PAYNE: Experimental studies in metal carcinogenesis: Chromium, nickel, iron, arsenic. Arch. environm. Hlth **5**, 445—462 (1962).
LAMY, P., R. SENAULT, P. SADOUL, R. HUTTIN, et J. GUILLERM: Les opacités massives chez les mineurs de fer. J. franç. Méd. Chir. thor. **13**, 283—292 (1959).
LUNDIN, P. M.: The carcinogenic action of complex iron preparation. Brit. J. Cancer **15**, 838—847 (1961).
KENNAWAY, E. L., and N. M. KENNAWAY: Further study on the incidence of cancer of the lung and larynx. Brit. J. Cancer **1**, 260—298 (1947).
McLAUGHLIN, A. I. G., and H. E. HARDING: Pneumoconisis and other causes of death in iron and steel foundry workers. Arch. industr. Hlth **14**, 350—378 (1956).
MONLIBERT, L., et ROUBILLE, R. HAYANGE: A propos du cancer bronchique chez le mineur de fer. J. franç. Méd. Chir. thor. **14**, 435—439 (1960).
MÜLLER, E., und W. EHRHARDT: Experimenteller Beitrag zur Frage der Carcinogenität des Eisenoxydstaubes. Z. Krebsforsch. **61**, 65—77 (1957).
OTTO, H.: Über Pneumokoniosen durch Erdfarben, insbesondere über Ockerlungen. Arch. Gewerbepath. **18**, 349—357 (1961).
RICHMOND, H. G.: Induction of sarcoma in the rat by iron-dextran complex. Brit. med. J. **1**, 947—949 (1959).
SAFFIOTTI, U., F. CEFIS, L. H. KOLB, and M. I. GROTE: Intratracheal injection of particulate carcinogens into hamster lungs. Proc. Amer. Ass. Cancer Res. **4**, 59 (1963).
SAGAIDAK, N. D.: Toxicology of radioactive iron. Gig. Tr. prof. Zabol. **6**, 22—28 (1959).
SCHNEIDER, H.: Über Siderose. Zbl. Arbeitsmed. **7**, 142—145 (1957).
SPREACACE, G. A.: Idiopathic pulmonary hemosiderosis. Amer. Rev. resp. Dis. **88**, 330—337 (1963).
STEWART, M. J., and J. S. FAULDS: The pulmonary fibrosis of haematite miners. J. Path. Bact. **39**, 233—241 (1934).
SUTHERLAND, C. L.: Review of gernez-Rieux-c et al.: Broncho-pneumopathies professionnelles. Paris: Masson & Cie 1961; Bull. Hyg. **37**, 457—458 (1962).
TODD, P. G., and D. RICE: Pneumoconiosis in boiler scaler. Lancet **1**, 309 (1944).
TURNER, H. M., and H. G. GRACE: An investigation into cancer mortality among males in certain Sheffield trades.. J. Hyg. **38**, 90 (1938).
VORWALD, A. J., and J. W. KARR: Pneumoconiosis and pulmonary malignancy. Amer. J. Path. **13**, 654 (1937).
ZOLLINGER, H. O.: Weichteiltumoren bei Ratten nach sehr massiven Eiseninjektionen. Schweiz. med. Wschr. **92**, 130—134 (1962); Path. et Microbiol. **25**, 296—300 (1962).

Beryllium

ARAKI, M., S. OKADA, and M. FUJITA: Experimental studies on beryllium-induced malignant tumors of rabbits. Gann **45**, 449—451 (1954).
AUB, J. C., and R. S. GRIER: Acute pneumonitis in workers exposed to beryllium oxide and beryllium metal. J. industr. Hyg. **31**, 123—133 (1949).

BARNES, J. M., and F. A. DENZ: Beryllium bone sarcomata in rabbits. Brit. J. Cancer 4, 212—222 (1950).

BRESLIN, A. J.: The control of beryllium oxide in the ceramic industry. Amer. Ceram. Soc. Bull. 30, 395—398 (1951).

—, and W. B. HARRIS: Health and safety laboratory. Health prodection in beryllium facilities, summary of ten years of experience. U. S. Atomic Energy Commission. New York: Operations Office 1958.

CAMPBELL, R. O.: A study of beryllium exposures at a high explosive assembly test facility. Am. industr. Hyg. Ass. J. 22, 385—391 (1961).

CHESNER, C.: Chronic pulmonary granulomatosis in residents of community near beryllium Plant. Ann. int. Med. 32, 1028—48 (1950).

CHOLAK, J., and D. M. HUBBARD: Spectrographic determination of beryllium in biological material and in air. Analyt. Chem. 20, 73—76 (1948).

COHEN, J. J.: Methods of handling and laundering beryllium-contaminated garments. Am. industr. Hyg. Ass. J. 24, 576—583 (1963).

Conference: Beryllium disease and its control. Arch. industr. Hlth 19, 91—266 (1959).

DeNARDI, J. M., H. S. VAN ORDSTRAND, and M. G. CARMODY: Acute dermatitis and pneumonitis in beryllium workers: A review of 405 cases in eight-year period with followup on recoveries. Ohio St. med. J. 45, 567—579 (1949).

— —, G. H. CURTIS, and J. ZIELINSKI: Berylliosis. Arch. industr. Hyg. 8, 1—24 (1953).

DUTRA, FR. R.: The pneumonitis and granulomatosis peculiar to beryllium workers. Amer. J. Path. 24, 1137—1165 (1948).

— Beryllium granulomas of the skin. Arch. Dermat. Syph. 60, 1140—1147 (1949).

— Experimental beryllium granulome of the skin. Arch. industr. Hyg. 3, 81—89 (1951).

— Pulmonary and cutaneous diseases caused by beryllium compounds. Postgrad. Med. 11, 383—386 (1952).

—, J. CHOLAK, and D. M. HUBBARD: Value of beryllium determinations in diagnosis of berylliosis. Amer. J. Clin. Path. 19, 229—232 (1949).

— —, D. M. HUBBARD, and J. L. ROTH: Persistence of beryllium oxide in lungs after inhalation of dust. Arch. industr. Hyg. 4, 65—73 (1951).

—, and E. J. LARGENT: Osteosarcoma induced by beryllium oxide. Amer. J. Path. 26, 197—209 (1950).

— —, and J. I. ROTH: Osteogenic sarcoma after inhalation of beryllium oxide. Arch. industr. Hyg. 4, 606 (1951).

— —, and J. L. ROTH: Osteogenic sarcoma after inhalation of beryllium oxide. Arch. Path. 51, 473—478 (1951).

EISENBUD, M., C. F. BERGOUT, and L. T. STEADMAN: Environmental studies in plant and laboratories using beryllium. The acute disease. J. industr. Hyg. 30, 281—285 (1948).

—, R. C. WANTA, C. DUSTAN, W. B. HARRIS, and B. S. WOLF: Non-occupational berylliosis. J. industr. Hyg. 31, 282—294 (1949).

FENN, G. K.: Chronic beryllium poisoning of long duration from fluorescent lamp manufacturing. Arch. industr. Hyg. 3, 571—574 (1951).

GARDNER, L. U.: Osteo-sarcoma from intravenous beryllium compounds in rabbits. Fed. Proc. 5, 221 (1946).

GRIER, R. S., P. NASH, and D. G. FREIMAN: Skin lesions in persons exposed to beryllium compounds. J. industr. Hyg. 30, 228—237 (1948).

HARDY, H. L.: The toxicity of beryllium. Lancet 261, 448 (1951).

— Case of chronic beryllium poisoning from atomic energy development. Arch. industr. Hyg. 3, 547—548 (1951).

— Beryllium disease: A continuing diagnostic problem. Amer. J. Med. Ski. 242, 150—158 (1961).

— Reaction to toxic beryllium compounds: Terminology. J. occup. Med. 53, 2—534 (1962).

— Beryllium case registry progress report: 1962. Arch. environm. Hlth 5, 265—268 (1962).

HELWIG, E. B.: Chemical (beryllium) granulomas of skin. Milit. Surg. 109, 540—544 (1952).

HEUSTIS, A. E.: Beryllium and its alloys. Mich. occup. Hlth 8, No. 4, 4. (1936).

HOAGLAND, M. B., R. S. GRIER, and M. B. HOOD: Beryllium and growth. I. Beryllium-induced osteogenic sarcomata. Cancer Res. 10, 629—635 (1950).

HUEPER, W. C.: A quest into the environmental causes of cancer of the lung. Publ. Health Monograph No. 36, U. S. Public Health Service Publ. 452, 1955, pp. 54.
— Methodologic explorations in experimental respiratory carcinogenesis. Arzneimittel-Forsch. 14, 814—822 (1964).
KAHLAU, G.: Der Lungenkrebs. Ergebn. allg. Path. Anat. 37, 258—419 (1954).
KLEMPERER, F. W., A. P. MARTIN, and J. VAN RIPER: Beryllium excretion in humans. Arch. industr. Hyg. 4, 251—256 (1951).
LEDERER, H., and J. SAVAGE: Beryllium granuloma of the skin. Brit. J. industr. Med. 11, 45—48 (1954).
LIEBEN, J., and Fr. METZNER: Epidemiological findings associated with beryllium extraction. Amer. industr. Hyg. Ass. J. 20, 494—499 (1959).
—, J. A. DATTOLI, and V. M. VOUGHT: Quantitative beryllium studies in postmortem lungs. Arch. environm. Hlth 7, 183—187 (1963).
LINDEKEN, C. L., and O. L. MEADORS: The control of beryllium hazards. Amer. industr. Hyg. Ass. J. 21, 245—251 (1960).
LISCO, H.: Discussion remark, proc. 9. international congress on industrial medicine 2, 614 (1948).
MACHLE, W.: Discussion. Symposium on industrial diseases. Radiology 50, 785 (1948).
—, E. C. BEYER, and H. TEDBROOK: Acute pneumonitis of beryllium workers and pulmonary granulomatosis of beryllium workers. Proc. 9th Internat. Congress Industrial Medicine, London, 1948, p. 615—629.
METZNER, Fr. N., and J. LIEBEN: Respiratory disease associated with beryllium refining and alloy fabrication. J. occup. Med. 3, 341—345 (1961).
Mineral Year Books. U. S. Bureau of Mines, Washington, D. C., 1947, p. 813.
MITCHELL, R. N., and E. C. HYAT: Beryllium. Amer. industr. Hyg. Ass. J. 18, 207—213 (1957).
MORGIS, G. G., and J. J. FORBES: Review of literature on health hazards of beryllium and its compounds. Bureau of Mines Information Circular 7574, 1950, p. 23.
NASH, P.: Experimental production of malignant tumors by beryllium. Lancet 1, 519 (1950).
—, R. S. GRIER, and D. G. FREIMAN: Granulomatous skin lesions produced by beryllium compounds. Proc. 9th Internat. Congress Industrial Medicine, London, 1948, p. 366—369.
NIEMÖLLER, H. K.: Spätcarcinome durch Berylliumaerosole beim Menschen. Int. Arch. Gewerbepath. 20, 180—186 (1963).
PASCUCCI, L. M.: Pulmonary disease in workers exposed to beryllium compounds: Its roentgen characteristics. Radiology 50, 23—30 (1948).
PERRY, K. M. A.: Pulmonary disease in relation to metallic oxide. Lancet 2, 463—468 (1955).
PRICE, C. H. G.: Experimental osteogenic sarcoma. 29th Ann. Rep. Brit. Emp. Cancer Camp. for the Year 1951, p. 219—221.
REEVES, A. L. A., and A. J. VORWALD: The humoral transport of beryllium. J. occup. Med. 3, 567—574 (1961).
REYNOLDS, P. W.: Beryllium disease from the ceramic industry. Arch. industr. Hyg. 3, 575—578 (1951).
RIZZUTI, A. B.: Beryllium granulomas of the anterior ocular structures. N. Y. J. Med. 51, 1065—1067 (1951).
SANDERS, O. A.: Chronic berylliosis in the neon sign industry. Arch. industr. Hyg. 3, 565—568 (1951).
SCHEPERS, G. W. H.: Recent observations on chronic pulmonary beryllium disease. Trans. 20th Ann. Meeting Industrial Hygiene Foundation, 1955, pp. 18. Pittsburgh: Mellon Institute.
— Neoplasia experimentally induced by beryllium compounds. Progr. exp. Tumor Res. (Basel) 2, 203—244 (1961).
— Chronic Berylliosis. Arch. Gewerbepath. 19, 1—26 (1962).
— Biological action of beryllium. Reaction of the monkeys to inhaled aerosols. Industr. Med. Surg. 33, 1—16 (1964).
—, Th. M. DURKAN, A. B. DELANANT, and Fr. T. CREEDON: The biological action of inhaled Beryllium Sulfate. Arch. industr. Hlth 15, 32—58 (1957).
SILSON, J. E., L. P. BENJAMIN, and S. C. WILSON: The use of beryllium in New York State. New York State Department of Labor Monthly Review. 28, No. 4, 13—16 (1949).

SISSONS, H. A.: Bone sarcomas produced experimentally in the rabbit, using compounds of Beryllium. Proc. 5th Congres Internat. Cancer, Paris, 1950, p. 50, Acta Un. int. Cancr. 7, 171—172 (1950).

STERNER, J. H., and M. EISENBUD: Epidemiology of beryllium intoxication. Arch. industr. Hyg. 4, 123—151 (1951).

TEPPER, L. B., H. L. HARDY, and R. I. CHAMBERLIN: Toxicity of beryllium compounds. Elsevier Monographs, 1961, pp. 190.

TIETZ, N. W., E. F. HIRSCH, and B. NEYMAN: Sppectrographic study of trace elements in cancerous and noncancerous human tissues. J. Amer. med. Ass. 165, 2187—2192 (1957).

VAN ORDSTRAND, H. S.: Berylliosis. Arch. industr. Hyg. 10, 232—234 (1955).

VIGLIANI, E. C.: Health hazards in a beryllium fabricating plant. Proc. 9th Interna. Congress Industrial Medicine, London, 1948, pp. 645—649.

VORWALD, A. J., and A. L. REEVES: Inhaled atmospheric pollutants in the genesis of lung cancer. Acta Un. int. Cancr. 15, 715—722 (1959).

WALKLEY, J.: A study of the Morin method for the determination of beryllium air samples. Amer. industr. Hyg. Ass. J. 20, 241—244 (1959).

WILLIAMS, W. J.: A histological study of the lungs in 52 cases of chronic beryllium disease. Brit. J. industr. Med. 15, 84—91 (1958).

WILSON, S. A.: Delayed chemical pneumonitis or diffuse granulomatosis of the lung due to beryllium. Radiology 50, 770—779 (1948).

YAMAGUCHI, S.: Study of beryllium-induced osteogenic sarcoma. Nagasaki Iggakai Zasshi 38, 127—138 (1963).

Mustard Gas

AXELROD, D. J., and J. G. HAMILTON: Radio-autographic studies of the distribution of lewisite and mustard gas in the skin and eye tissue. Amer. J. Path. 23, 389—411 (1947).

BAADER, E. W.: Berufskrankheiten. 5. Aufl. München: Urban & Schwarzenberg 1960.

BEEBE, G. B.: Lung cancer in World War I veterans: possible relation to mustard-gas injury and 1918 influenza epidemic. J. nat. Cancer Inst. 25, 1231—1252 (1960).

BOYLAND, E.: Biochemical reactions of chemical warfare agents. Nature 161, 225 (1948).

—, and E. S. HORNING: Induction of tumours with nitrogen mustard. Brit. J. Cancer 3, 118—123 (1949).

BRANDT, E. L., and A. C. GRIFFIN: Reduction of toxicity of nitrogen mustards by cysteine. Cancer 4, 1030—1035 (1951).

BROCK, N.: Zur pharmakologischen Charakterisierung zyklischer N-Lost-Phosphamidester als Krebs-Chemotherapeutika. Arzneimittel-Forsch. 8, 1—9 (1958).

BROCKBANK, W.: Occupational incidence of primary lung cancer. Quart. J. Med. 1, 31—40 (1932).

CASE, R. A. M., and A. J. LEA: Mustard gas poisoning, chronic bronchitis, and lung cancer. Brit. J. prev. soc. Med. 9, 62—72 (1955).

Department of health, education and welfare: Effects of chemical warfare agents. July, 1955, p. 17.

DERISCHANOFF, J. M.: Zur Statistik und Genese des Lungenkrebses. Z. Krebsforsch. 35, 481—491 (1932).

FUJITO, T.: Studies of Danis' test and indican in gas poisoning patients. Med. J. mutual Aid Ass. 12, 155—156 (1963).

GILMAN, A.: Therapeutic applications of chemical warfare agents. Fed. Proc. 5, 285—292 (1946).

—, and Fr. S. PHILIPS: The biological actions and therapeutic applications of b-chloroethyl amines and sulfides. Science 103, 409—416 (1946).

GRAEF, E., D. KARNOFSKY, V. B. JAGER, B. KRICHESKY, and H. W. SMITH: The clinical and pathologic effects of the nitrogen and sulfur mustards in laboratory animals. Amer. J. Path. 24, 1—47 (1948).

GRIFFIN, A. C., E. L. BRANDT, and E. L. TATUM: Nitrogen mustards as cancer inducing agents. J. Amer. med. Ass. 144, 571 (1950).

HADDOW, A., and G. M. TIMMIS: Bifunctional sulphonic acid esters with radiomimetic activity. Acta Un. int. Cancr. 7, 469—471 (1951).

HESTON, W. E.: Induction of pulmonary tumors in strain a mice with methyl-bis(beta-chloro-ethyl)amine hydrochloride. J. nat. Cancer Inst. 10, 125—130 (1949).
— Carcinogenic action of the mustards. J. nat. Cancer Inst. 11, 415—423 (1950).
— Occurrence of tumors in mice injected subcutaneously with sulfur mustard and nitrogen mustard. J. nat. Cancer Inst. 13, 131—140 (1954).
HUEPER, W. C.: A quest into the environmental causes of cancer of the lung. Publ. Health Monograph No. 36, U. S. Public Health Service Publ. No. 452, Washington, 1955, p. 54.
— Berufskrebse. Handbuch der gesamten Arbeitsmedizin. Bd. 2. Hrsg. E. W. Baader. München: Urban & Schwarzenberg. 1961.
HÜNERMANN, T.: Kehlkropfkrebs nach Gelbkreuzvergiftung. Z. Laryng. 17, 369—376 (1929).
KARNOFSKY, D. A., I. GRAEF, and H. W. SMITH: Studies on the mechanism of action of the nitrogen and sulfur mustards in vivo. Amer. J. Path. 24, 275—291 (1948).
KELLNER, B., and L. NEMETH: Biological effect of 1:6-dimethane-sulfonyl-D-mannitol in animal experiments. Brit. J. Cancer 13, 469—476 (1959).
KIKUTH, W.: Über das Lungencarcinom. Virchows Arch. path. Anat. 255, 107—128 (1925).
KINDRED, J. E.: The blood cells and the hematopoietic and other organs of dogs given intravenous injections of 2-chloroethyl vesicants. Arch. Path. 47, 378—398 (1949).
— Histologic changes occurring in the hematopoietic organs of albino rats after single injections of 2-chloroethyl vesicants. Arch. Path. 43, 253—295 (1947).
KLOTZ, M. O.: Association of silicosis and carcinoma of the lung. Amer. J. Cancer 35, 38—49 (1939).
KOELSCH, E.: Lungenkrebs und Beruf. Acta Un. int. Cancr. 3, 243—251 (1958).
LINDQUIST, P. A.: Chemical and biological warfare. J. Amer. med. Ass. 169, 356—358 (1959).
MACKLIN, M.: Has a real increase in lung cancer been proved? Ann. int. Med. 17, 308—324 (1942).
MACY, R., G. N. JARMAN, A. MORRISON, and E. E. REID: The polysulfides in Levinstein process Mustard Gas. Science 355—359 (1947).
MATZ, P. B.: Incidence of primary bronchiogenic carcinoma. J. Amer. med. Ass. 111, 2086—2092 (1938).
MONGELI, N. S.: Infortunio colletivo da solfure di etile boclorurato un gruppo di pescatori. Rass. Med. industr. 29, 441—454 (1960).
OSBORNE, E. D., J. W. JORDON, Fr. C. HOAK, and Fr. J. PSCHIERER: Nitrogen mustard therapy in cutaneous blastomatous disease. J. Amer. med. Ass. 135, 1123—1128 (1947).
PHILPOTT, O. S., A. R. WOODBURNE, and G. A. WALDNIFF: Nitrogen mustard in the treatment of mycosis fungoides. J. Amer. med. Ass. 135, 631—633 (1947).
RHOADS, C. P.: Nitrogen mustards in the treatment of neoplastic disease. J. Amer. med. Ass. 131, 656—658 (1946).
ROCHE, L., E. GRUNWALD, et J. ROUANET: Emphysème professionnel dû l'yperite. Arch. Mal. prof. 18, 339—342 (1957).
ROGERS, St.: The in vitro initiation of pulmonary adenomas in mouse lung tissue with nitrogen mustard. J. nat. Cancer Inst. 15, 1379—1390 (1955).
SARTORELLI, E., M. GIUBILEO, e E. BARTALINI: Contributo allo studio della bronchite cronico asmatiforme con enfysema polmonare quale po stumo di intossicazione professionale da iprete. Med. d. Lavoro 48, 336—346 (1957).
SHULLENBERGER, C. C., C. H. WATKINS, and R. R. KIERLAND: Experience with nitrogen mustard therapy. J. Amer. med. Ass. 139, 773—777 (1949).
SPAMER, E.: Ein Fall von Primärkarzinom der Epiglottis bei Vergiftung durch französisches Kampfgas. Z. Laryngol. 10, 44—60 (1921).
SPITZ, S.: The histological effects of nitrogen mustards on human tumors and tissues. Cancer 1, 383—398 (1958).
TILLEY, cited by F. LICKINT: Ätiologie und Prophylaxe des Lungenkrebses. Dresden: Steinkopff 1952.
URAM, H., B. FISHER, and E. R. FISHER: The hepatotoxic effect of nitrogen mustard after direct intraportal injection. Cancer 8, 144—147 (1956).
VISSER, J., and R. E. J. TEN SELDAM: Over de „carcinogene" en anticarcinogene eigenschappen von verschillende huidirritantia. Geneesk. T. Nederland. Indie. 78, 3280—3291 (1938).

WADA, S., A. YAMADA, Y. NISHIMOTO, S. TOKUOKA, M. MIYANISHI, S. KATSUTA, and H. UMISA: Neoplasmus of the respiratory tract among poison gas workers. J. Hiroshima med. Ass. 16, 728—745 (1963).

WINTROBE, M. M., and C. M. HUGULEY: Nitrogen-mustard therapy for Hodgkin's disease, lymphosarcoma, the leukemias, and other disorders. Cancer 1, 357—382 (1948).

WOLFSON, S, and M. B. OLNEY: Accidental ingestion of a toxic dose of chlorambucil. J. Amer. med. Ass. 165, 239—240 (1957).

YAMADA, A.: Patho-anatomical studies on respiratory cancers developed in workers with occupational exposure to mustard gas. J. Hiroshima med. Ass. 7, 719—761 (1959).

— On the late injuries following occupational inhalation of mustard gas, with special references to carcinoma of the respiratory tract. Acta path. jap. 13, 131—155 (1963).

—, F. HIROSE, and M. MIYANISHI: An autopsy case of bronchial carcinoma found in a patient succumbed to occupational mustard gas poisoning. Gann 44, 216—218 (1953).

— —, M. NAGAI, and T. NAKAMURA: Five cases of cancer of the larynx found in persons who suffered from occupational mustard gas poisoning. Gann 48, 366—368 (1957).

—, M. NAGAI, M. KAMIMATSUNE, Y. NAKAHARA, and I. HORINO: A case of cancer of the pharynx developed in a worker suffering from occupational mustard gas and lewisite poisoning. J. Hiroshima med. Ass. 8, 1107—1112 (1960).

—, Y. NISHIMOTO, S. TOKUOKA, M. MIYANISHI, S. KATSUTA, and H. UMISA: Neoplasmus of the respiratory tract among poison gas workers. J. Hiroshima med. Ass. 16, 728—745 (1963).

—, A. OSHITA, and K. TABA: A case of occupational mustard gas cancer of the larynx. J. Hiroshima med. Ass. 7, 2711—2715 (1959).

YOKORO, K., I. OHARA, et al.: Two cases of mustard gas cancer of the respiratory tract. Gann. 49 (Suppl.), 351—352 (1948).

Isopropyl Oil

BAADER, E. W.: Die Gefahr des Berufskrebses bei der Isopropylalkoholfabrikation. Zbl. Arbeitsmed. 1, 90 (1951).

DOLL, R.: Occupational lung cancer: A review. Brit. J. industr. Med. 16, 181—190 (1959).

ECKARDT, R. R.: Industrial carcinogens. New York: Grune & Stratton 1959.

ECKARDT, R. E., N. V. HENDRICKS, and C. BERRY: Epidemiological study of potential cancer problem in an alcohol plant. Unpublished information received from Dr. J. P. Holt (1949).

FOWLER, P. B. S.: Printers' asthma. Lancet 1, 755 (1952).

HUEPER, W. C.: Occurrence of cancers of the respiratory system among workers of an isopropanol operations. Unpublished report (1946).

— A quest into the environmental causes of cancer of the lung. Publ. Health Monograph No. 36. PHS Publ. No. 452. USGPO, Washington, D. C., 1955, pp. 54.

KEESER, E.: Über den Isopropylalkohol und seine gewerbetoxikologische Beurteilung. Zbl. Arbeitsmed. 1, 25—26 (1951).

— Entgegnung zu den vorstehenden Ausführungen über die Gefahr des Berufskrebses bei der Isopropylalkoholfabrikation. Zbl. Arbeitsmed. 1, 90—91 (1951).

LEHMAN, A. J., and H. F. CHASE: The acute and chronic toxicity of isopropyl alcohol. J. Lab. clin. Med. 29, 561—567 (1944).

WEIL, C. S., H. F. SMYTH, and Th. W. NALE: Quest for a suspected industrial carcinogen. Arch. industr. Hyg. 5, 535—547 (1952).

Coal Tar, Tar Oils, Soot, and Other Combustion Products of Coal

ASK-UPMARK, E.: Bronchial carcinoma in printing workers. Dis. Chest 27, 427—435 (1955).

BINI, G.: Su di un case tumore polmonare di sospetta origine professionale. Ateneo parmense 28, 37—52 (1957).

BLAHA, K.: Pachydermia of the larynx in relation to certain noxious industrial substances. Acta Univ. Carol. Med. (Praha) 10, 248—254 (1960).

BLÜMLEIN, H.: Kehlkopfkrebs und berufliche Inhalationsnoxen. Münch. med. Wschr. 99, 1333—1335 (1957).

BONNET, J.: Quantitative analysis of benzo(a)pyrene in vapors coming from melted Tar. NCI Monogr. 9, 221—223 (1962).

BRESLOW, L.: Occupational factors in lung cancer. A Preliminary Report. Publ. Hlth Rep. 68, 286—288 (1953).

—, L. HOAGLIN, G. RASMUSSEN, and H. K. ABRAMS: Occupations and cigarette smoking as factors in lung cancer. Amer. J. Publ. Hlth 44, 171—181 (1954).

BRUUSGAARD, A.: Occurrence of certain forms of cancer in gasworkers. T. norsk Laegeforen 79, 755—756 (1959).

BUELL, P., J. E. DUNN, Jr., and L. BRESLOW: The occupational-social class risks of cancer mortality in Men. J. chron. Dis. 12, 600—621 (1960).

CAMPBELL, J. A.: Note on the experimental production of cancer by dust obtained from tarred roads. Lancet 1, 233 (1934).

— Cancer of the skin and increase in incidence of primary tumors of lung in mice exposed to dust obtained from tarred road. Brit. J. exp. Path. 15, 287—294 (1934).

— Lung tumors in mice and man. Brit. med. J. 1, 179—183 (1943).

COHART, E. M.: Socioeconomic distribution of cancer of the lung in New Haven. Cancer 8, 1126—1129 (1955).

CURWEN, M. P., E. L. KENNAWAY, and N. M. KENNAWAY: Cancer of the lung and larynx in town and country. Acta Un. int. Cancr. 10, 104—109 (1954).

DIKUN, P. P., L. M. SHABAD, and V. L. NORKIN: Pollution of the atmosphere of industrial towns by 3:4-benzpyrene. Gigiena 1, 6—11 (1956).

DOIG, A. T.: Dust diseases, excluding fibrotic pneumoconiosis. In E. R. A. Merewether: Industrial medicine and hygiene. Vol. III. London: Butterworth & Co. 1956.

DOLL, R.: The causes of death among gas-workers with special reference to cancer of the lung. Brit. J. industr. Med. 9, 180—185 (1952).

— Occuppational lung cancer: A review. Brit. J. industr. Med. 16, 181—190 (1959).

EPSTEIN, A. A.: Zur Frage des professionellen Krebses der Hände. Zbl. Gewerbehyg. 17, 256—263 (1930).

— Zur Frage des Berufskrebses der Hände. Zbl. Haut- u. Geschl.-Kr. 37, 373 (1931).

FALK, H. L., P. KOTIN, and A. MEHLER: The carcinogenicity of certain polycyclic aromatic hydrocarbons for man. Arch. environm. Hlth 8, 721 (1964).

—, and P. E. STEINER: The identification of aromatic polycyclic hydrocarbons in carbon blacks. Cancer Res. 12, 30—39 (1952).

— — The adsorption of 3, 4-benzpyrene and pyrene by carbon blacks. Cancer Res. 12, 40—43 (1952).

FISCHER-WASELS, B.: Die Ursachen des primären Lungencarcinoms. Frankf. Z. Path. 49, 145 (1936).

FISHER, R. E. W.: Occupational skin cancer in tar workers. Arch. industr. Hyg. 7, 12—18 (1953).

GÄRTNER, H., and F. W. BRAUSS: Untersuchungen zur Frage der Rußlunge und zur Schädlichkeit des reinen Kohlenstaubanteiles im Staub der Kohlenbergwerke. Med. Welt. 20, 235—268 (1951).

GARSCHIN, W. G., and J. A. PIGALEW: Experimentelle Untersuchungen über atypische Epithelwucherungen. Atypische Epithelwucherungen in den Lungen bei Entzündungen, die durch intrapulmonale Steinkohlenteerinjektionen hervorgerufen werden. Z. Krebsforsch. 33, 631—653 (1931).

GORHAM, E.: On the correlation of lung cancer with tar in air pollution. Med. Offr 101, 178 (1959).

GORSKI, T.: Experimental investigations on the carcinogenic properties of some pitches and tars produced from Silesian pit coal. Med. Pracy 10, 309—317 (1959).

GRAHAM, S., M. LEVIN, and A. M. LILIENFELD: The socioeconomic distribution of cancer of various sites in Buffalo, N. Y., 1948—1952. Cancer 13, 180—191 (1960).

GRIFFITH, G. W.: Atmospheric pollution and lung cancer. In R. W. RAVEN (Ed.): Cancer, Progr. Vol. London: Butterworth 1963.

GRUSHKO, Y. M., P. P. DIKUN, L. M. SHABAD, T. I. RUKAVISHNIKOVA, L. M. ZAK, and O. M. VLASENKO: Comparative investigations of air pollution with a cancerogenic substance (3:4-benzpyrene) in Irkutsk and Angarsk. Gig. i Sanit. 4, 7—10 (1958).

HAENSZEL, W.: Cancer mortality among the foreign-born in the United States. J. nat. Cancer Inst. 26, 37—132 (1961).

HARDING, H. E.: Carcinogenic potency of carbon black. 30th Ann. Rep., Brit. Emp. Cancer Campaign, 1952, pp. 202—203.

HELLER, I.: Occupational cancers. J. industr. Hyg. 12, 169—197 (1930).

HENRY, S. A.: Occupational cutaneous cancer attributable to certain chemicals in industry. Brit. med. Bull. 4, 387—401 (1947).

HEUSTIS, A. E.: How to keep a foundry clean: Part II. Mich. occup. Hlth 9, 1—8 (1964).

HUEPER, W. C.: Occupational tumors and allied diseases. Springfield, Ill.: C. C. Thomas 1942.

— Experimental studies on cancerigenesis of synthetic liquid fuels and petroleum substitutes. I. American shale oils. II. Bergius oils. III. Fischer-Tropsch oils. Arch. industr. Hyg. 8, 307—327 (1953).

— Recent developments in environmental cancer. A review. Arch. Path. 58, 360—399; 475—523; 645—682 (1954).

— A quest into the environmental causes of cancer of the lung. Publ. Health Monogr. No. 36, DHEW, PHS Publn. No. 452, Washington, D. C., USGPO, 1955, pp. 54.

— Experimental carcinogenic studies on hydrogenated coal oils. II. Fischer Tropsch oils. Industr. Med. Surg. 25, 459—463 (1956).

— Experimental carcinogenic studies on hydrogenated coal oils. I. Bergius oils. Industr. Med. Surg. 25, 51—55 (1956).

— Environmental factors in the production of human cancer. In Vol. I. Raven, R. W. (Ed): Cancer. London: Butterworth 1957.

— Environmental cancer of the lung. Acta Un. int. Cancr. 13, 97—140 (1957).

— Role of occupational and environmental air pollutants in production of respiratory cancers. Arch. Path. 63, 427—450 (1957).

— Berufskrebse. Handbuch für die gesamte Arbeitsmedizin. Vol. 2. Baader, E. W. (Ed.). München: Urban & Schwarzenberg, 1961.

— Chemically induced skin cancers in man. Nat. Cancer Inst. Monogr. 10, 377—391 (1963).

— Directions and directives of occupational cancer research. Acta Un. int. Cancr. 19, 461—464 (1963).

— Methodologic explorations in experimental respiratory carcinogenesis. Arzneimittel-Forsch. 14, 814—822 (1964).

— Unpublished medicolegal evidence.

—, and W. D. CONWAY: Chemical carcinogenesis and cancers. Springfield, Ill.: C. C. Thomas 1965.

—, P. KOTIN, E. C. TABOR, W. W. PAYNE, H. FALK, and E. SAWICKI: Carcinogenic bioassays on air pollutants. Arch. Path. 74, 89—116 (1962).

—, and M. KURATSUNE: Polycyclic aromatic hydrocarbons in coffee soots. J. nat. Cancer Inst. 20, 37—51 (1958).

— — Polycyclic aromatic hydrocarbons in roasted coffee. J. nat. Cancer Inst. 24, 463—469 (1960).

—, and W. W. PAYNE: Carcinogenic studies on soot of coffee roasting plants. Arch. Path. 69, 716—727 (1960).

— — Carcinogenic studies on petroleum asphalt, cooling oil, and coal tar. Arch. Path. 70, 372—384 (1960).

HUSTED, E., and G. BILLMANN: Primary cancer of lung. Hospitalstidende 79, 325 (1935).

INGALLS, T. H.: Incidence of cancer in the carbon black industry. Arch. industr. Hyg. 1, 662—676 (1950).

—, and R. RISQUEZ-IRABBAREN: Periodic search for cancer in the carbon black industry. Arch. environm. Hlth 2, 429—433 (1961).

KAWAHATA, K.: Über die berufliche Entstehung des Lungenkrebses bei der Generatorgas-Fabrikation. Gann 30, 341—344 (1936).

— Über die gewerblich hervorgerufenen Lungenkrebse bei Generator-Gas-Arbeitern in den Stahlwerken. Gann 32, 367—388 (1938).

KAWAI, M., T. MATSUYAMA, and H. AMAMOTO: A study on occupational lung cancer of the gas producer workers in Yawata Iron & Steel Works. J. Labour Hyg. in Iron & Steel Industry 10, 5—9 (1961).

KENNAWAY, E. L.: The anatomical distribution of the occupational cancers. J. industr. Hyg. 7, 69—93 (1925).

KENNAWAY, N. M., and E. L. KENNAWAY: A study of the incidence of cancer of the lung and larynx. J. Hyg. 36, 236 (1936).

KIMINA, S. N.: Cancerogenic substances in the atmosphere and the incidence and mortality of lung cancer in the vicinity of aluminium mills. Abstr. 8th internat. Cancer Congr. Moscow, 1962, p. 183.

KIMURA, N.: Artificial production of a cancer in the lungs following the intrabronchial insufflation of coal tar. Jap. med. Wld 3, 45 (1923); Gann 17, 15 (1923).

KOELSCH, Fr.: Arch. Gewerbepath. 5, 454 (1934).

KOLOMAZNIK, L., J. ZDRAZIL, and F. PICHA: Incidence of benign neoplasms and precancerous and cancerous conditions in the respiratory passages of foundry workers laboring in an athmosphere with a high content of 3,4-benzpyrene. Cesk. Otolaryng. 12, 1—11 (1963).

KOTIN, P.: The role of atmospheric pollution in the pathogenesis of pulmonary cancer: A review. Cancer Res. 16, 375—393 (1956).

KURODA, S., and K. KAWAHATA: Z. Krebsforsch. 45, 36 (1936).

— — Clinical study of primary pulmonary cancer in workers of steel factory. Jap. J. med. Sc. VIII, Int. Med., Pediat. Psychiat. 5, 41—43 (1938).

Lancet: 1927, Mar. 12, 582. Cancer. Tar Cause Pulmonary Cancer.

LEITER, J., M. B. SHIMKIN, and M. J. SHEAR: Production of subcutaneous sarcomas in mice with tars extracted from atmospheric dusts. J. nat. Cancer Inst. 3, 155—165 (1942).

LINK, K.: Ein Fall von Teerkrebs des Fingers (und des Magens?) bei einem Feuermann eines Gaswerks. Zbl. allg. Path. path. Anat. 99, 556—572 (1959).

LISTER, W. B.: Carbon pneumoconiosis in a synthetic graphite worker. Brit. J. industr. Med. 18, 114—116 (1961).

LOCKHART, R.: Investigation of warts prevalent among workers in reduction works of aluminium industry. Brit. J. industr. Med. 11, 296—300 (1954).

MAISEL, B., C. PEARCE, J. CONNOLLY, and J. PEARCE: Carbon-black carcinoma of Stensen's duct. Arch. Surg. 78, 331—339 (1959).

MALY, E., and E. MADER: The contamination of the atmosphere with tar-like substances during the electrolytic production of aluminium. Pracov. Lék. 11, 367—368 (1959).

MANCUSO, T. E., and E. J. COULTER: Methodology in industrial health studies. Arch. environm. Hlth 6, 515—524 (1963).

—, E. MACFARLANE, and J. D. PORTERFIELD: The distribution of cancer mortality in Ohio. Amer. J. publ. Hlth 45, 58—70 (1955).

MCLAUGHLIN, A. I. G.: Health risks of the various foundry occupations. Chap. IX. Industrial lung diseases of iron and Steel Foundry workers. Ministry of Labour & National Service, London: H. M. Stat. Off. 1950.

—, W. B. LAWRIE, and H. WOODS: Foundry processes. Chap. II. Industrial lung diseases of iron and steel foundry workers. Ministry of Labour & National Service, London: H. M. Stat. 1950.

MENZ, M.: Über Berufsschädigungen bei Gaswerkarbeitern inbesondere der Gaskokerei Kleinhüningen. Schweiz. med. Wschr. 77, 895—899 (1947).

MESTITZOVA, M.: Experimental study on the chronic exposure of inbred mice to tar vapours. Pracov. Lék. 13, 55—62 (1961).

—, and P. KOSSEY: Experimental contribution to the problem of the genesis of lung cancer. Neoplasma (Bratisl.) 8, 27—39 (1961).

MILLER, A. A., and F. RAMSDEN: Carbon pneumoconiosis. Brit. J. industr. Med. 18, 103—113 (1961).

MILLS, C. A.: Occupation as a factor in the community health hazards of air pollution. Amer. J. med. Sci. 226, 177—178 (1953).

MÖLLER, P.: Primärer Lungenkrebs bei mit Teer gepinselten Ratten. Acta path. microbiol. scand. 1, 412—437 (1924).

MORRISON, S. L.: Occupational mortality in Scotland. Brit. J. industr. Med. 14, 130—132 (1957).

MÜLLSCHITZKY, A.: Bronchial carcinoma in tar worker with skin cancer; case. Dermat. Wschr. 109, 973—975 (1939).

MURPHY, J. B., and E. STURM: Primary lung tumors in mice following the cutaneous applications of coal tar. J. exp. Med. 42, 693 (1925).

NAU, C. A., J. NEAL, and V. STEMBRIDGE: A study of the physiological effects of carbon black. I. Ingestion. Arch. industr. Hlth 17, 21—28 (1958).

— — — A study of the physiological effects of carbon black. II. Skin contract. Arch. industr. Hlth 18, 511—520 (1958).

— — — A study of the physiological effects of carbon black. III. Adsorption and elution potentials; subcutaneous injections. Arch. environm. Hlth 1, 512—533 (1960).

— — —, and R. N. COOLEY: Physiological effects of carbon black. IV. Inhalation. Arch. environm. Hlth 4, 415—531 (1962).

NEAL, J., M. THORNTON, and C. A. NAU: Polycyclic hydrocarbon elution from carbon black or rubber products. Arch. environm. Hlth 4, 598—606 (1962).

OPPENHEIMER, M.: Ein noch nicht beschriebenes berufliches Kennzeichen an der Haut der Schuhmacher. Arch. Dermat. Syph. 147, 359—361 (1924).

OSHIMA, T., K. TAKEMOTO, and K. NAMIE: Experimental study on carcinogenicity of hydrocarbons in pulmonary carcinoma. Nippon Eiseigaku Zasshi (Jap. J. Hyg.) 18, 142 (1963).

PASSEY, R. D.: Experimental soot cancers. Brit. med. J. 2, 1112—1113 (1922).

PATCH, I. L.: Pitch and pulmonary carcinoma. Brit. J. Tuberc. 47, 145—150 (1953).

PEACOCK, P. R.: An aetiological study of lung tumours in mice. In Severi, L. (Ed.): The morphological precursors of cancer. Perugia: Div. Cancer Res. 1962.

POCHE, R., O. MITTMANN, and O. KNELLER: Statistische Untersuchungen über das Bronchialcarcinom in Nordrhein-Westfalen. Z. Krebsforsch. 66, 87—108 (1964).

REID, D. D., and C. BUCK: Cancer in coking plant workers. Brit. J. industr. Med. 13, 265—269 (1956).

ROESCH, H.: Drei verschiedene Carcinome bei einem Paraffinarbeiter. Virchows Arch. path. Anat. 245, 1 (1923) (cited by Patch).

SAMSSONOW, M.: Über den experimentellen Lungenkrebs. Z. Krebsforsch. 49, 525—559 (1939/40).

SARUTA, N., S. YAMAGUCHI, N. TSUTSUMI, and Y. KODAMA: Effects of air pollution on the health of people of Northern Kyushu. Japan. first report. Kyushu J. med. Sci. 12, 167—176 (1961).

SAWICKI, E., F. T. FOK, W. ELBERT, T. R. HAUSER, and J. MEEKER: Polynuclear aromatic hydrocarbon composition of air polluted by coal tar pitch fumes. Amer. industr. Hyg. Ass. J. 23, 482—486 (1962).

SCHABAD, L. M.: Les tumeurs primitives du poumon chez les souris badigeonnées au goudron. C. R. Soc. Biol. 99, 1497 (1928).

— Studien über primäre Lungengeschwülste bei Mäusen und ihr Verhalten bei Steinkohlenteer als cancerogenem Faktor. Z. Krebsforsch. 30, 24—59 (1929).

— Experimentelle atypische Epithelialwucherungen nach intratracheobronchialer Einführung des Steinkohlenteers in die Lungen. Z. Krebsforsch. 38, 154 (1932).

— Quelques données expérimentales sur les tumeurs du poumon. Acta int. Cancer (Paris) 3, 189—196 (1938).

SCHNURER, L., and S. R. HAYTHORNE: The effects of coal smoke of known composition on rabbits lungs. Amer. J. Path. 13, 676 (1937).

SEELIG, M. G., and E. L. BENIGNUS: Coal smoke soot and tumors of the lung in mice. Amer. J. Cancer 28, 96—111 (1936).

— — The production of experimental cancer of the lung in mice. Amer. J. Cancer 33, 549—554 (1938).

— — Lung tumor revelopment in a resistant strain of mice subjected to inhalation of soot. Amer. J. Cancer 34, 391—398 (1938).

SHABAD, L. M.: Some aspects of lung cancer aetiology and pathogenesis. Vop. Onkol. 3, 387—393 (1957).

— Experimental cancer of the lung. J. nat. Cancer Inst. 28, 1305—1332 (1962).

SIMONDS, J. P., and J. S. CURTIS: Lesions induced in the lungs by the intravenous injection of tar. Arch. Path. 19, 287 (1935).

STEINBRUCK, C., und CARL: Künstliche Krebserzeugung durch Druckerschwärze. Berl. tierärztl. Wschr. 45, 525 (1929).

STEINER, P. E.: The conditional biological activity of the carcinogens in carbon blacks, and its elimination. Cancer Res. 14, 103—110 (1954).

STOCKS, P.: Air pollution and cancer mortality in Liverpool hospital region and North Wales. Int. J. Air Pollut. 1, 1—13, 1958.

— The epidemiology of cancer. Practitioner 182, 667—672 (1959).

TEDESCHI, C.: Lesioni da catrame plivia cudovenosa. Tumori 16, 101 (1930).

TÖPPNER, R.: Roentgenography of the soot lung. Fortschr. Röntgenstr. 76, 722—728 (1952); Radiology 60, 613 (1953).

TURNER, H. M., and H. G. GRACE: Reported high incidence of lung cancer among metal grinders, engineers, foundry workers. J. Hyg. 38, 90 (1938).

VON HAAM, E., and F. S. MALLETTE: Studies on the toxicity and skin effects of compounds used in the rubber and plastics industries. Arch. industr. Hyg. 6, 237—242 (1952).

—, H. L. TITUS, I. CAPLAN, and G. Y. SHINOWARA: Effect of carbon blacks on carcinogenic compounds. Proc. Soc. exp. biol. Med. 98, 95—98 (1958).

WATSON, A. J., J. BLACK, A. T. DOIG, and G. NAGELSCHMIDT: Pneumoconiosis in carbon electrode makers. Brit. J. industr. Med. 16, 274—285 (1959).

WILDER, C. S.: Environmental cancer in Connecticut: II. Differences in incidence of cancer among areas. Conn. Hlth Bull. 70, 6 (1956).

YAMAGOWA, K., and K. ICHIKAWA: Experimentelle Studie über die Pathogenese der Epithelgeschwülste. Mitt. med. Fak. Tokyo. 15, 295—344 (1915).

Petroleum — Mineral Oil — Wax — Asphalt — Petroleum Carbon — Carbon Black — Methylated Naphthalene — Combustion Products — Shale Oil Derivatives

ANDERVONT, H. B.: Studies of methylated naphthalene derivatives. Nat. Res. Council Insect Control Comm. Rep. 183, 1948.

AULD, S. J. M.: Environmental cancer and petroleum. J. Inst. Petroleum 36, 235—253 (1950).

AYER, H. E.: Sampling methods for oil mist in industry. Med. Bull. 24, 122—134 (1964).

BAKER, E. G.: Origin and migration of oil. Science 129, 871—874 (1959).

BALDWIN, R. W., G. J. CUNNIMGHAM, and D. PRATT: Studies on carcinogenic action of motor engine oil additives. Brit. J. Cancer 15, 123 (1961).

BATTIGELLI, M. C.: Air pollution from diesel exhaust. Med. Bull. 23, 187—192 (1963).

BERNDT, H.: Krebs und Beruf. Eine statistische Untersuchung über das Magen- und das Bronchialkarzinom. Krebsarzt 18, 289—296 (1963).

BONSER, G. M., E. BOYLAND, E. R. BUSBY, D. B. CLAYSON, P. L. GROVER, and J. W. JULL: A further study of bladder implantation in the mouse as a means of detecting carcinogenic activity: Use of crushed paraffin wax or stearic acid as the vehicle. Brit. J. Cancer 17, 127—136 (1963).

—, D. B. CLAYSON, and J. W. JULL: The potency of 20-methylcholanthrene relative to other carcinogens on bladder implantation. Brit. J. Cancer 17, 235—241 (1963).

— — —, and L. N. PYRAH: The carcinogenic properties of 2-amino-1-naphthal hydrochloride and its parent amine 2-naphthylamine. Brit. J. Cancer 6, 412—424 (1952).

— — — — The induction of tumours of the bladder epithelium in rats by the implantation of paraffin wax pellets. Brit. J. Cancer 7, 456—459 (1953).

BOYD, J. T., and R. DOLL: Gastro-intestinal-cancer and the use of liquid paraffin. Brit. J. Cancer 8, 231—237 (1954).

BROCKBANK, E. M.: Industrial epithelioma, especially in cotton operatives. Clin. J. 71, 180 (1942).

— Letter to the editor: Cancer of the respiratory system. Brit. med. J. 2, 417 (1950).

CALBIANI, M.: Rischio di intossicazione nelle sale prova motori e collaudo dei motoscotter. Med. d. Lavoro 53, 344—352 (1962).

CHRISTIAN, H. A.: Cancer of the lung in employees of a public utility. A fifteen-year-study (1946—1960). J. occup. Med. 4, 133—139 (1962).

CLEMO, G. R.: Chimney smoke and diesel fumes. 34th Ann. Rep. for the Year 1956, British Empire Cancer Campaign, p. 313.

COLOMB, D.: L'avenir des paraffinomes. A propos d'une observation de reticulolymphoblastosarcomatose avec anémie hémolytique acquise par auto-anticorps froids et cryoglobulinémie, ayant compliqué un paraffinome ayant 50 ans d'évolution. Ann. Derm. Syph. 89, 36—46 (1962).

COMMINS, B. T.: Polycyclic hydrocarbons in rural and urban air. Int. J. Air Pollut. 1, 14—17 (1958).
—, WALLER, R. E., and P. J. LAWTHER: Smoke in a London diesel bus garage. An interim report. Brit. med. J. 2, 753—754 (1956).
— — — Air pollution in diesel bus garages. Brit. J. industr. Med. 14, 232—239 (1957).
Committee on Medical Science, Education, and Research of the British Medical Association: Air pollution. J. Amer. med. Ass. 180, 84 (1962).
COOK, J. W., W. CARRUTHERS, and D. L. WOODHOUSE: Carcinogenicity of mineral oil fractions. Brit. med. Bull. 14, 132—140 (1958).
COOPER, R. L.: A study in atmospheric pollution. Acta Un. int. Cancer 10, 102—103 (1954).
CROOK, A. E.: Observations on the effect of locomotive haulage on environmental conditions in mines. Trans. Inst. Mining Engineers 109, 147 (1949).
CRUICKSHANK, C. N. D., and A. GOUREVITCH: Skin cancer of the hand and forearm. Brit. J. industr. Med. 9, 74—79 (1952).
—, and J. R. SQUIRE: Skin cancer in the engineering industry from the use of mineral oil. Brit. J. industr. Med. 7, 1—11 (1950).
DANIEL, J. W., A. C. FRAZER, J. M. FRENCH, and H. G. SAMMONS: The intestinal absorption of liquid paraffin in the rat. Biochem. J. 54, 32—33 (1953).
DAVIS, B. F.: Paraffin cancer. Coal tar and petroleum products as causes of chronic irritation and cancer. J. Amer. med. Ass. 62, 1716 (1914).
DIKUN, P. P.: The presence of 3:4-benzpyrene in indoor Air. Vopr. Onkol, 6, 84—86 (1960).
Division of Air Pollution, Dept. Health, Education & Welfare. P. H. S.: Publn. No. 763, Atmospheric emissions from petroleum refineries. Washington, D. C., U. S. Govt. Print. Off. 1960, pp. 56.
DOOLEY, A. E.: Toxicity of petroleum product additives. Arch. environm. Hlth 6, 324—328 (1963).
DRUCKREY, H., D. SCHMÄHL, and R. PREUSSMANN: Fluoreszierende Verunreinigungen bei Paraffinum liquidum und organischen Lösungsmitteln. Arzneimittel-Forsch. 9, 600—604 (1959).
EBY, L. T., W. PRIESTLEY, J. REHNER, Jr., and M. E. HALL: Properties of high boiling petroleum products. Non-biological laboratory methods for predicting carcinogenicity. Anal. Chem. 25, 1500—1507 (1953).
ECKARDT, R. E.: Carcinogenicity of petroleum products with particular reference to the automotive industry. Industr. Med. Surg. 26, 396—398 (1957).
Editorial: Liquid paraffin risks. Brit. med. J. 4562, 1141 (1948).
EICHHOFF, H. J., and G. TITSCHACK: Die Kennzeichen von Kohlenwasserstoffwachsen durch Fluoreszenzspektroskopie. Erdöl und Kohle 11, 705—708 (1958).
— — Nachweis und Bestimmung von aromatischen, polycyklischen Kohlenwasserstoffen in Paraffin. Arzneimittel-Forsch. 7, 376—379 (1958).
EICKHOFF, W.: Statistische Erhebungen zur Frage des Berufskrebses von Textilarbeitern. Arch. Hyg. Bakt. 132, 313—323 (1950).
ENGEBRIGTSEN, J. N.: Dermatoses caused by gas-oil among workers in an asbestos-cement factory. Nord. hyg. T. 520, (1951).
FALK, H. L., P. KOTIN, and A. MILLER: Milk as an eluant of polycyclic aromatic hydrocarbons added to wax. Nature 183, 1184—1185 (959).
— —, and A. MEHLER: Polycyclic hydrocarbons as carcinogens for man. Arch. environm. Hlth 8, 721—730 (1964).
FIFE, J. G.: Carcinoma of the skin in machine tool setters. Brit. J. industr. Med. 19, 123—125 (1962).
FITTON, A.: Exhaust gases from motor vehicles. The composition of exhaust gases from motor vehicles. Roy. Soc. Prom. Hlth J. 76, 664—687 (1956).
FOE, R. B. and R. S. BIGHAM, Jr.: Lipid pneumonia following occupational exposure to oil spray. J. Amer. med. Ass. 155, 33—34 (1954).
FREDDE, B. A.: Queries and minor notes. Exposure to oils. J. Amer. med. Ass. 140, 1374 (1949).
GILMAN, J. P. W., and S. D. VESSELINOVITCH: Cutting oils and squamous-cell carcinoma: Part. II. An experimental study of the carcinogenicity of two types of cutting oils. J. industr. Med. 12, 244—248 (1955).

GILMAN, J. P. W., and S. D. VESSELINOVITCH: An evaluation of the relative carcinogenicity of two types of cutting oil. Arch. industr. Hlth. 14, 341—345 (1956).

GOLDFIELD, J., and R. G. MCANLIS: Low-voltage electrostatic precipitators to collect oil mists from roofing felt asphalt saturators and stills. Amer. industr. Hyg. Ass. J. 24, 411—416 (1963).

HARINGTON, J. S., and M. SMITH: Studies of hydrocarbons on mineral dusts. The elution of 3:4-benzpyrene and oils from asbestos and coal dusts by serum. Arch. environm. Hlth 8, 453—458 (1964).

—, and P. D. TOENS: Natural occurrence of amino-acids in dolomitic limestones containing algal growths. Nature 200, 947—948 (1963).

HECHT, G.: Personal communication.

HENDRICKS, N. V.: Some industrial hygiene problems in the petroleum industry. Industr. Hyg. Quarterly 11, 111—115 (1950).

—, C. M. BERRY, J. G. LIONE, and J. J. THORPE: Cancer of the scrotum in wax pressmen. I. Epidemiology. Arch. industr. Hlth 19, 524—529 (1959).

—, G. H. COLLINGS, A. E. DOOLEY, J. T. GARRETT, and J. B. RATHER: A review of exposures to oil mist. Arch. environm. Hlth 4, 139—145 (1962); Med. Bull. 22, 199—209 (1962).

HENRY, S. A.: Cancer of the scrotum in relation to occupation. London: Oxford Univ. Press 1946.

HIEGER, I.: The carcinogenicity of minerals oils. 29th Ann. Rep. Brit. Emp. Cancer Campaign for Year 1951.

—, and D. L. WOODHOUSE: The value of the rabbit for carcinogenicity tests on petroleum fractions. Brit. J. Cancer 6, 293—295 (1952).

HOLT, J. P.: 1949 (unpublished). Report covering the study of the cancer problem in a paraffin department.

HOLTZ, J. C.: Safety with mobile diesel-powered equipment underground. U. S. Dept. Interior, Bureau of Mines R. I. 5616, 1960.

HORTON, A. W., D. T. DENMAN, and R. P. TROSSET: Carcinogenesis of the skin. II. The accelerating properties of aliphatic and related hydrocarbons. Cancers Res. 17, 758—766 (1957).

HUEPER, W. C.: Über die histologischen Veränderungen im menschlichen Gewebe nach Injektion von Paraffin. Frankfurt. Ztschr. Path. 29, 268—286 (1923).

— Experimental studies on cancerigenesis of synthetic liquid fuels and petroleum substitutes. I. American shale oils. II. Bergius oils. III. Fischer-Tropsch oils. Arch. industr. Hyg. 8, 307—327 (1953).

— A quest into the environmental causes of cancer of the lung. Publ. Health Monog. No. 36, Dept. H. E. W., PHS Publn. No. 542, Washington, D. C., USGPO, 1955, pp. 54.

— Experimental carcinogenic studies on hydrogenated coal oils. I. Bergius oils. Industr. Med. Surg. 25, 51—55 (1956).

— Experimental carcinogenic studies on hydrogenated coal oils. II. Fischer-Tropsch oils. Industr. Med. Surg. 25, 459—462 (1956).

— Experimental carcinogenic studies in asphalts. Amer. industr. Hyg. Ass. J. 26, 95 (1965).

—, and H. J. CAHNMANN: Carcinogenic bioassay of benzo(a)-pyrene-free fractions of american shale oils. Arch. Path. 65, 608—614 (1958).

—, and W. D. CONWAY: Chemical carcinogenesis and cancers. Publn. No. 585, American Lecture Series. I. N. KUGELMASS, (ed.). Springfield, Ill.: C. C. Thomas 1965.

—, and W. W. PAYNE: Carcinogenic studies on soot of coffee roasting plants Arch. Path. 69, 716—727 (1960).

— — Carcinogenic Studies on petroleum asphalt, cooling oil, and coal tar. Arch. Path. 70, 372—384 (1960).

HUGUENIN, R., J. FAUVET, et J. BOURDIN: Rôle éventuel des nébulisations de certaines huiles industrielles dans l'étiologie du cancer bronchopulmonaire. Bull. Soc. Med. Paris 65, 1020—1022 (1949).

— — — Industrial oils and bronchopulmonary cancers. Foreign Letter. J. Amer. med. Ass. 142, 501 (1950).

HUGUENIN, R., J. FAUVET, et M. MAZABRAUD: Rôle éventuel des nébulisations d'huilles industrielles dans la pathogénic des cancers bronchopulmonaires. Arch. Mal. prof. 11, 48 (1950).
— — — Papel eventual de las nebulaciones de aceites industriales en la patogenia del cáncer broncopulmonar. Bol. espan. Cancerol. 3, 53—54 (1952).
HUMPERDINCK, K.: Diseases of respiratory tract in printers and their assistants who work on machines with spraying apparatus. Arch. Gewerbepath. 9, 559—565 (1939).
IRVING, C. C., H. R. GUTMANN, and D. M. LARSON: Evaluation of the carcinogenicity of aminofluorenols by implantation into the bladder of the mouse. Cancer Res. 23, 1782—1791 (1963).
JAMPOLIS, R. W., J. R. McDONALD, and O. T. CLAGETT: Mineral oil granuloma of the lungs: an evolution of methods for identification of mineral oil in tissue. Surg. Gynec. Obstet 97, 105—119 (1953).
JONES, J. G.: An investigation into the effects of exposure to an oil mist on workers in a mill for the cold reduction of steel strip. Ann. occup. Hyg. 3, 264—271 (1961).
JULSRUD, A. C.: Bronchial cancer following massive inhalation of gasoline. Nord. Med. 49, 136—137 (1953).
KAPLAN, I.: Relationship of noxious gases to carcinoma of the lung in railroad workers. J. Amer. med. Ass. 171, 2039—2043 (1959).
KATZ, M.: Carcinogenic hazards of aromatic polycyclic hydrocarbons in the polluted atmosphere. Occup. Hlth Rev. 14, 3—10 (1962).
KOTIN, P., and H. L. FALK: Production of tumors in C 57 BL mice with atmosphere-extracted aliphatic hydrocarbons. Proc. Amer. Ass. for Ca. Res. 2, (April) (1955).
— — II. The experimental induction of pulmonary tumors in strain-A mice after their exposure to an atmosphere of ozonized gasoline. Cancer 9, 910—917 (1956).
— — Air pollution and lung cancer. Proc. Natl. Conf. Air Pollution. Dec. 10—12, 1962. Washington, D. C., U. S. P.H.S. Publ. No. 1022, USGPO, 1963, 436 pp.
— Atmospheric factors in pathogenesis of lung cancer. Adv. Cancer Res. 7, A. HADDOW, and S. WEINHOUSE: (eds.). New York: Academic Press Inc. 1963.
— — Polluted urban air and related environmental factors in the pathogenesis of pulmonary cancer. Dis. Chest 45, 236—246 (1964).
— —, and C. J. McCAMMON: III. The experimental induction of pulmonary tumors and changes in the respiratory epithelium in C 57 BL mice following their exposure to an atmosphere of ozonized gasoline. Cancer 11, 473—481 (1958).
— —, and M. THOMAS: Aromatic hydrocarbons. II. Presence in the particulate phase of gasoline-engine exhausts and the carcinogenicity of exhaust extracts. Arch. ind. Hyg. 9, 164—177 (1954).
— — — Aromatic hydrocarbons. III. Presence in the particulate phase of diesel-engine exhausts and carcinogenicity of exhaust extracts. Arch. industr. Hlth 11, 113—120 (1955).
— — — I. Production of skin tumors in mice with oxidation products of aliphatic hydrocarbons. Cancer 9, 905—909 (1956).
KÜHN, M.: Motor- und Feuerungsabgase als Ursachen der Luftverunreinigung. Zbl. biol. Aerosol-Forsch. 6, 431—447 (1961).
KURATSUNE, M., and W. C. HUEPER: Polycyclic aromatic hydrocarbons in coffee soots. J. nat. Cancer Inst. 20, 37—51 (1958).
LAMPE, K. F., and W. B. DEICHMANN: The identification of nitro-olefins in the combustion products of hydrocarbons. Industr. Med. Surg. 33, 281—283 (1964).
LARSON, R. H.: Query. Fumes from casting iron. J. Amer. med. Ass. 149, 622 (1952).
LEITCH, A.: Paraffin cancer and its experimental production. Brit. med. J. 2, 1104 (1922).
LIJINSKY, W.: Separation of polycyclic aromatic hydrocarbons in complex mixtures. Chromatographic determination of trace amounts in petroleum waxes. Anal. Chem. 32, 684—687 (1960).
—, I. DOMSKY, G. MASON, H. Y. RAMAHI, and T. SAFAVI: The chromatographic determination of trace amounts of polynuclear hydrocarbons in petroleum, mineral oil, and coal tar. Anal. Chem. 35, 952—956 (1963).
— —, and C. R. RAHA: A short method of testing petroleum waxes for the presence of polycyclic aromatic hydrocarbons. J. Assoc. Official Agric. Chem. 46, 725—731 (1963).

LIONE, J. G., and J. S. DENHOLM: Cancer of the scrotum in wax pressmen. II. Clinical observations. Arch. industr. Hlth 19, 530—539 (1959).

LONGMUIR, J.: Epithelial cancer in paraffin oil workmen. Edinb. med. J. 29, 542 (1883).

LUSHBAUGH, C. C.: Infiltrating adenomatous lesions of the stomach, cecum, and rectum of monkeys similar to early human carcinoma and carcinoma *in situ*. Cancer Res. 9, 385—394 (1949).

—, J. W. GREEN, and C. F. REDEMANN: Effects of prolonged inhalation of oil fogs on experimental animals. Arch. industr. Hyg. 1, 237—247 (1950).

—, and A. HACKETT: An infiltration adenomatous lesion of the colon of rats ingesting motor lubricating oil (S. G. F. No. 1 oil). J. nat. Cancer Inst. 9, 159—172 (1948).

LYONS, M. J.: Vehicular exhausts: Identification of further carcinogens of the polycyclic aromatic hydrocarbon class. Brit. J. Cancer 13, 126—131 (1959).

—, and H. JOHNSTON: Aromatic hydrocarbons from vehicular exhausts. Brit. J. Cancer 11, 60—66 (1957).

MACKENNA, R. M. B., and S. HORNER: Occupational skin diseases. In MEREWETHER, E. R. A. Industr. Med. 2, 1—101 (1954).

MASTROMATTEO, E.: Cutting oils and squamous-cell carcinoma. Part I. Incidence in a plant with a report of six cases. Brit. J. industr. Med. 12, 240—243 (1955).

MEYER-BRODNITZ, F. K.: Zur gewerbehygienischen Bedeutung des Paraffin-Spritzverfahrens. Arch. Gewerbehyg. 3, 523 (1932).

MEYERS, J. B., and R. L. GRIFFITH: Lipoid pneumonia due to prolonged ingestion of mineral oil. Dis. Chest. 27, 677—684 (1955).

MIESCHER, G., and F. SCHWARZ: Wirkt der Ruß von Ölfeuerungen carcinogen? Schweiz. med. Wschr. 72, 1081 (1942).

MILLS, C. A.: Motor exhaust cases and lung cancer in Cincinnati. Amer. J. med. Sci. 239, 316—319 (1960).

MITTLER, S.: Cancer from the highway. The Frontier (Armour Res. Fdtn.) 11—13 (1956).

—, and S. NICHOLSON: Carcinogenicity of atmospheric pollutants. Industr. Med. Surg. 26, 135—138 (1957).

NEUKOMM, S.: The newt test in relation to investigation on carcinogenic and cocarcinogenic substances. NCI Monogr. No. 9, 71—73 (1962).

NULIK, J. D., and J. G. ERDMAN: Genesis of hydrocarbons of low molecular weight in organic-rich aquatic systems. Science 141, 806—807 (1963).

PAGE, R. C., J. P. HOLT, N. V. HENDRICKS, R. E. ECKARDT, C. L. STANTON, W. E. SMITH, D. A. SUNDERLAND, K. SUGIURA, H. G. M. FISCHER, W. PRIESTLEY, Jr., L. T. EBY, G. G. WANLESS, J. REHNER, Jr., F. H. BLANDING, and W. H. KING, Jr.: Symposium on a cancer control program for high-boiling catalytically cracked oils. Arch. industr. Hyg. 4, 297—345 (1951).

POTTER, M., and C. L. ROBERTSON: Development of plasma-cell neoplasms in BALB/c mice after intraperitoneal injection of paraffin-oil adjuvant, heat-killed staphylococcus mixtures. J. nat. Cancer Inst. 25, 847—861 (1960).

PROKHOROVA, E. K., and N. N. ZNAMENSKY: The 3:4-benzpyrene contents of paraffin of Soviet make. Vopr. Onkol. 9, 72—76 (1963).

PROUDFIT, J. P., H. S. VAN ORDSTRAND, and C. W. MILLER: Chronic lipid pneumonia following occupational exposure. Arch. industr. Hyg. 1, 105—111 (1950).

RÖSCH, H.: Drei verschiedene Carcinome bei einem Paraffinarbeiter. Virchow's Arch. path. Anat. 245, 1—8 (1923).

SANTE, L. R.: The fate of oil particles in the lung and their possible relationship to the development of bronchiogenic carcinoma. Amer. J. Roentgenol. 62, 788—797 (1949).

SCHMÄHL, D., and A. REITER: Versuche zur Krebserzeugung mit flüssigem Paraffin, gelber Vaseline und Wollfett. Arzneimittel-Forsch. 3, 403—406 (1953).

SCHMIDTMANN, M.: Über chronische Autogasschäden. Untersuchungen am Dieselmotor. Arch. Gewerbepath. 8, 1 (1937).

SCHNEIDER, L.: Pulmonary hazard of the ingestion of mineral oil in apparently health adult. New Engl. J. Med. 240, 284 (1949).

SCHOCH, E. O.: Zur Frage der Schädlichkeit paraffin- und vaselinehaltiger Präparate. Mschr. Krebsbekämpf. 11, 31—33 (1943).

SCHULTE, H. F.: Does mist cooling risk operator. Amer. Mach. 99, 122—124 (1955).

SCHWARTZ, L., L. TULIPAN, and J. BIRMINGHAM: Occupational diseases of the skin. 3rd Ed. Philadelphia, Pa.: Lea & Febiger 1957.

SHUBIK, P., and U. SAFFIOTTI: The carcinogenic and promoting action of low boiling catalytically cracked oils. Proc. Amer. Ass. Cancer Res. 1, 45 (1954).

— —, W. LIJINSKY, G. PIETRA, H. RAPPAPORT, B. TOTH, C. R. RAHA, L. TOMATIS, R. FELDMAN, and H. RAMAHI: Studies on the toxicity of petroleum waxes. Toxicol. appl. pharmacol. 4, 62 (1962).

SIMMERS, M. H., E. PODOLAK, and R. KINOSITA: Carcinogenic effects of petroleum asphalt. Proc. Soc. exp. Biol. (N. Y.) 101, 266—268 (1959).

SMITH, P. V., Jr.: The occurrence of hydrocarbons in recent sediments from the Gulf of Mexico. Science 116, 437—439 (1952).

SMITH, W. E., D. A. SUNDERLAND, and K. SUGIURA: Experimental analysis of the carcinogenic activity of certain petroleum products. 5th Internat. Congr. on Cancer, Paris, July 1950, p. 47.

— — — Experimental analysis of the carcinogenic activity of certain petroleum products. Arch. industr. Hyg. 4, 299—314 (1951).

SOUTHAM, A. H.: Mule-spinner's cancer. Report internat. Conf. on Cancer, London, 1928. Bristol: John Wright & Sons, Ltd.

SPINK, M. S., A. H. BAYNES, and J. B. L. TOMBLESON: Skin carcinoma in the process of ‚Standford Jointing'. Brit. J. industr. Med. 21, 154—157 (1964).

SQUIRE, J. R., C. N. D. CRUICKSHANK, and E. TOPLEY: Occupational skin disease. Brit. med. Bull. 7, 2841 (1950).

STEINBRÜCK, C., and CARL: Künstliche Krebserzeugung durch Druckerschwärze. Berl. tierärztl. Wschr. 45, 525 (1929).

SULA, J. P.: The carcinogen 3,4-benzpyrene in the living environment and human organism. Neoplasma (Bratisl.) 10, 571—579 (1963).

SULLIVAN, J. L., and G. J. CLEARY: A comparison of polycyclic aromatic hydrocarbon emissions from diesel- and petrol-powered vehicles in partially segregated traffic lanes. Brit. J. industr. Med. 21, 117—134 (1964).

SUNDERLAND, D. A., W. E. SMITH, and K. SUGIURA: The pathology and growth behavior of experimental tumors induced by certain petroleum products. Cancer 4, 1232—1245 (1951).

TEBBENS, B. D., J. F. THOMAS, and M. MUKAI: Aromatic hydrocarbon production related to incomplete combustion. Arch. industr. Hlth 14, 413—425 (1956).

— — — Hydrocarbon synthesis in combustion. Arch. industr. Hlth 13, 567—573 (1956).

THOMAS, D. W., and M. BLUMER: Pyrene and fluoranthene in manganese nodules. Science 143, 39 (1964).

TOUREINE, A., and H. BOUR: Lubricating oils and pulmonary disease. Rev. méd. franç. 20, 285 (1939).

TSUCHIYA, K.: The relation of occupation to cancer especially cancer of the lung. Cancer 18, 136—144 (1965).

TWORT, C. C., and J. D. FULTON: Experiments on the nature of the carcinogenic agents in mineral oil. J. Path. Bact. 32, 149 (1929).

—, and J. M. TWORT: Induction of cancer by cracked mineral oils. Lancet 2, 1226 (1935).

— — Prevention of mineral oil and tar dermatitis and cancer. Lancet 1, 286 (1934).

VAN FAROWS, D. E.: Occupational health studies in the investment casting industry. Environmental aspects. Arch. industr. Hlth 15, 223—244 (1957).

VOSAMAE, A.: On the blastomagenic-action of the Estonian shale oil soot and the soot of liquid fuel obtained from the processing of shale oil. Acta Un. int. Cancr. 19, 739—741 (1963).

WADE, L.: Observations on skin cancer among refinery workers. Arch. environm. Hlth 6, 730—735 (1963).

WAGNER, W. D., P. G. WRIGHT, and H. E. STOKINGER: Inhalation toxicology of oil mists. I. Chronic effects of white mineral oil. Med. Bull. 24, 135—152 (1964).

WALLER, R. E., B. T. COMMINS, and P. J. LAWTHER: Air pollution in road tunnels. Brit. J. industr. Med. 18, 250 (1961).

WATSON, A. J., J. BLACK, A. T. DOIG, and G. NAGELSCHMIDT: Pneumoconiosis in carbon electrode makers. Brit. J. industr. Med. 16, 274—285 (1959).

WHITEHEAD, W. L., and I. A. BREGER: The originn of petroleum: effects of low temperature pyrolysis on the organic extract of a recent marine sediment. Science 111, 335—337 (1950).

WOOD, E. H.: Unusual case of carcinoma of both lungs associated with lipoid pneumonia. Radiology 40, 193—195 (1943).

WOOD, H. B.: The noncarcinogenic nature of purified mineral oils. J. Amer. med. Ass. 94, 1641 (1930); Cancer Res. 5, 720 (1930); Z. Krebsforsch. 33, 134 (1931); Amer. J. Cancer 15, 319 (1931).

WOODHOUSE, D. L.: The carcinogenic activity of some petroleum fractions and extracts. Comparative results in tests on mice repeated after an interval of eighteen months. J. Hyg. 47, 121—134 (1950).

— The carcinogenic activity of mineral oils. 29th Ann. Rep. Brit. Emp. Cancer Campeign for Year 1951, pp. 170—171.

WYNDER, E. L.: Industrial aspects of skin cancer. Bull. Amer. inst. Chemists 30, 23 (1953).

—, and D. HOFFMANN: A study of air pollution carcinogenesis. III. Carcinogenic activity of gasoline engine exhaust condensate. Cancer 15, 103—108 (1962).

ZEGLIO, P.: Le alterazioni delle vie respiratorie da vie respiratorie da vapori di bitume. Rass. Med. industr. 19, 268—273 (1950).

— Changes in the respiratory tract from the vapours of bitumen. Bull. Hyg. 26, 621 (1951).

Ionizing Radiations

ABRAHAMSON, L., M. H. O'CONNOR, and M. L. ABRAHAMSON: Bilateral alveolar lung carcinoma, associated with the injection of thorotrast. Irish. J. med. Sci. 6, 229—235 (1950).

Advisory Committee on Health Hazards in Uranium Mining and Milling Industry. Arch. industr. Hlth 14, 212—214 (1956).

AGRICOLA, G.: De re metallica. Basel 1597.

ALERCIO, J. S., G. A. WELFORD, and R. S. MORSE: A radiochemical determination of alpha exposure from enriched uranium in urine. Amer. industr. Hyg. Ass. J. 22, 443—447 (1961).

ALTMANN, H.-W., W. HUNSTEIN, and E. STUTZ: Strahleninduzierte (Sr⁹⁰) Lungencarcinome bei Ratten. Naturwissenschaften 46, 85—86 (1959).

— — — Über Lungenveränderungen und Lungentumoren bei Ratten nach Bestrahlung mit radioaktivem Strontium (Sr⁹⁰). Beitr. path. Anat. 124, 145—175 (1961).

—, R. LICK, and E. STUTZ: Über die Histogenese strahleninduzierter (Sr⁹⁰) Plattenepithelcarcinome in der Rattenlunge. 1. Die Veränderungen am Bronchialepithel. Beitr. path. Anat. 125, 403—426 (1961).

— — — Über die Histogenese strahleninduzierter (Sr⁹⁰) Plattenepithelcarcinome in der Rattenlunge. 2. Die Rolle des Alveolarepithels Beitr. path. Anat. 125, 427—444 (1961).

ARCHER, V. E., H. J. MAGNUSON, D. A. HOLADAY, and P. A. LAWRENCE: Hazards to health in uranium mining and milling. J. occup. Med. 4, 55—60 (1962).

—, and C. L. SIMPSON: Semi-quantitative relationship of radiation and neoplasia in man. Health physics (Pergamon Press) 9, 56—67 (1963).

ARNSTEIN, A.: Über den sogenannten „Schneeberger Lungenkrebs". Verh. dtsch. path. Ges. 16, 332—342 (1913).

— Sozialhygienische Untersuchungen über die Bergleute in den Schneeberger Kobaltgruben, insbesondere über das Vorkommen des sogenannten „Schneeberger Lungenkrebses". San.-Wes., Wiem. 25, 64—83 (1913).

AUB, J. C., R. D. EVANS, L. H. HEMPELMANN, and H. S. MARTLAND: The late effects of internally-deposited radioactive materials in man. Medicine 31, 221—329 (1952).

AUCKE: Der Lungenkrebs in den Schneeberger Kobaltgruben. Ein Fall von Lymphosarcoma. Inaug. Diss. München 1884.

AURAND, K., U. FEINE, W. JACOBI, and A. SCHRAUB: Investigation of radiation dose in the lungs caused by radon bearing atmosphere. Strahlentherapie 104, 345—354 (1957).

AWAAD, H., A. F. EL-SHERBINI, E. HAMMOUD, I. HAZAA, M. KHARADLY, and F. VALIC: Radiation hazards in Red Sea phosphate mines. J. Egypt. med. Ass. 36, 1—14 (1961).

BAADER, E. W.: Personal communication, 1951.

BATZENSCHLAGER, A., M. DORNER, et M. WEILL-BOUSSON: La pathologie tumorale du thorotrast chez l'homme. Oncologia 16, 28—63 (1963).

BAUDISCHE, E.: Zu den Strahlenreaktionen der Lungen und Pleura bei Brustkrebs-Patienten. Strahlentherapie 114, 135—146 (1961).

BAUER, J. T., and P. H. SCHRAER: Late pathologic effect of high voltage Roentgen rays on the human lung: Report of two cases. Amer. J. Path. 16, 651 (1940).

BEHOUNEK, F.: Über die Verhältnisse der Radioaktivität im Uranpecherzbergbaurevier von St. Joachimsthal in Böhmen. Physik. Zschr. 28, 333—344 (1927).

— Cited by J. STOCKLASA: Die Bedeutung der Luftradioaktivität für die Entstehung der Joachimsthaler und Schneeberger Bergkrankheit. Dtsch. med. Wschr. 59, 1199 (1933).

—, und M. FORT: Joachimsthaler Bergmannskrankheit. Strahlentherapie 70, 487—498 (1941).

BELT, T. H.: Über tödliche Lungenfibrose bei gewerblicher Radiumschädigung. Frankfurt. Z. Path. 42, 170—187 (1931/32).

BERGMANN, M, and E. A. GRAHAM: Pneumonectomy for severe irradiation damage of the lung. J. thorac. Surg. 22, 549 (1951); Surg. Gynec. Obst. 94, 535—536 (1952).

BERMAN, I. L., and E. P. ERNEST: Use of radioactive static eliminators in a printing plant. Industr. Med. Surg. 19, 229 (1950).

BEUTEL, A., und A. WOLDRICH: Klinische und röntgenologische Beobachtungen über die Entwicklung des Joachimsthaler Bronchialcarcinoms. Z. Krebsforsch. 34, 109 (1931).

BEYREUTHER, H.: Multiplicität von Carcinomen bei einem Fall von sog. „Schneeberger" Lungenkrebs mit Tuberkulose. Virchows. Arch. path. Anat. 250, 230—243 (1924).

BLACK, C. E.: Commercial lead as a possible inciting factor in bronchiogenic carcinoma. Report of two cases. Arch. Path. 35, 366—372 (1943).

BRANDT, A.: Bericht über die im Schneeberger Gebiet auf Veranlassung des Reichsausschusses für Krebsbekämpfung durchgeführten Untersuchungen. Z. Krebsforsch. 47, 108 (1938).

BUDA, J. A., J. J. CONLEY, and R. RANKOW: Carcinoma of the maxillary sinus following thorotrast instillation. Amer. J. Surg. 106, 868—871 (1963).

CAMPBELL, J. A.: Lung tumours in mice; incidence as affected by inhalation of certain carcinogenic agents and some dusts. Brit. Med. J. 1, 217—221 (1942).

CARMICHAEL, H., and P. R. TUNNICLIFFE: Measurement of alpha-active dust in the atmosphere. J. industr. Hyg. 30, 211—227 (1948).

CEMBER, H.: Further studies on lung cancer from Ce ^{144} F$_3$. Hlth Physics 9, 539—544 (1963).

— Radiogenic lung cancer. Progr. exp. Tumor Res. (Basel) 4, 251—303 (1964).

—, and K. STEMMER: Lung cancer from radioactive cerium chloride. Hlth Physics 10, 43—48 (1964).

—, and J. A. WATSON: Carcinogenic effects of strontium 90 beads implanted in the lungs of rats. Amer. industr. Hyg. Ass. J. 19, 36—42 (1958).

— — Bronchogenic carcinoma from radioactive barium sulfate. Arch. industr. Hlth 17, 230—235 (1958).

— —, and T. B. GRUCCI: Pulmonary effects from radioactive thallium-activated clay particles. Arch. industr. Hlth 15, 449—450 (1957).

— —, and M. E. NOVAK: The influence of radioactivity and lung burden on the pulmonary clearance rate of barium sulfate. Amer. industr. Hyg. Ass. J. 22, 27—32 (1961).

— —, and A. A. SPRITZER: Bronchogenic carcinoma from radioactive cerium fluoride. Arch. industr. Hlth 19, 14—23 (1959).

CHU, F. C. H., R. PHILLIPS, J. J. NICKSON, and J. G. MCPHEE: Pneumonitis following radiation therapy of cancer of the breast by tangential technic. Radiology 64, 642—654 (1955).

COREY, R. C., H. PERRY, and C. H. SCHWARTZ: Off-site disposal of radioactive incinerator residues by solid fluxes. Amer. industr. Hyg. Ass. J. 12, 52—57 (1951).

DAWSON, K. B.: Radioactive material in the atmosphere. Brit. J. Cancer 6, 22—31 (1952).

Department of Health, Education & Welfare: Control of radon and daughters in uranium mines and calculations on biologic effects. Publ. Hlth Serv. Publn. No. 494, 1957, Washington, D. C. U. S. Govt. Print. Off. 81 pp.

DE VILLIERS, A. J., and J. P. WINDISCH: Lung cancer in a fluorspar mining community. I. Radiation, dust, and mortality experience. Brit. J. industr. Med. 21, 94—109 (1964).

DINGWALL-FORDYCE, I., and R. E. LANE: A follow-up study of lead workers. Brit. J. industr. Med. 20, 313—315 (1963).

DOENECKE, F.: Über tödliche Lungenfibrose bei gewerblicher Radiumschädigung. Frankfurt. Z. Path. 42, 161—169 (1931).

DÖHNERT, H. R.: Experimentelle Untersuchungen zur Frage des Schneeberger Lungenkrebses. Z. Krebsforsch. 47, 209 (1938).

DOYLE, H. N.: Uranium mining and milling. A current study. Occup. Hlth 13, 37 (1953).

DUNHAM, C. L.: Radioactive fallout. Its significance for the practitioner. J. Amer. med. Ass. 183, 50—53 (1963).

Editorial: Atmospheric carcinogens. Lancet 2, 30 (1952).

Editorial: Gold, uranium, and sulfuric acid in South Africa. Chem. Eng. News 32, 1364—1365 (1954).

EICKEN: Larynxkarzinom nach alter Röntgenschädigung. Zbl. Hals-, Nas.- u. Ohrenheilk. 35, 392—398 (1932).

EISENBUD, M., and J. H. HARLEY: Radioactive Dust from nuclear detonations. Science 117, 141—147 (1953).

ENGELBRECHT, F. M., B. F. THIART, and A. CLAASSENS: Fibrosis and collagen in rats' lungs produced by radioactive mine dust. Ann. occup. Hyg. 2, 257—266 (1960).

ESCHENBRENNER, A. B., and E. MILLER: Effects of lung-continued total body gamma irradiation on mice, Guinea pigs, and rabbits. In R. E. ZIRKLE: Biological effects of external X- and gamma-radiation. Part I. McGraw-Hill Book Co 1954.

EVANS, R. D.: Quantitative aspects of radiation carcinogenesis in humans. Acta Un. int. Cancer 6, 1229—1237 (1950).

—, and C. GOODMAN: Determination of the thoron content of air and its bearing on lung cancer hazards in industry. J. industr. Hyg. 22, 89—99 (1940).

FISCHER-WASELS, B.: Die Ursachen des primären Lungencarcinoms. Frankfurt. Z. Path. 49, 145 (1936).

FLEMING, J. A. C., J. F. FILBEE, and G. WIERNIK: Sequelae to radical irradiation in carcinoma of the breast. An inquiry into the incidence of certain radiation injuries. Brit. J. Radiol. 34, 713—719 (1961).

FREID, J. R., and H. GOLDBERG: Postirradiation changes in lungs and thorax. Am. J. Roentg. 43, 877 (1940).

FRUHLING, L., C.-M. GROS, A. BATZENSCHLAGER, et M. DORNER: La maladie du thorotrast. Ann. Méd. 57, 132 (1956).

GARRETT, M.: Eight further cases of radiation-induced cancer. Brit. med. J. 5133, 1329—1331 (1959).

GATES, O., and S. WARREN: Histogenesis of lung carcinoma in mice. Arch. Path. 71, 693 (1961).

GELLER, E. I., F. X. WORDEN, G. CASSIDY, and C. Y. BARTHOLOMEW: Personnel protection program for industrial use of krypton-85. Amer. industr. Hyg. Ass. J. 22, 403—415 (1961).

GLUCKSMANN, A., L. F. LAMERTON, and W. V. MAYNEORD: Carcinogenic effects of radiation. In RONALD W. RAVEN (ed.): Cancer, Vol. 1. London: Butterworth & Co. 1957.

GOOLDEN, A. W. G.: Radiation cancer: a review with special reference to radiation tumours in the pharynx, and thyroid. Brit. J. Radiol. 30, 626—640 (1957).

Governors' Conference on Health Hazards in Uranium mines. A summary report. Puplic Health Service Publn. No. 843, Washington. D. C. U. S. Govt. Print. Off., 1961, 13 pp.

GUIMARAES, J. P., L. F. LAMERTON, and W. R. CHRISTENSEN: The late effects of thorotrast administration. A review and an experimental study. Brit. J. Cancer 11, 253—267 (1955).

HÄRTING, F. H., and W. HESSE: Der Lungenkrebs, die Bergkrankheit in den Schneeberger Gruben. Vjschr. Med. gerich. K. 30, 296—309 (1879); 31, 102—132 (1879); 31, 313—337 (1879).

HAMPERL, H.: Akute und chronische Strahlenschädigung beim Menschen. Arch. Gewerbepath. 7, 699—706 (1936/37).

HARRIS, S. J.: Radon levels found in mines in New York State. Mthly Rev. N. Y. St. Dept. Labor. 33, 37—40 (1954).

HARRIS, W. B., and I. KINGSLEY: The industrial hygiene of uranium fabrication. Arch. industr. Hlth 19, 540—565 (1959).

HASTERLIK, R. J., C. E. MILLER, and A. J. FINKEL: Carcinoma of the mastoid and paranasal sinuses in radium-bearing patients. Abstr. 8th Internat. Congr. Moscow, 1962, p. 238.

HELD, B. J.: Planning ventilation for nuclear reactor facilities. Amer. industr. Hyg. Ass. J. 23, 83—87 (1962).

HESTON, W. E., E. LORENZ, and M. K. DERINGER: Occurrence of pulmonary tumors in strain A mice following total-Body X-radiation and injection of nitrogen mustard. Cancer Res. 13, 573—577 (1953).

HOFER, O.: Kieferhöhlenkarzinom durch radiumhaltiges Kontrastmittel hervorgerufen. Dtsch. zahnärztl. Z. 7, 736—741 (1952).

HOLINGER, P. H., and W. F. RABBETT: Late devolopment of laryngeal and pharyngeal carcinoma in previously irradiated areas. Laryngoscope 63, 105—112 (1953).

HOLLISTER, H.: Radioactive fallout in peace and war. Arch. environm. Hlth 8, 590—597 (1964).

HOPMANN: Erkrankungen durch Röntgenstrahlen und andere strahlende Energie. In Fabrikärzte der deutschen Industrie. Ärztliche Merkblätter über berufliche Erkrankungen. Berlin: Springer 1930.

HUBACHER, O.: Are the uranium-bearing lodes of coal and marl in Bleiken and Blapbach of medical significance? Schweiz. med. Wschr. 93, 733—737 (1963).

HUBER, P.: Luftkontamination durch Atombombentests. Oncologia 16, 221—229 (1963).

HUECK: Foreign letter - Berlin - pulmonary carcinomas in Schneeberg miners. J. Amer. med. Ass. 113, 2436—2437 (1939).

— Kurzer Bericht über Ergebnisse anatomischer Untersuchungen. Z. Krebsforsch. 49, 312—315 (1939-1940).

HUEPER, W. C.: Macromolecular substances as pathogenic agents. Arch. Path. 33, 267—290 (1942).

— Memorandum: Proposed occupational cancer survey of Colorado. Nov. 30, 1948.

— Environmental lung cancer. Industr. Med. Surg. 20, 49—62 (1951).

— Environmental cancer problems in Colorado. Unpublished report to Colorado State Medical Society 1952.

— Recent developments in environmental cancer. Arch. Path. 58, 360—399; 475—523; 645—682 (1954).

— Potential cancer hazards from cosmetics to producers and consumers. W. WERBLE (ed.): Drug research reports. Washington, D. C., 1960.

—, J. H. ZUEFLE, A. M. LINK, and M. G. JOHNSON: Experimental studies in metal cancerigenesis. II. Experimental uranium cancers in rats. J. nat. Cancer Inst. 13, 291—305 (1952).

HUG, O.: Die karzinogenen Wirkungen ionisierender Strahlen. Strahlentherapie 102, 546—558 (1957).

INGRAM, M.: Health hazards in radiation work. Science 111, 103—109 (1950).

IRMSCHER, G.: Über einen Todesfall an chronischer Pneumonie nach Inhalation von alpha- und beta-strahlenaktivem ‚Industriestaub‘ vor rund 20 Jahren. Dtsch. Gesundh.-Wes. 13, 1732—1735 (1958).

JACOBS, F.: Industrie du radium. Editorial. Paris Méd. 60, 114—119 (1926).

JACOE, P. W.: The occurrence of radon in non-uranium mines in Colorado. Arch. industr. Hyg. 8, 118—124 (1953).

— Occurrence of radon in non-uranium mines in Colorado. Occup. Hlth 13, 104 (1953).

JACQUES, P.: Cancer du larynx chez la femme après irradiation thyroidienne prolongée. Otorhino-laring. int. 19, 277 (1935).

JECH, C.: Retention of radon decay products in human lungs. Arch. industr. Hlth 13, 475—479 (1956).

KAHLAU, G.: Experimentelle Erzeugung von Lungentumoren durch Radiumemanation. Klin. Wschr. 27, 551—552 (1949).

— Experimentelle Erzeugung von Lungentumoren durch Radiumemanation. Verh. dtsch. Ges. Path. 32, 379—385 (1950).

KALBFLEISCH, H. H.: Tödliche Lungenfibrose infolge gewerblicher Schädigung durch Radium. Arch. Gewerbepath. 7, 699—706 (1936).

— Tödliche Lungenfibrose infolge gewerblicher Schädigung durch Radium. Samml. Vergiftungsf. 8, 27—30 (1937).

KILHAM, L., R. J. LOW, S. F. CONTI, and F. D. DALLENBACH: Intranuclear inclusions and neoplasms in the kidey of wild rats. J. nat. Cancer Inst. 29, 863—885 (1962).

KING, E. R., W. S. COLE, A. HORWITZ, and C. T. KLOPP: Carcinoma of the larynx occurring in a patient receiving therapeutic doses of I[131]. Arch. Otolaryngol. 59, 333—338 (1954).

KOTSCHETKOWA, T. A., and G. AWRUNINA: Veränderungen in den Lungen und in anderen Organen bei intratrachealer Einführung einiger Radio-Isotope (Na^{24}, P^{32}, Au^{198}). Arch. Gewerbepath. 16, 24—33 (1957).

KOCHETKOVA, T. A., G. A. AVRUNINA, and H. V. SAGAIDAK: Experimental lung cancer induced by some radioactive compounds of P^{32}, Au^{198}, and Fe^{59}. Abstr. 8th int. Cancer Cong. Moscow 1962.

— —, and N. D. SAGAIDAK-CHERNYAK: Experimental lung cancer induced with radioactive compounds, P^{32}, Au^{198}, and Fe^{59}. Acta Un. int. Cancr. 19, 684—686 (1963).

KURSHAKOVA, N. N., and A. E. IVANOV: A model of experimental lung cancer caused by intratracheal introduction of radioactive cerium. Biull. eksp. Biol. Med. 54, 787—789 (1963).

KUSCHNER, M.: Radiation induced bronchogenic carcinoma in rats. Amer. J. Path. 34, 554 (1958).

LANGE, K.: Krebserkrankungen und geologische Verhältnisse im Erzgebirge. Z. Krebsforsch. 42, 306—310 (1935).

LASKIN, S., M. MUSCHNER, N. NELSON, B. ALTSHULER, J. H. HARLEY, and M. DANIELS: Carcinoma of the lung in rats exposed to the B-radiation of intrabronchial ruthenium ^{106} pellets. J. nat. Cancer Inst. 31, 219—231 (1963).

LISCO, H.: Radiation and carcinogenesis. Int. Forum 2, 13—16 (1954).

— Autoradiographic and histopathologic studies in radiation carcinogenesis of the lung. Lab. Invest. 8, 162—170 (1959).

—, and M. P. FINKEL: Observations on lung pathology following the inhalation of radioactive cerium. Fed. Proc. 8, 360—361 (1949).

LITTLE, J. B., E. P. RADFORD, Jr., H. L. McCOMBS, V. R. HUN, and C. NELSON: Polonium-210 in lungs and soft tissues of cigarette smokers. Radiat. Res. 22, 209 (1964).

LOCKHART, L. B., Jr.: Concentrations of radioactive materials in the air during 1957. Science 128, 1139 (1958).

LÖWY, J.: Der Bronchialkrebs als Berufskrankheit. Med. Klinik 24, 1784 (1928).

— Über die Joachimstaler Bergkrankheit; vorläufige Mitteilung. Med. Klinik 25, 141—142 (1929).

— Report: The Joachimsthal miners' disease. Translation: 4th Int. Congr. Occup. Dis., Lyons, April 1929.

— Die Wirkung der Joachimsthaler Pechblende im Tierversuch. Med. Klinik 18, 619 (1936).

— Der Bronchialkrebs als Berufskrankheit. Acta Un. int. Cancr. 3, 182—188 (1938).

— Occupational tumors. Suppl. to Occup. Hlth. Int. Labour Office, Geneva, 1939.

LORENZ, E.: Radioactivity and lung Cancer; a critical review of lung cancer in the miners of Schneeberg and Joachimsthal. J. nat. Cancer Inst. 5, 1—15 (1944).

— Effects of long continued total-body gamma irradiation on mice, guinea pigs and rabbits. VI. Conclusions and applicability of results to the problem of human protection. In R. E. ZIRKLE: Biologic effects of external X- and gamma-radiation. 1st ed. New York: McGraw-Hill Book Co., Inc. 1954.

—, A. B. ESCHENBRENNER, W. E. HESTON, and M. K. DERINGER: Increase in incidence of lung tumors in strain A mice following long-continued irradiation with gamma rays. J. nat. Cancer Inst. 6, 349—353 (1946).

—, W. E. HESTON, A. B. ESCHENBRENNER, and M. K. DERINGER: Biological studies in the tolerance range. Radiol. 49, 274—285 (1947).

LOUGHEED, M. N. and G. H. MAGUIRE: Irradiation pneumonitis in the treatment of carcinoma of the breast. J. Canad. Ass. Radiol. 11, 1—10 (1960).

LOUTIT, J. F.: The effects of ionizing radiations. In E. R. A. MEREWETHER (ed.): Industrial medicine and hygiene. Vol. 2. London: Butterworth & Co. Ltd. 1954.

LOVE, R. A.: Lung carcinoma in an industrial population at an atomic pile site. AECU-1620. Technical Information Service, Oak Ridge, Tenn. U. S. A. E. C., 1951.

LOWRY, P. H.: The theoretical ground-level dose-rate from the radioargon emitted by the Brookhaven reactor stack. Arch. industr. Hyg. 4, 617 (1951).

LUDEWIG, P., and E. LORENSER: Untersuchung der Grubenluft in den Schneeberger Gruben auf den Gehalt an Radiumemanation. Strahlentherapie 17, 428 (1924).

Machis, A., and J. C. Geyer: Burning radioactive wastes in institutional incinerators. Amer. industr. Hyg. Ass. J. 13, 199—210 (1952).

Mahler, et R. Ziel: Quelques considérations sur l'état sanitaire et les mesures techniques de salubrité prises dans les mines d'uranium-radium de Jachymov, en ce qui touche tout particulièrement le cancer professionnel. Société des Nations (League of Nations), Health Organization Commission on Cancer, Geneva, May 1930.

— Bibliog. Tech. Work of the Health Organization of the League of Nations, 1920—1945, Bull. Hlth Org. Geneva 11, 35 (1945).

— League of Nations, Bull. Helth Org. 11—12, (1945—1946).

Majoros, M., K. D. Devine, and E. M. Parkhill: Malignant transformation of benign laryngeal papillomas in children after radiation therapy. Surg. Clin. N. Amer. 43, 1049—1061 (1963).

Martland, H. S.: The occurrence of malignancy in radioactive persons. Amer. J. Cancer 15, 2435—2516 (1931).

McAdams, W. A.: Radiation protection laws and codes — a scramble for action. Amer. industr. Hyg. Ass. J. 20, 246—248 (1959).

Medical Research Council: The hazards to man of nuclear and allied radiations. London: H. M. Stationery Office 1956.

— The hazards to man of nuclear and allied radiations. 2nd Rep. London: H. M. Stationery Office 1960.

Melnikov, R. A.: The induction of tumors in monkeys and rabbits by chemical and radiation agents. Acta Un. int. Cancr. 19, 708—709 (1963).

Miller, S. E., D. A. Holaday, and H. N. Doyle: Health protection of uranium miners and millers. Arch. industr. Hlth 14, 48—55 (1956).

Morrill, E. E., Jr.: Radioactive dust and gas in the uranium mines of Utah. Amer. industr. Hyg. Ass. J. 15, 269—276 (1954).

Morris, J. P.: Hazards in the radium and mesothorium refining plant at the University of Missouri. J. industr. Hyg. 20, 36 (1938).

Moshman, J., and A. H. Holland, Jr.: On the incidence of cancer in Oak Ridge, Tenn. Cancer 2, 567—575 (1949).

Murray, E. F.: Radium dial work claims 43d victim. N. Y. Times 1959.

Neitzel, E.: Berufsschädigungen durch radioactive Substanzen. Arbeitsmedizin Heft 1 (1935).

Neuman, W. F.: Urinary uranium as a measure of exposure hazard. Industr. Med. Surg. 19, 185—191 (1950).

Nielsen, G., and J. Kracht: Zur Cancerogenese nach diagnostischer Thorotrastanwendung. Frankfurt. Z. Path. 68, 661—667 (1958).

Official Report from Czechoslovakian Commission: Untersuchungen über die Gesundheit der Bergarbeiter auf den staatlichen Radiumgruben im Joachimstal in der Tschechoslowakei. Münch. med. Wschr. 82, 1666 (1935).

Park, J. F., W. J. Bair, and W. J. Clarke: Chronic toxicity of inhaled plutonium in dogs. Radiat. Res. 22, 222—223 (1964).

Parsons, W. D., A. J. de Villiers, L. S. Bartlett, and M. R. Becklake: Lung cancer in a fluorspar mining community. II. Prevalence of respiratory symptoms and Disability. Brit. J. industr. Med. 21, 110—116 (1964).

Peller, S.: Lung cancer among mine workers in Joachimsthal. Hum. Biol. 11, 130—143 (1939).

Pirchan, A., and H. Sikl: Cancer of the lung in the miners of Jáchymov (Joachimstal). Report of cases observed in 1929—1930. Amer. J. Cancer 16, 681—722 (1932).

Rajewsky, B.: Untersuchungen zum Problem der Radiumvergiftung; toxische Mengen des in den menschlichen Körper eingeführten Radiums. Strahlentherapie 56, 703 (1936).

— Bericht über die Schneeberger Untersuchungen. Z. Krebsforsch. 49, 315 (1939).

— Physikalische Diagnostik der Radiumvergiftungen. Strahlentherapie 69, 438—502 (1941).

—, A. Schraub, und G. Kahlau: Experimentelle Geschwulsterzeugung durch Einatmung von Radiumemanation. Naturwissenschaften 31, 170—171 (1943).

— —, and E. Schraub: Toxic dose of inspired radium emanation. Naturwissenschaften 30, 489—492 (1942).

RISEL, cited by A. THIELE: Die Schneeberger Lungenkrankheit, in Fabrikärzte der chemischen Industrie. Ärztl. Merkbl. über berufliche Erkrankungen. 3. Auflage Berlin: Springer 1930.

RÖSSLE, R.: Aussprache zu den Vorträgen. Z. Krebsforsch. 32, 686 (1930).

ROSTOSKI, O.: Clinical and radiological study of Schneeberg lung cancer. Rep. Int. Conf. on Cancer, London 1928.

—, and E. SAUPE: Gewerbehygienische und klinisch-röntgenologische Untersuchungen an den Erzbergleuten des Johanngeorgenstadter Grubenbezirkes in Sachsen. Arch. Gewerbepath. 1, 731 (1931).

— —, and G. SCHMORL: Die Bergkrankheit der Erzbergleute in Schneeberg in Sachsen (Schneeberger Lungenkrebs). Z. Krebsforsch 23, 360 (1926).

ROTH, F.: Thorotrastcarcinom der Bronchien. Zbl. Path. 96, 417—418 (1957).

SAUPE, E.: Bericht über eine roentgenologische Reihenuntersuchung in Joachimsthaler Bergleuten. Fortschr. Roentgenstr. 60, 163—171 (1939).

SCHEFFLER, C. L.: Die Gesundheit der Bergleute. Chemnitz 1770.

SCHLUNDT, H., W. McGAVOCK, Jr., and M. BROWN: Dangers in refining radioactive substances. J. industr. Hyg. 13, 117 (1931).

SCHMIDTMANN, M.: Experimentelle Untersuchungen über die Wirkung der Schneeberger Staubs auf das Bronchialepithel. Z. Krebsforsch. 32, 677 (1930).

SCHMOERL, G.: Über den Schneeberger Lungenkrebs. Verh. dtsch. path. Ges. 19, 192 (1923).

— Pathological study of Schneeberg lung cancer. Rep. Int. Conf. on Cancer, London 1928. Bristol: John Wright & Sons, Ltd., p. 272.

SEPKE, G.: Zum Schneeberger Lungenkrebs. Zbl. Arbeitsmed. 7, 114—116 (1957).

SETTER, L. R., C. E. ZIMMER, D. S. LICKING, and E. C. TABOR: Air-borne particulate beta radioactivity measurements of the national air sampling network — 1953—1959. Amer. industr. Hyg. Ass. J. 22, 192—200 (1961).

SHAPIRO, J.: An evelution of the pulmonary radiation dosage from radon and its daughter products. UR-298 Atomic Energy Project W-7401-University of Rochester Atomic Energy Project, 1954.

— Radiation dosage from breathing radon and its daughter products. Arch. industr. Hlth 14, 169—177 (1956).

SHERWOOD, R. J., and J. BEDFORD: A lead hazard in boiler cleaning. Arch. industr. Hlth 14, 92—95 (1956).

SIENKO, C., and G. COCCONI: Contamination of photographic emulsion caused by beta-active dust. Science 119, 422—423 (1954).

SIKL, H.: Über den Lungenkrebs der Bergleute in Joachimstal (Tschechoslowakei). Z. Krebsforsch. 32, 609—613 (1930).

— The present status of knowledge about the Jachymov disease (cancer of the lungs in the miners of the radium mines). Acta Un. int. Cancr. 6, 1366—1375 (1950).

STEIN: Radiumstrahlen und Lungenkrebs. Zbl. allg. Path. path. Anat. 103, 138 (1962).

STOCKLASA, J.: Die Bedeutung der Luftradioaktivität für die Entstehung des Joachimsthaler und Schneeberger Bergkrankheit. Dtsch. med. Wschr. 59, 1199—1200 (1933).

SULTZER, M., and J. B. HURSH: Polonium in urine of miners exposed to radon. Atomic Energy Proj. W-7401-eng.-49, UR-266, University of Rochester, N. Y. 1953.

— — Polonium in urine of miners exposed to radon. Arch. industr. Hyg. 9, 89—100 (1954).

TAJIAMA, E., and T. DOKE: Airborne radioactivity. Science 123, 211—214 (1956).

TELEKY, L.: Berufliche Radiumschädigungen. Wien. klin. Wschr. 16, 910 (1937); Wien. klin. Wschr. 50, 619—623 (1937).

— Occupational cancer of the lung. J. industr. Hyg. 19, 73—85 (1937).

— Der berufliche Lungenkrebs. Acta Un. int. Cancr. 3, 253—273 (1938).

TEMPLE, L. A., D. H. WILLARD, S. MARKS, and W. J. BAIR: Induction of lung tumours by radioactive particles. Nature 183, 408—409 (1959).

—, S. MARKS, and W. J. BAIR: Tumours in mice after pulmonary deposition of radioactive particles. Int. J. Radiat. Biol. 2, 143—156 (1960).

THIELE, A., O. ROSTOSKI, E. SAUPE, and G. SCHMORL: Über den Schneeberger Lungenkrebs. Münch. med. Wschr. 71, 24 (1924).

Tönges, E., and H. K. Kalbfleisch: Ein zweiter Fall von tödlicher Lungenfibrose infolge gewerblicher Radiumeinwirkung. Frankfurt. Z. Path. 50, 100 (1937).

Torrey, J. D., and P. W. Jacoe: Uranium mining operations on the Colorado plateau. Arch. industr. Hlth 12, 37—377 (1955).

Tschelnitz, H.: Physikalische Bemerkungen zur Ätiologie des St. Joachimsthaler Lungenkarzinoms. Strahlentherapie 53, 269—275 (1935).

Tsivoglou, E. C., and H. E. Ayer: Emanation of radon in uranium mines and control by ventilation. Arch. industr. Hyg. 8, 125—132 (1953).

Tullis, J. L.: Delayed effects of ionizing radiations in man. Arch. Path. 66, 403—417 (1958).

Uhlig, M.: Über den Schneeberger Lungenkrebs. Virchows Arch. path. Anat. 230, 76 (1921).

Ulmer, W. T., R. Nicolas, H. Muth, E. Oberhausen, and C. Onstead: Untersuchungen über den ^{40}K- und ^{138}Cs-Gehalt von Bergarbeitern. Int. Arch. Gewerbepath. 19, 571—580 (1962).

Unnewehr, F.: Durch Radoninhalation hervorgerufene Tumorbildung und Gewebsveränderung. (Tierexperimentelle Untersuchungen an Mäusen.) Strahlentherapie 108, 421—427 (1959).

van Esch, G. J., H. van Genderen, H. H. Vink: The induction of renal tumours by feeding of basic lead acetate to rats. Brit. J. Cancer 16, 289—297 (1962).

van Nieuwenhuyse, B.: Cancers du larynx aprés radiothérapie pour goître. Ann. Oto-laryng. 69, 230—232 (1952).

Vesin, M. S.: Cancer pulmonaire provoqué par les émanations radioactives. Arch. Mal. prof. 9, 280—283 (1948).

Vögtlin, J., and W. Minder: Über Thorotrastschäden nach Bronchographie, retrograder Pyelographie, Salpingographie und Arteriographie. Radiol. Clin. (Basel) 21, 96—115 (1952).

Waelsch, J. H.: Czechoslovak medical publications during the German occupation. I. Industrial diseases. Bull. Hyg. 21, 341—344 (1946).

Wagoner, J. K., V. E. Archer, B. E. Carroll, D. A. Holaday, and P. A. Lawrence: Cancer mortality patterns among U. S. uranium miners and millers, 1950 through 1962. J. nat. Cancer Inst. 32, 787—801 (1964).

—, R. W. Miller, F. E. Lundin, Jr., J. F. Fraumeni, Jr., and M. E. Haij: Unusual cancer mortality among a group of underground metal miners. New Engl. J. Med. 269, 284—289 (1963).

Warren, S.: Effects of radiation on normal tissues. Arch. Path. 34 (1942) and 35 (1943): 443—450; 562—608; 749—787; 917—931; 1070—1084; 121—139; 304—353.

—, and O. Gates: Radiation pneumonitis, experimental and pathologic observations. Arch. Path. 30, 440—460 (1940).

— — Production of bronchial carcinomas in mice. Amer. J. Path. 35, 669—1197 (1933).

—, and J. Spencer: Radiation reaction in lung. Amer. J. Roentgenol. 43, 682 (1940).

Warschowski, S.: Radium mines and miners in the Belgian Congo. Presse méd. 41, 1195—1197 (1933).

Watanabe, K.: The influence of radioactive dust on experimental pneumoconiosis. Tohoku J. exp. Med. 66, 131—143 (1957).

Weber, F. A.: Die Bergkrankheit der Erzbergleute in Schneeberg in Sachsen (Schneeberger Lungenkrebs). Arb. a. d. Reichsgesundheitsamt 57, 179—188 (1926).

Wegst, A. V., C. A. Pelletier, and G. H. Whipple: Detection and quantitation of fallout particles in a human lung. Science 143, 957—959 (1964).

Ziel, R.: Gesundheitstechnische Vorkehrungen bei der Radiumgewinnung in Joachimsthal. Med. Klinik 26, 623 (1930).

— La maladie minière à Joachimsthal. Bull. off. int. d'Hyg. publique. 26, 701—701 (1934).

— Zur Frage des Lungenkrebs bei den Bergleuten Joachimsthals. Med. Klinik 31, 1535 (1935).

Zuppinger, A.: Die Gefährdung durch ionisierende Strahlungen. Schweiz. med. Wschr. 88, 1171—1179 (1958).

Miscellaneous Respiratory Carcinogens
Isonicotinic Acid Hydrozide (Isoniacid)

Balo, J.: Lungenkarzinom und Lungenadenom. Budapest: Ungarische Akademie der Wissenschaften 1957.

—, E. Juhasz, and J. Temes: Pulmonary infarcts and pulmonary carcinoma. Cancer 9, 918—922 (1956).

BIANCIFIORI, C., E. BUCCIARELLI, F. E. SANTILLI, and R. RIBACCHI: Lung carcinogenesis by isonicotinic acid hydrazide and its metabolites in CBA/Cb/Se mice. Lav. Ist. Anat. Univ. Perugia 23, 209—220 (1963).
—, and R. RIBACCHI: The induction of pulmonary tumors in BALB/c mice by oral administration of isoniazid. In L. SEVERI (ed.): The morphological precursors of cancer. Perugia, 1962.
— — Pulmonary tumours in mice induced by oral isoniazid and its metabolites. Nature 194, 488—489 (1962).
— —, E. BUCCIARELLI, F. P. DI LEO, ed U. MILIA: Cancerogenesi polmonare da idrazina solfato in topi femmine BALB/c. Lav. Ist. Anat. Univ. Perugia, 23, 115—128 (1963).
— — — — — Lung cancerogenesis by hydrazine sulfate in female BALB/c mice. Lav. Ist. Anat. Perugia 23, 115—128 (1963).
BOYSEN, J. E.: Health hazards associated with selected propellants. Arch. environ. Health 7, 71 (1963).
DEICHMANN, W. B., W. E. MACDONALD, W. A. D. ANDERSON, and E. BERNAL: Adenocarcinoma in the lungs of mice exposed to vapors of 3-nitro-3-hexene. Toxicol. appl. Pharmacol. 5, 445—456 (1963).
DI LEO, F. P., and U. MILIA: Problemi biochimici nella tumorioenesi polmonare sperimentale da isoniazide e idrazina. Lav. Ist. Anat. Univ. Perugia 23, 129—143 (1963).
HUEPER, W. C.: Über die intravenöse Kampferölinjektion auf Grund pathologisch-anatomischer Untersuchungen. Med. Klinik 12, 8 (1922).
— Methodologic explorations in experimental respiratory carcinogenesis. Arzneimittel-Forsch. 14, 814—822 (1964).
JUHASZ, J., J. BALO, and G. KENDREY: Über die geschwulsterzeugende Wirkung des Isonicotinsäurehydrazid (INH). Z. Krebsforsch. 62, 188—196 (1957).
— — — Experimental investigation of the cancerogenic action of isonicotinic acid hydrazide (INH). Tuberk. Kérd. 10, 49—54 (1957).
— —, and B. SZENDE: Neue experimentelle Angaben zur geschwulsterzeugenden Wirkung des Isonicotinsäurehydrazid (INH). Z. Krebsforsch. 65, 434—438 (1963).
MORI, K.: Induction and transplantation of cancer of the lung in rats. Gann 54, 415—525 (1963).
—, A. YASUNO, and K. MATSUMOTO: Induction of pulmonary tumours in mice with iso nicotinic acid hydrazide. Gann 51, 83—89 (1960).
PANSA, E., A. PICCO, and M. GNAVI: Sul problema del supposto effetto carcinogenetico dell'acido isonicotinico (IAI). Minerva med. 53, 3162—3168 (1962).
RIBACCHI, R., C. BIANCIFIORI, U. MILIA, F. P. DI LEO, and E. BUCCIARELLI: Cancerogenesi polmonare da idrazide dell'acido isonicotinico in topi maschi BALB/c, con e senza MTV. Lav. Ist. Anat. Univ. Perugia 23, 103—114 (1963).
RÖSSLE, R.: Schweiz. med. Wschr. 73, 1200 (1943).
SCHWAN, S.: Isonicotinic acid hydrazide (INH) as a cancerogenic agent in mice. Pat. pol. 12, 53—56 (1961).
STANTON, M. F., and C. J. BLACKWELL: Induction of epidermoid carcinoma in lungs of rats: A "new" method based upon deposition of methylcholanthrene in areas of pulmonary infarction. J. nat. Cancer Inst. 27, 375—407 (1961).
STRAUSS, F. H., E. DORDAL, and A. KAPPAS: The problem of pulmonary scar tumors. A case report and brief review. Arch. Path. 76, 693—699 (1963).
VIALLIER, J., et F. CASANOVA: L'isoniazide a-t-il des propriétés cancérigènes? Essai sur l'animal. C. R. Soc. Biol. 154, 985—987 (1960).
WEINSTEIN, H. J., and R. KINOSITA: Isoniazid and pulmonary tumors in mice. Amer. Rev. resp. Dis. 88, 124—125 (1963).

Nitrosamines

ARGUS, M. F., and C. HOCH-LIGETI: Comparative study of the carcinogenic activity of nitrosamines. J. nat. Cancer Inst. 27, 695—709 (1961).
— — Induction of malignant tumors in the Guinea pig by oral administration of diethylnitrosamine. J. nat. Cancer Inst. 30, 533—551 (1963).

ARNDT, F., B. EISTERT, and W. WALTER: The question of the physiological activity, including carcinogenicity of alkylnitrosamides used in the manufacture of diazoalkanes. Naturwissenschaften 50, 379—380 (1963).

BOYSEN, J. E.: Health hazards of selected rocket propellants. Arch. environm. Hlth 7, 71—75 (1963).

DONTENWILL, W., and U. MOHR: Carcinome des Respirationstractus nach Behandlung von Goldhamstern mit Diäthylnitrosamin. Z. Krebsforsch. 64, 305—312 (1961).

— — Die organotrope Wirkung der Nitrosamine. Z. Krebsforsch. 65, 166—167 (1962).

— — Vergleichende Untersuchungen an metaplastischen und malignen Epithelwucherungen des Respirationstraktes im Tierexperiment. Z. Krebsforsch. 65, 168—170 (1962).

— —, and M. ZAGEL: Über die unterschiedliche Lungencarcinogene Wirkung des Diäthylnitrosamin bei Hamster und Ratte. Z. Krebsforsch. 64, 499—502 (1962).

DRUCKREY, H., S. IVANKOVIC, and R. PREUSSMANN: Selective production of brain tumors in rats by methylnitrosourea. Naturwissenschaften 51, 144 (1964).

—, and R. PREUSSMANN: Erzeugung von Lungenkrebs durch subcutane Injektion von N,N-Diamylnitrosamin an Ratten. Naturwissenschaften 49, 111—112 (1962).

— — Zur Entstehung carcinogener Nitrosamine am Beispiel des Tabakrauchs. Naturwissenschaften 49, 498—499 (1962).

— — N-Nitroso-N-methyl-urethane: A potent carcinogen. Nature 195, 1111 (1962).

— —, J. AFKHAM, and G. BLUM: Erzeugung von Lungenkrebs durch Methylnitrosourethan bei intravenöser Gabe an Ratten. Naturwissenschaften 49, 451—452 (1962).

— —, G. BLUM, and S. IVANKOVIC: Carcinogenic effect of diazomethane ethylacetate and an ester of N-nitrososarcosine as an example of the transport-form, active-form principle. Naturwissenschaften 50, 100—101 (1963).

— —, and D. SCHMÄHL: Carcinogenicity and chemical structure of nitrosamines. Acta Un. int. Cancr. 19, 510—512 (1963).

— — —, and M. MÜLLER: Erzeugung von Blasenkrebs an Ratten mit N,N-Dibutylnitrosamin. Naturwissenschaften 49, 19 (1962).

—, A. SCHILDBACH, D. SCHMÄHL, R. PREUSSMANN, und S. IVANKOVIC: Quantitative Analyse der carcinogenen Wirkung von Diäthylnitrosamin. Arzneimittel-Forsch. 13, 841—851 (1963).

—, D. STEINHOFF, R. PREUSSMANN, and S. IVANKOVIC: Krebserzeugung durch einmalige Dosis von Methylnitrosoharnstoff und verschiedenen Dialkyl-nitrosaminen. Naturwissenschaften 50, 735 (1963).

— — — — Erzeugung von Krebs durch eine einmalige Dosis von Methylnitroso-Harnstoff und verschiedenen Dialkylnitrosaminen an Ratten. Z. Krebsforsch. 66, 1—10 (1964).

GRUNDMANN, E., and H. SIEBURG: Die Histogenese und Cytogenese des Lebercarcinoms der Ratte durch Diäthylnitrosamin im lichtmikroskopischen Bild. Beitr. pat. Anat. 126, 57—90 (1962).

HENSCHLER, D., and W. ROSS: Zur Frage der Bildung cancerogener Nitrosamine aus Gewebsaminen und inhalierten Stickstoffoxyden. Naturwissenschaften 50, 503 (1963).

HERROLD, K. McD., and L. J. DUNHAM: Effects of subcutaneous injection of diethylnitrosamine in the Syrian hamster. Proc. Amer. Assoc. Cancer Res. 4, 28 (1963).

— — Induction of tumors in the Syrian hamster with diethylnitrosamine (N-Nitrosodiethylamine). Cancer Res. 23, 773—777 (1963).

MAGEE, P. N.: Carcinogenesis by nitrosocompounds with special reference to alkylation of nucleic acids. 8th Internat. Cancer Congr., Moscow, 1962, p. 19.

—, and J. M. BARNES: Induction of kidney tumours in the rat with dimethylnitrosamine (N-nitrosodimethylamine). J. Path. Bact. 84, 19—31 (1962).

SCHOENTAL, R.: Carcinogenic action of diazomethane and of nitroso-N-methyl urethane. Nature 188, 420—421 (1960).

— Experimental induction of squamous carcinoma of the lung, oesophagus and stomach. 8th Internat. Cancer Congr. Moscow, 1962, p. 175—176.

— Experimental induction os spuamous carcinoma of the lung, oesophagus, and stomach. The mode of their induction. Acta Un. int. Cancr. 19, 680—683 (1963).

— Induction of tumours of the stomach in rats and mice by N-nitroso-N-alkylurethanes. Nature 199, 190 (1963).

SCHOENTAL, R., and P. N. MAGEE: Induction of squamous carcinoma of the lung and of the stomach and oesophagus by diazomethane and N-methyl-N-nitroso-urethane, respectively. Brit. J. Cancer 16, 92—100 (1962).

TAKAYAMA, S., and K. OOTA: Malignant tumours induced in mice fed with N-nitroso-dimethylamine. Gann 54, 465—472 (1963).

THOMAS, C.: Zur Morphologie der durch Diäthylnitrosamin erzeugten Leberveränderungen und Tumoren bei der Ratte. Z. Krebsforsch. 64, 224—233 (1961).

—, and G. KERSTING: Morphology of cerebral tumors of rats induced by methylnitrosourea. Naturwissenschaften 51, 144—145 (1964).

—, and D. SCHMÄHL: Zur Morphologie der durch intravenöse Injektion von Nitrosomethyl-urethan erzeugten Lungentumoren bei der Ratte. Z. Krebsforsch. 65, 294—302 (1963).

ZAK, F. G., J. H. HOLZNER, E. J. SINGER, and H. POPPER: Renal and pulmonary tumors in rats fed dimethylnitrosamine. Cancer Res. 20, 96—99 (1960).

Nitroquinolines and Related Nitro- and Amino-Compounds

CHINO, T.: Experimental production of labial and lingual carcinoma by local application of 4-nitroquinoline N-oxide. Fukuoka Acta med. 53, 1053—1070 (1963).

ENDO, H., and F. KUME: Induction of sarcoma in rats by subcutaneous injection of 4-hydro-xylaminoquinoline N-oxide. Naturwissenschaften 50, 525—526 (1963).

HAYASHI, Y., N. KANIZAWA, and G. IDE: Histochemical study on experimental inhalation of p-benzoquinone. I. Lung tissue of mice, with emphasis on peripheral bronchioles. Jap. J. Cancer. Clin. 9, 167—168 (1963).

KISHIZAWA, F.: Para-benzochinon. Carcinogenic action of para-benzoquinone on the lung of mice by the experimental inhalation. Gann 45, 389—391 (1954).

LACASSAGNE, A., N. P. BUU-HOI, and F. ZAJDELA: Inégale efficacité du 4-nitroquinoléine-N-oxyde, dans la production d'épithéliomas de la peau chez deux lignées différentes de souris. C. R. Soc. Biol. 155, 444—446 (1961).

— — — Production de sarcomes, chez la souris, par injections de 4-nitroquinoléine-N-oxyde et de 4-nitroquinaldine-N-oxyde. C. R. Soc. Biol. 154, 528—530 (1960).

MORI, K.: Induction of pulmonary tumors in rats by subcutaneous injections of 4-nitro-quinoline 1-oxide. Gann 53, 303—308 (1952).

— Preliminary note on adenocarcinoma of the lung in mice induced with 4-nitroquinoline N-oxide. Gann 52, 265—270 (1961).

— Experimental induction of pulmonary tumors in mice. J. Showa med. Ass. 22, 51—52 (1962).

—, and A. YASUNO: Induction of pulmonary tumors in mice by subcutaneous injection of 4-nitroquinoline N-oxide. Gann 52, 149—154 (1961).

NAKAHARA, W., and F. FUKUOKA: Study of carcinogenic mechanism based on experiments with 4-nitroquinoline N-oxide. Gann 50, 1—15 (1959).

— —, and S. SAKAI: The relation between carcinogenicity and chemical structure of certain quinoline derivatives. Gann 49, 33—41 (1958).

SHIRASU, Y.: Further studies on carcinogenic action of 4-hydroxyaminoquinoline 1-oxide. Gann 54, 487—495 (1963).

—, and A. OHTA: A preliminary note on the carcinogenicity of 4-hydroxaminoquinoline 1-oxide. Gann 54, 221—228 (1963).

TAKAYAMA, S.: Skin carcinogenesis with a single painting of 4-nitroquinoline N-oxide. Gann 51, 139—145 (1960).

— Effect of 4-nitroquinoline N-oxide painting on azo dye hepatocarcinogenesis in rats, with note on induction of skin fibrosarcoma. Gann 52, 165—172 (1961).

— Carcinogenic action of 6-chloro-4-nitroquinoline 1-oxide on the rat skin. Gann. 52, 167 (1962).

TAKIZAWA, N.: Über die experimentelle Erzeugung der Haut- und Lungenkrebse bei der Maus durch Bepinselung mit Chinone. Gann 34, 158—160 (1940).

— On the carcinogenic action of certain quinones. Preliminary report. Proc. Imperial Academy (Tokyo) 16, 309—312 (1940).

—, and S. KANIZAWA: Experimental induction of pulmonary carcinoma. Jap. J. Cancer Clin. 9, 172—173 (1963).

URI, J., R. BOGNAR, and I. BEKESI: Fungicidal effect of methyl derivatives of 8-hydro-oxyquinoline on dermatophytes. Acta microbiol. Acad. Sci. Hung. 4, 279—287 (1957).

Carbamates

BALL, J. N., and P. N. COWEN: Urethane as a carcinogen and as an anaesthetic for fishes. Nature 18, suppl. 6, 370 (1959).

BALO, J.: Lungenkarzinom und Lungenadenom. Budapest: Ungarische Akademie der Wissenschaften 1957.

BARTALINI, E.: L'azione dello Zineb (etilenbisditiocarbammato di zinco) sull'uomo. Med. d. Lavoro 53, 45—59 (1962).

CRAMER, H. J.: Berufliche Kontaktekzeme bei Masseuren durch Allylthiocarbamid. Berufsdermatosen 10, 148—154 (1962).

ESKOLA, O.: Case of aleukia haemorrhagica (Frank) and pammyelophthisis after urethane treatment in leukemia. Acta med. scand. 133, 261 (1949).

FIORE-DONATI, L., L. CHIECO-BIANCHI, G. DE BENEDICTIS, and G. MAIORANO: Leukaemogenesis by urethan in new-born Swiss mice. Nature 190, 278—279 (1961).

—, G. DE BENEDICTIS, G. MAIORANO, and L. CHIECO-BIANCHI: Development of pulmonary adenomas in mice suckled by mothers receiving urethan. Naturwissenschaften 48, 409—410 (1961).

FUKUI, K., C. NAGATA, A. IMAMURA, and Y. TAGASHIRA: On the relation between electronic structure and carcinogenic activity of urethan (ethylcarbamate) and related compounds. Gann 52, 127—134 (1961).

GUYER, M. F., and P. E. CLAUS: Tumor of the lung in rats following injections of urethane (ethyl carbamate). Cancer Res. 7, 342—345 (1947).

HADDOW, A., W. A. SEXTON: Influence of carbamic esters (urethanes) on experimental animal tumours. Nature 157, 500—503 (1946).

HENSHAW, P. S.: Minimal number of anesthetic treatments with urethane required to induce pulmonary tumours. J. nat. Cancer Inst. 4, 523—525 (1944).

HUEPER, W. C.: Carcinogenic studies on isopropyl-N-phenyl carbamate. Industr. Med. Surg. 21, 71—74 (1952).

— Carcinogenic studies on water-insoluble polymers. Path. microbiol. (Basel) 24, 77—106 (1961).

JAFFE, W. G.: Carcinogenic action of ethyl urethane on rats. Cancer Res. 7, 107—112 (1947).

KLEIN, M.: The transplacental effect of urethane on lung tumorigenesis in mice. J. nat. Cancer Inst. 12, 1003—1010 (1952).

— Lung adenomas in offspring following injection of pregnant mice with urethan. Cancer Res. 12, 275 (1952).

— Influence of urethan on lung tumorigenesis in immature, newborn, and fetal mice. Proc. Amer. Ass. Cancer Res. 1, 26 (1954).

KYLE, R. A., R. S. SCHWARTZ, H. L. OLINER, and W. DAMESHEK: Syndrome clinically resembling adrenal cortical insufficiency associated with long term Busulfan (myleran) therapy. Blood 18, 497 (1961).

LARSEN, C. D.: Evaluation of the carcinogenicity of a series of esters of carbamic acid. J. nat. Cancer Inst. 8, 99—101 (1947).

— Pulmonary-tumor induction with alkylated urethans. J. nat. Cancer Inst. 9, 35 (1948).

— Pulmonary-tumor induction by transplacental exposure to urethane. J. nat. Cancer Inst. 8, 63—70 (1947).

—, and W. E. HESTON: Induction of pulmonary tumors in mice by anesthetic agents. Cancer Res. 5, 592 (1945).

MOSTOFI, F. K., and C. D. LARSEN: Pulmonary lesions induced in Wistar rats by urethane. Amer. J. Path. 25, 807—808 (1949).

NETTLESHIP, A., and P. S. HENSHAW: Induction of pulmonary tumors in mice with ethyl carbamate (urethane). J. nat. Cancer Inst. 4, 309—319 (1943).

NISHIMURA, H., and M. KUGINUKI: Congenital malformations induced by ethyl-carbamate in mouse embryos. Okajima Fol. anat. Jap. 31, 1—10 (1958).

RITCHIE, A. C.: Epidermal carcinogenesis in the mouse by intraperitoneally administered urethane followed by repeated applications of croton oil. Brit. J. Cancer 11, 206—211 (1957).

ROSIN, A.: Early changes in the lungs of rats treated with urethane (ethyl carbamate). Cancer Res. 9, 583—588 (1949).

SALAMAN, M. H., and F. J. C. ROE: Incomplete carcinogens: ethyl carbamate (urethane) as an initiator of skin tumour formation in the mouse. Brit. J. Cancer 7, 472—481 (1953).

SCHOENTAL, R.: Carcinogenic action of diazomethane and of nitroso-N-methyl urethane. Nature 188, 420—421 (1960).

SHABAD, L. M., and L. P. NAUMOVA: Investigation of the posssible blastomogenic action of certain substances inhibiting sprouting of vegetables in storage. Vop. Pitan. 15, 27—32 (1956).

TANNENBAUM, A., and C. MALTONI: Neoplastic response of various tissues to the administration of urethan. Cancer Res. 22, 1105 (1962).

VAN ESCH, G. J., H. VAN GENDEREN, and H. H. VINK: The production of skin tumours in mice by oral treatment with urethane, isopropyl-N-phenyl-carbamate or isopropyl-N-chlorophenyl-carbamate in combination with skin painting with croton oil and Tween 60. Brit. J. Cancer 12, 355—362 (1958).

Chlorinated Hydrocarbons

DAVIS, K. J., and O. G. FITZHUGH: Tumorigenic potential of aldrin and dieldrin. Toxicol. appl. Pharmacol. 4, 187—189 (1962).

DELLA PORTA, G., B. TERRACINI, and P. SHUBIK: Induction with carbon tetrachloride of liver cell carcinomas in hamsters. J. nat. Cancer Inst. 26, 857—863 (1961).

EDWARDS, J. E., E. H. HESTON, and A. J. DALTON: Induction of the carbon tretrachloride hepatoma in strain L mice. J. nat. Cancer Inst. 3, 297—301 (1942).

FITZHUGH, O. G., and A. A. NELSON: The chronic oral toxicity of DDT. J. Pharm. exp. Ther. 89, 18—30 (1947).

GARDNER, W. U., and J. BODDAERT: Testicular interstitial cell tumors in hybrid mice given tri-p-anisyl-chloroethylene. Arch. Path. 50, 750—764 (1950).

HARGRAVE: cited by R. CARSON, in *Silent Spring*.

HUEPER, W. C.: Unpublished information.

NELSON, A. A.: Carcinogenic substances in food. Int. Rec. Med. 169, 47—49 (1956).

— Personal communication on "Liver tumors in dogs".

POPPER, H., S. S. STERNBERG, D. L. OSER, and H. OSER: The carcinogenic effect of aramite in rats. Cancer 13, 1035—1046 (1960).

RANDIG, K.: Lungenkrebs bei einem Jugendlichen Chemielaboranten. Zbl. Arbeitsmed. 6, 110—111 (1956).

STERNBERG, S. S., H. POPPER, B. L. OSER, and H. OSER: Gallbladder and bile duct adenocarcinomas in dogs after long term feeding of aramite. Cancer 13, 780—789 (1960).

TULLNER, W. W.: Uterotrophic action of the insecticide methoxychlor. Science 33, 647 (1961).

Formaldehyde

BOURNE, H. G., Jr., and S. SEFERMANN: Wrinkle-proofed clothing may liberate toxic quantities of formaldehyde. Industr. Med. 28, 232—233 (1959).

FISHER, A. A., N. B. KANOF, and E. M. BIONDI: Free formaldehyde in textiles and paper. Arch. Derm. 86, 753 (1962).

GARSCHIN, W. G., and L. M. SHABAD: Atypical growth of bronchial epithelium after the introduction of formalin int the lung. Z. Krebsforsch. 43, 137—145 (1935).

GLASS, W. I.: An outbreak of formaldehyde dermatitis. N. Z. med. J. 60, 423—427 (1961).

HENSON, E. V.: The toxicology of some aliphatic aldehydes. J. occup. Med. 1, 457—462 (1959).

HORTON, A. W., R. TYE, and K. L. STEMMER: Experimental carcinogenesis of the lung. Inhalation of gaseous formaldehyde or an aerosol of coal tar by C3H mice. J. nat. Cancer Inst. 30, 31—43 (1963).

LUTZ, G.: Formalinekzeme bei Buchdruckern. Zbl. Gewerbehyg. 17, 266—268 (1930).

WATANABE, F., T. MATSUNAGA, T. SOEJIMA, and Y. IWATA: Study on the carcinogenicity of aldehyde. First report. Experimentally produced rat sarcomas by repeated injections of aqueous solution of formaldehyde. Gann 45, 451—452 (1954).

—, and S. SUGIMOTO: Study on the carcinogenicity of aldehyde. Second report. Seven cases of transplantable sarcomas of rats appearing in the areas of repeated subcutaneous injections of urotropin. Gann 46, 365—366 (1955).

Natural and Man-Made Polymers

BERGMANN, M., I. J. FLANCE, and H. T. BLUMENTHAL: Thesaurosis following inhalation of hair spray. A clinical and experimental study. N. Engl. J. Med. **258**, 471—476 (1958).

— —, P. T. CRUZ, N. KLAM, P. R. ARONSON, R. A. JOSHI, and H. T. BLUMENTHAL: Thesaurosis due to inhalation of hair spray. Report of twelve new cases, including three autopsies. N. Engl. J. Med. **266**, 750—755 (1962).

BRESLOW, L.: Occupational factors in lung cancer. A preliminary report. Publ. Hlth Rep. **68**, 286—288 (1953).

BRUNNER, M. J., R. P. GIOVACCHINI, J. P. WYATT, F. E. DUNLAP, and J. C. CALANDRA: Pulmonary disease and hair spray polymers: A disputed relationship. J. Amer. med. Ass. **184**, 851—857 (1963).

CARES, R. M.: Thesaurosis from inhaled hair spray? Arch. environm. Hlth **11**, 80—85 (1965).

DOYLE, J. A., M. GOLONBEK, and M. R. RAMIREZ: Experimental study. Arch. Histol. Norm. Pat. **8**, 290—296 (1963).

DRAIZE, J. H., A. A. NELSON, S. H. NEWBURGER, and E. A. KELLEY: Inhalation toxicity studies of six types of aerosol hair sprays. Proc. Sci. Section Toilet Goods Assoc. **31**, 5 (1959).

EDELSTON, B. G.: Thesaurosis following inhalation of hair spray. Lancet. **1959**, 112—113.

Editorial: Thesaurosis following inhalation of hair spray. Lancet. **1959**, 412.

— Thesaurosis caused by hair spray. J. Amer. med. Ass. **176**, 1055—1056 (1961).

— Hair sprays and health. J. Amer. med. Ass. **181**, 632 (1962).

HUEPER, W. C.: Macromolecular substances as pathogenic agents. Arch. Path. **33**, 267—290 (1942).

— Experimental carcinogenic studies in macromolecular chemicals. I. Neoplastic reactions in rats and mice after parenteral introduction of polyvinyl pyrrolidones. Cancer **10**, 8—18 (1957).

— Carcinogenic studies on water-soluble and insoluble macromolecules. Arch. Path. **67**, 589—617 (1959).

— Macromolecular agents as benign and malignant cell proliferants. Nat. Cancer. Inst. Monogr. **14**, 357—377 (1964).

— Cancer induction by polyurethane and polysilicone plastics. J. nat. Cancer Inst. (In press.)

JOHN, H. H.: Thesaurosis: A survey of those at risk. The med. Officer **109**, 399—400 (1963).

QUESTIONS and ANSWERS: Hair spray and blood dyscrasias. J. Amer. med. Ass. **188**, 197 (1964).

Subject Index

2-Acetylaminofluorene lung cancers 10, 150
Acid workers 7
Air Pollutants, arsenic 31
— —, asbestos 41, 50
— —, 3,4-benzpyrene 27, 81, 94, 112, 114
— —, beryllium 99
— —, carbon black 113
— —, chromium 72, 75, 81, 83
— —, coal tar 113, 114
— —, iron 94
— —, nickel 86
— —, radioactive chemicals 145
Aliphatic epoxides 118
Alkali workers 7
Anthracosis 2
Arsenic 8, 9, 11, 22, 24, 25, 28, 30—38
—, carcinogenic dose 33, 36
— cancer 32
— —, experimental 36
— —, occupations 33—35
— content air 31
— — biologic material 37
— — food 31
— — water 31
— — soil 32
— — tobacco 31
—, occupational larynx cancer 34, 35
—, — lung cancer 33
—, — paranasal sinus cancer 34, 35
— poisoning animals 32
Asbestos 8, 9, 11, 14, 22, 23, 38—56
—, anticarcinogenic action 53
— cancers 40, 41
— —, causative mechanisms 55
— —, cigarette smoking 54
— —, age distribution 52
— —, experimental 54—55
— —, latent period 54
— —, sex distribution 53
— —, syncarcinogenesis 54
— carcinoma lung 42—50
— —, lung, pathology 47—50
— chrysotile 39, 50
— crocidolite 39, 50
— exposure stigmata 40
— nonoccupational exposures 40, 41
— occupational exposures 40

— products 40
— technologic data 38
— mesothelioma, epidemiology 50—52
— —, peritoneum 39, 40, 41, 45, 50—53
— —, pleura 39, 41, 42, 50—53
— warts 40
Asbestosis 40, 41
—, epidemiology 41, 42—47
Asphalt, native 120
Atmospheric pollutants 12, 23
Atomic energy plants lung cancers 142
Automobile exhaust 123—125

Bagassosis 2, 6
—, lung cancer hazard 152
Benzidin 9, 10, 151
3,4-Benzpyrene air 11, 81, 97, 112, 114
— asbestos cancers 56
Beryl 99, 100
Berylliosis, nonoccupational 100
—, occupational 100
Beryllium 9, 10, 23
—, technologic data 99
— cancer, experimental bone 100
— —, — lung 100
— content biologic material 102
—, exposure non-occupational 100
—, — occupational 100
— lung cancer 101
— — —, allergy 102
— — —, beryllium-protein complex 102
— — —, causal mechanism 102
— — —, smoking 101
Boiler scalers 94, 96
Bronchitis, chronic 1, 3, 7

Cabinet makers 7
Carbamate 10, 11
Carbon polymers 11
— —, water insoluble lung cancer hazard 153
— —, water soluble lung cancer hazard 153
— black 113, 118
Carnotite 138
Carcinogenic symptom complex 21
Chlorinated hydrocarbons lung cancer hazard 151

Chromates 7—9, 12, 13, 15, 22, 24, 25, 28, 79, 81
Chrome cancer hazards intraplant 59
— — — periplant 58, 64, 72
— cancers, clinical aspects 70
— —, chromate proceducers 57, 59
— —, experimental 68—70
— —, former workers 62
— —, larynx 59
— —, latent period 64
— —, lung epidemiology 59—64
— —, — histologic types 65—70
— —, mesothelioma 65
— —, nasal sinus 59
— —, negroes 63
— pigments 58, 59, 77
— — cancers 58, 59
Chromitosis 68
Chromite ore 57, 60, 76
Chromium 56—85
—, air pollution 83
—, plant air 73, 74, 75
— products 57
—, technologic data 57
—, water pollution 83
— carcinogenesis 80—82
— —, allergy 82
— —, biologic availability 81
— —, fuel products 81
— —, valence 81
— content, biologic materials 70—72
— exposure, nonoccupational 57, 58
— —, occupational 57, 58
— —, stigmata 56—57, 63
— lung cancer, colored workers 75
— — —, experimental 76—80
— — —, medical prophylaxis 84
— — —, prevention 82—84
— — —, smoking 75
Cigarette makers 6
— tar cancers, lung 108
— — —, skin 108
Coal combustion products 107
— distillation products, paraffin 107, 108
— — —, tar oils 107, 108
— economy 108
— miners 2
— pitch 107
— soot 107
— tar, air pollution 113
— — exposure, occupational 108—114
— — fumes 8, 9, 11, 14, 16, 21, 22, 24, 28
— — —, 3,4-benzpyrene content 112
— — oils 107, 108
— —, respiratory cancer hazards 108, 109
— —, technologic data 107
— — workers, larynx cancers 109

Coal tar workers, lung cancers 109
— — —, paranasal sinus cancers 109
— — cancers, experimental 113, 114
— — —, skin 108
— — —, multicentric 112
— — lung cancers, incidence 110
— — — —, epidemiology 109—111
Cobalt miners 127
Coke oven workers lung cancer 109—112
Colorado plateau lung cancers 133, 138
Cutting oil additive 125
— — cancers, experimental 125
— oils 118, 119

DDT, lung cancer hazard 152
Diesel engine exhaust 123, 124
Dust, mineral 2
—, vegetable 6

Electrometallurgical workers, lung cancer 113
Epoxides, aliphatic and aromatic 10, 11
Ethyl carbamate, lung cancer 151

Fluorspar miners 131
Food contaminants 12, 23, 31
Formalaldehyde, lung cancer hazard 152
Foundry workers 94, 96, 112

Gas house workers, lung cancer 109—111
Gasoline 118
— additive 124
—, oxidized 10, 11
Glass 5
Grain dockers 6

Hair lacquer 12, 153
Hard rock miners 133
Hematite miners 94
Hydrogenated coal oils 118
8-Hydroxyquinoline 12

Iatrogenic carcinogens 12
Infarct, lung 1
Ionizing radiations 125
— — generators 125
Iron, asbestos cancers 55
— -carbohydrate complex 98
—, exposure non-occupational 94
—, — occupational 94, 96
—, technologic data 93
— larynx cancer 96, 98
— lung cancer, 3,4-benzpyrene 97
— — —, causal mechanism 98
— — —, epidemiology 94—96
— — —, experimental 97
— — —, incidence 96
— — —, smoking 96

Iron oxide 9, 10
— —, carcinogenic carrier 98
— polishers 94
Irritants, industrial 1, 3, 8
Isoniacid 10, 13
—, lung cancer 148
Isonicotinic acid hydrazide 148
Isopropyl alcohol 104—106
— oil 8, 9, 22
— —, chemical composition 106
— —, polymers 107
— —, technologic data 105
— — cancers, epidemiology 106
— — larynx cancer 106
— — lung cancer 106
— — nasal sinus cancer 106
— — respiratory cancers, experimental 107

Larynx cancer 8, 16, 22, 24, 30, 34, 35, 56, 59, 96, 104, 106, 109, 145
Lost see mustard gas 103
Luminous dial painters paranasal sinus cancers 143
Lung cancer, anthracosis 2
Lung cancers, epidemiology demographic distribution 26
— — —, emigrants 26
— —, experimental silica 5
— —, former workers 15, 61, 62
— —, infarct 1, 148
— —, occupational age distribution 24
— — —, attack rates 24
— — —, coal tar workers 109
— — —, epidemiology 14
— — —, exposure period 27
— — —, histologic types 28
— — —, household 21, 23, 100
— — —, intraplant spread 23
— — —, lag period 27
— — —, latent period 27
— — —, medicolegal aspects 15
— — —, neighborhood cancers 23, 41, 72, 81, 100
— — —, nuclear energy installations 142
— — —, radiation workers 142
— — —, radioactive wastes 142
— — —, radium laboratories 142
— — —, regional industries 17, 18
— — —, sex distribution 22
— — —, socioeconomic classes 16
— — —, trades and professions 16
— — —, women 21
— —, pneumoconiosis 2—7
— —, scar 1, 3, 6, 129
— —, silicosis 2—6
— —, traumatic 2
— —, tuberculous scar 148

Mesothelioma asbestos 25, 27, 40, 41
—, chromates 65
Metal ore miners 133
— smelter workers 7
Methylated naphthalene 118
Mineral oil 7—9, 11, 12, 16, 22, 24, 25
— oils see petroleum
Motor exhaust 10
Mustard gas 8, 9, 22
— —, anticarcinogen 105
— —, poisoning 103
— —, technologic data 103
— — cancer, causal mechanism 105
— — —, experimental 105
— — —, larynx 104
— — —, lung 103
— — —, nasal sinus 104
— — exposure, occupational 103, 104
— — —, non-occupational 103, 104
— — respiratory cancer, incidence 104

Negroes, chromium lung cancer 75
Newfoundland, lung cancers 131
Nickel 8, 9, 11, 22
— content, biologic material 90
—, gasoline additive 86, 93
—, technologic data 85
— cancer, experimental 91, 92
— carbonyl 85, 86
— exposure, nonoccupational 86
— —, occupational 86
— —, smoking 86
— larynx cancer 87
— lung cancer, incidence 87
— paranasal sinus cancer, incidence 87
— refinery workers 86, 87
— respiratory cancer, allergy 89
— — —, alkali 88—90
— — —, arsenic 88, 89
— — —, causative mechanism 93
— — —, exposure time 88
— — —, latent period 88
— — —, pathology 89
— — —, prevention 93
— — —, sequential appearance 88
Nitro-olefins 118
Nitroquinolines lung cancer 150
4-Nitroquinoline-1-oxide 10
Nitrosamines 10, 11, 29
—, lung cancer 150
—, paranasal sinus cancers 150

Ocher miners 97
Oil economy 108
— pneumonitis 121
Oils, vegetable oxidized and polymerized, lung cancer hazard 152

Painters 7
Paranasal sinus cancer 8, 22, 24, 25, 28, 34,
    35, 56, 59, 104, 106, 109, 143, 146
Pesticides 6
Petroleum, natural sources 118, 120
—, technologic data 118
— asphalt 118
— oil 118
— —, uses 120, 21
— — cancers, larynx 121
— — —, lung 120
— — —, skin 118
— paraffins 118
— wax 118
— — cancers, man 122
— — —, experimental 122
Pluripotentiality, respiratory carcinogens
    21, 29
Pneumoconiosis 2—7
Pneumonitis, chemical 7
Polyetiology, respiratory cancers 29
Polymer cancers, asbestos 55, 56
— —, isopropyl oil 107
Polypropylenes 106
Polyurethanes, lung cancer hazard 151

Quartz 5

Radioactive chemicals 8, 9, 22, 125
— exposures, nonoccupational 126
— —, occupational 126
— fallout 125, 126
— mines global aspects 135
— ore miners 127
— — —, Joachimsthal 137
— — —, New Foundland 133
— — —, Non-Uranium Miners 127
— — —, Rocky Mountains 135
— — —, Schneeberg Miners 127
— respiratory cancer, hazards 126
Radiation cancers 126
— larynx cancers, X-radiation medication
    145
— lung cancer, Colorado plateau metal ore
    mines 133
— — —, Colorado plateau mines incidence
    135
— — —, experimental 144, 146
— — —, Joachimsthal miners exposure time
    137
— — —, Joachimsthal miners lag period 137
— — —, Joachimsthal miners silicosis 137
— — —, Joachimsthal mines 136
— — —, Joachimsthal mines radioactivity
    137
— — —, Joachimsthal radium plant 136

Radiation lung cancers, lead workers 141
— — —, metal ore miners, smoking 135
— — —, New Foundland, age distribution
    133
— — — —, fluorspar mine 131, 133
— — — —, incidence 131
— — — —, mine radioactivity 132
— — — —, smoking 133
— — —, non-uranium ore miners 127—135
— — —, Rocky Mountain Uranium Miners,
    exposure time 139
— — —, Rocky Mountain Uranium Miners,
    incidence 139
— — —, Rocky Mountain Uranium Miners,
    smoking 140
— — —, Rocky Mountain Uranium Mines
    138
— — —, Rocky Mountain Uranium Mines,
    radioactivity 140, 141
— — —, Schneeberg, cobalt ore 127
— — — —, exposure time 128
— — — —, inbreeding 128, 130
— — — —, incidence 127, 128
— — — — —, mine, radioactivity 129, 130
— — — —, pathology 128, 129
— — — —, silicosis 128
— — —, thorium dioxide medication 144
— — —, uranium ore mines 136
— — — hazards, radioactive water 143
— paranasal sinus cancers, thorium dioxide
    medication 144
— respiratory cancer hazards, air pollution
    145
— pneumonitis X-radiation medication 145
Respiratory cancer, see Lung cancer, Larynx
    cancer, Paranasal sinus cancer
— —, compensation laws 154
— —, polyetiology 29
— — hazards, control laws 154
— — —, social aspects 155
— carcinogens, classification 9
— —, exposure routes 11, 29
— —, exposure types 12
— —, extrapulmonary cancers 11
— —, nonspecific 1
— —, pattern of dissemination 23
— —, peri- and extraplant spread 23, 41, 50,
    58, 59, 75, 81, 86, 94, 100, 112, 114,
    123
— —, pluripotentiality 21
— —, potency 24
— —, potential 147
— —, smoking 9, 10, 12—14, 16, 21, 29, 32,
    54, 75, 86, 96, 101, 133, 135, 140
— —, specific 7
— —, systemic effects 8, 21, 24, 25
Rubber workers lung cancer 113

Scar cancer, lung 1, 3, 6
Schneeberg miners, lung cancer 127
Shale oils 118
Shellac pneumoconiosis 6, 7
Sideroma 98
Siderosis, lung idiopathic 94, 97
— — occupational 94
Silastic 39
Silicones 39
Silicosis 2—6
—, anticancerous effect 4
—, hematite miners 4
—, Schneeberg miners 4
Smudge pots 125
Soot 8, 9, 10

Tabacosis 6
Tobacco contaminants 6, 32
— Dust 6
Trauma, lung cancer 2

Uranium economy 108
— ore miners 136—141
Urethane 10, 11

Water pollutants 31, 143
Wax pressers, scrotal cancers 119

X-Radiation, lung cancer 125

Ynerite see Mustard gas 103

Monographs already published

SCHINDLER, R., Lausanne: Die tierische Zelle in Zellkultur (Volume 1).

Neuroblastomas — Biochemical Studies. Edited by C. BOHUON, Villejuif (Volume 2, Symposium).

In production

HUEPER, W. C., Bethesda: Occupational and Environmental Cancers of the Respiratory System (Volume 3).

GOLDMAN, L., Cincinnatti: Laser Cancer Research (Volume 4).

METCALF, D., Melbourne: The Thymus. Its Role in Immune Responses, Leukemia Development and Carcinogenesis (Volume 5).

Malignant Transformation by Viruses. Edited by W. H. KIRSTEN, Chicago (Volume 6, Symposium).

MOERTEL, CH. G., Rochester: Multiple Primary Malignant Neoplasms: Their Incidence and Significance (Volume 7).

New Trends in the Treatment of Cancer. Edited by P. RENTCHNICK, Genève (Volume 8, Symposium).

LINDENMANN, J., Zürich / A. KLEIN, Gainesville, Florida: Immunity to Transplantable Tumors following Viral Oncolysis (Volume 9).

In preparation

DENOIX, P., Villejuif: Le traitement des cancers du sein.

FISHER, E. R., Pittsburgh: Ultrastructure of Human Normal and Neoplastic Prostate.

FREEMAN, R. G., Houston: Treatment of Skin Cancer.

FUCHS, W. A., Bern: Lymphography and Tumordiagnosis.

GRUNDMANN, E., Wuppertal-Elberfeld: Morphologie und Cytochemie der Carcinogenese.

HALPERN, B., Paris / PEJSACHOWICZ, Paris: L'agrégation des cellules cancéreuses in vitro.

HAYWARD, J. L., London: Cancer of the Breast: Hormonal Changes.

KERN, G., Köln: Carcinoma in situ.

MARTZ, G., Zürich: Hormonbehandlung der Tumoren.

MATHÉ, G., Villejuif: Les essais d'éradication des leucémies aiguës.

NELSON, R. S., Houston: Radioactive Phosphorus in the Diagnosis of Gastrointestinal Cancer.

NEWMAN, M. K., Detroit: Neuropathies and Myopathies associated with Occult Malignancies.

214

Pack, G. T., New York: Clinical Aspects of Cancer Immunity and Cancer Susceptibility.

Pack, G. T., New York / A. H. Islami, New York: Tumors of the Liver.

Ritzman, S. E., Galveston / W. C. Levin, Galveston: The Syndrome of Macroglobuli-
nemia.

Steward, J. K., Manchester: Tumors in Children.

Weil, R., Lausanne: Biological and structural properties of polyoma virus and its
DNA.

Zilber, L. A., Moskva: Virogenetic Theory of Cancer Origin.

Herstellung: Konrad Triltsch, Graphischer Betrieb, Würzburg